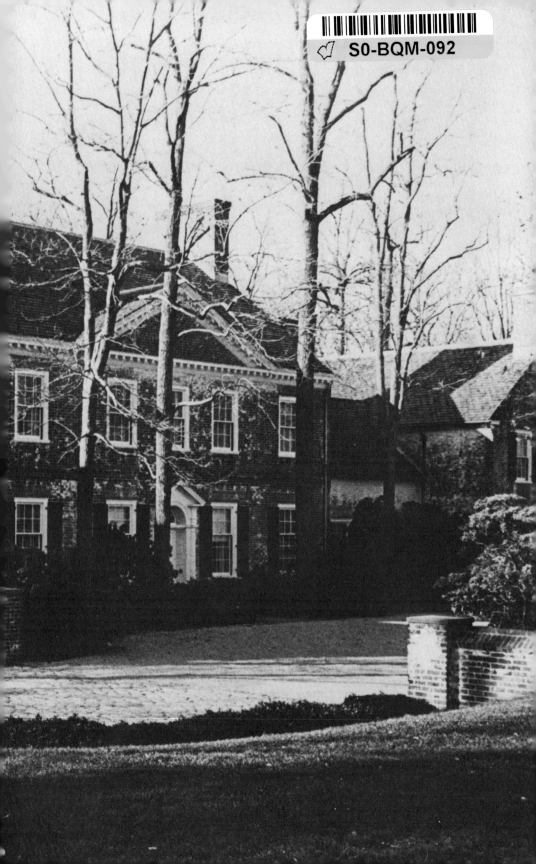

Carcinogen Risk Assessment: New Directions in the Qualitative and Quantitative Aspects

Banbury Report Series

Carcinogen Risk Assessment: New Directions in the Qualitative and Quantitative Aspects

Edited by

RONALD W. HART
National Center for Toxicological Research

FRED D. HOERGER
The Dow Chemical Company

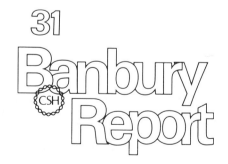

COLD SPRING HARBOR LABORATORY
1988

Banbury Report 31: Carcinogen Risk Assessment: New Directions in the Qualitative and Quantitative Aspects

© 1988 by Cold Spring Harbor Laboratory
All rights reserved
Printed in the United States of America
Cover and book design by Emily Harste

Library of Congress Cataloging-in-Publication Data

Carcinogen risk assessment: new directions in the qualitative and
  quantitative aspects/edited by Ronald W. Hart, Fred D.
  Hoerger.

    p. cm.—(Banbury report; 31)
  Bibliography: p.
  Includes index.
  ISBN 0-87969-231-6
  1. Carcinogenicity testing. 2. Health risk assessment.
3. Carcinogens—Structure-activity relationships. I. Hart, Ronald
W. II. Hoerger, Fred D. III. Series.
RC268.65.C366 1988
616.99'4071—dc19

                    88-1702
                    CIP

All Cold Spring Harbor Laboratory publications may be ordered directly from Cold Spring Harbor Laboratory, Box 100, Cold Spring Harbor, New York 11724. (Phone: 1-800-843-4388) In New York State (516) 367-8325.

BANBURY PROGRAM SPONSORS

Corporate Sponsors

Core Supporters

Special Program Support

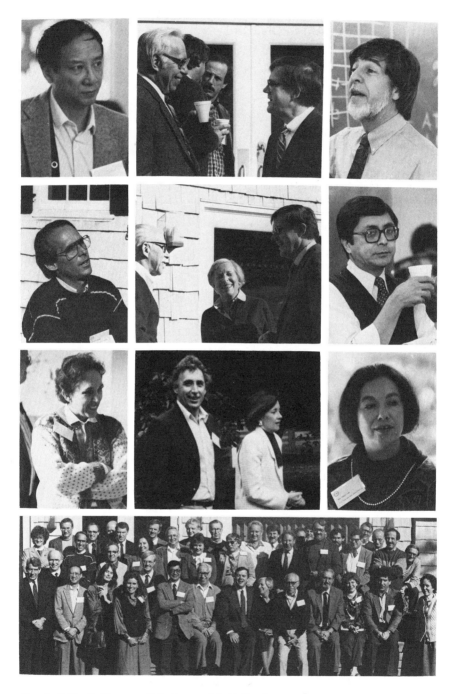

Row 1: P. Fu; F. Hoerger, F.P. Guengerich; J. Trosko
Row 2: F. Beland; R. Setlow, B. Singer, R. Hart; A.K. Ahmed
Row 3: M. Poirier; C. Travis, K. Deasy; M.F. Lowe

Participants

A. Karim Ahmed, Natural Resources Defense Council, New York, New York

Elizabeth Anderson, Clement Associates, Inc., Washington, D.C.

Deborah Barsotti, Agency for Toxicology, Substance and Disease Registry, Atlanta, Georgia

Frederick A. Beland, Division of Biochemical Toxicology, National Center for Toxicological Research, Jefferson, Arkansas

Robert Benson, Center for Veterinary Medicine, U.S. Food and Drug Administration, Rockville, Maryland

David B. Clayson, Sir Frederick G. Banting Research Centre, Health and Welfare Canada, Ottawa, Ontario

Murray S. Cohn, U.S. Consumer Product Safety Commission, Washington, D.C.

Kenny S. Crump, Clement Associates, Inc., Ruston, Louisiana

Karen M. Deasy, Centers for Disease Control, National Institute for Occupational Safety and Health, Washington, D.C.

Paul F. Deisler, Jr., Houston, Texas

Kurt Enslein, Health Designs, Inc., Rochester, New York

Ronald W. Estabrook, Department of Biochemistry, University of Texas Health Science Center, Dallas

William Farland, U.S. Environmental Protection Agency, Washington, D.C.

W. Gary Flamm, Center for Food Safety and Nutrition, U.S. Food and Drug Administration, Washington, D.C.

Peter Fu, Division of Biochemical Toxicology, National Center for Toxicological Research, Jefferson, Arkansas

John D. Graham, Department of Health Policy and Management, Harvard University School of Public Health, Boston, Massachusetts

F. Peter Guengerich, Department of Biochemistry, Vanderbilt University School of Medicine, Nashville, Tennessee

Ronald W. Hart, National Center for Toxicological Research, U.S. Food and Drug Administration, Jefferson, Arkansas

Fred D. Hoerger, The Dow Chemical Company, Midland, Michigan

Mary Elizabeth Jacobs, Center for Devices and Radiological Health, U.S. Food and Drug Administration, Rockville, Maryland

Kenneth Kraemer, National Cancer Institute, Bethesda, Maryland

Daniel Krewski, Health Protection Branch, Health and Welfare Canada, Ottawa, Ontario

William Lijinsky, NCI-Frederick Cancer Research Facility, Frederick, Maryland

Mary Frances Lowe, U.S. Food and Drug Administration, Rockville, Maryland

Robert W. Mason, Division of Biomedical and Behavioral Science, National Institute for Occupational Safety and Health, Cincinnati, Ohio

Christopher J. Michejda, NCI-Frederick Cancer Research Facility, Frederick, Maryland

Ian C. Munro, Canadian Center for Toxicology, Guelph, Ontario

Robert A. Neal, Chemical Industry Institute of Toxicology, Research Triangle Park, North Carolina

Frederica Perera, Division of Environmental Sciences, Columbia University School of Public Health, New York, New York

Emil A. Pfitzer, Department of Toxicology and Pathology, Hoffmann-La Roche, Inc., Nutley, New Jersey

Miriam C. Poirier, National Cancer Institute, Bethesda, Maryland

Richard B. Setlow, Department of Biology, Brookhaven National Laboratory, Upton, New York

B. Singer, Lawrence Berkeley Laboratory, University of California, Berkeley

Randall Smith, Division of Standards, Development and Technology Transfer, National Institute for Occupational Safety and Health, Cincinnati, Ohio

Donald E. Stevenson, Department of Health, Safety and Environmental Toxicology, Shell Oil Company, Houston, Texas

Catherine St. Hilaire, ILSI Risk Science Institute, Washington, D.C.

Raymond W. Tennant, Cellular and Genetic Toxicology Branch, National Institute of Environmental Health Sciences, Research Triangle Park, North Carolina

Dhiren Thakker, NIDDK, National Institutes of Health, Bethesda, Maryland

Todd Thorslund, Clement Associates, Inc., Washington, D.C.

Curtis C. Travis, Health and Safety Research Division, Oak Ridge National Laboratory, Tennessee

James E. Trosko, Department of Pediatrics and Human Development, Michigan State University, East Lansing

Wendell Weber, Department of Pharmacology, University of Michigan, Ann Arbor

Elizabeth K. Weisburger, National Cancer Institute, Bethesda, Maryland

James D. Wilson, Environmental, Safety and Health Staff, Monsanto Company, St. Louis, Missouri

Preface

From 1983 to 1986, several initiatives by the federal government related to the policy aspects of risk assessment, with particular emphasis on carcinogens. These included a study by the National Academy of Science on managing the risk assessment process, an interagency report compiled by the Office of Science and Technology Policy relating to the state of the science of carcinogens, a major policy statement by Health and Human Services, and risk assessment guidelines by the Environmental Protection Agency. In establishing a framework for risk assessment in regulatory agencies, these policy statements reflected the state of the science during the early part of this decade but could only generally anticipate that there would be advances in scientific information and thought that would have policy implications.

During the past five years, there have been significant advances in scientific research that provided new insights for the evaluation of human risks from carcinogenic agents. These included development and use of pharmacokinetic information for characterization of target organ dose, insights into the mechanism of carcinogenic action by specific agents, advances in molecular biology, and compilation of structure-activity relationships.

Experience with regulatory policies on risk assessment and the emergence of more research findings have led to much recent discussion on ways for improving the basis of risk assessment. Constructive questions have been raised. Is there a basis for revising some of the key assumptions used in the risk assessment process? What research directions will be most effective? Can diverse biological findings, e.g., pharmacokinetics or mechanism of action, be integrated into the assessment, either qualitatively or quantitatively? Can qualitative factors and weight-of-the-evidence judgments be addressed in evaluating the human relevancy of animal or in vitro data?

These proceedings were planned to address the above questions through contributions from leading researchers, leaders in formulation of government policy, and scientists from the private sector involved in research and assessments. The proceedings represent examination of advances in structure-activity relationships, pharmacokinetics and metabolism, molecular biology, integration of information in the assessment, and discussion of the implications of these advances for research and policy formation. In designing the first three sections, authors' papers are presented, dealing with recent advances. A "bridging" discussant focuses commentary on application of the science, followed by a panel discussion of the topics raised. An open question and answer period concludes each panalist's presentation. Section IV consists of authors' papers representing new approaches for integrating diverse types of information into the overall risk assessment. Each paper addresses either qualitative evaluation or new models to quantify pharmacokinetic and mechanistic information and is followed by comments by conference participants. Concluding Section V addresses the implications of the preceding sections for future direction in research and policy formation for improving the basis of risk assessments. Two introductory papers categorize current efforts. Conclusions and recommendations for future directions are drawn from two panels of the conference participants.

Financial support from the Food and Drug Administration, the National Institute of Occupational Safety and Health, the American Industrial Health Council, and The Dow Chemical Company is gratefully acknowledged. Also, Karim Ahmed, Elizabeth Andersen, John Doull, and the late Steve Prentis were instrumental in planning the conference.

The administrative effort of Bea Toliver of the Banbury Center was essential for the success of the conference. The gracious hospitality of Katya Davey, hostess of Robinson House, is acknowledged, and the diligent effort of Ralph Battey, Banbury editor, and Inez Sialiano, editorial assistant, are responsible for the timely publication of the proceedings.

R.W. Hart
F.D. Hoerger

Contents

Introduction

RONALD W. HART AND ANGELO TURTURRO
National Center for Toxicological Research
Food and Drug Administration
Jefferson, Arizona 72079

OVERVIEW

One of the greatest archeological finds of modern times was the discovery of the third millenium B.C. capital of Mari in northern Syria by a nomad searching for funerary stones. In a ruined room of the palace on small pillowlike clay tablets, there were found thousands of cunieform-inscribed letters in Akkadian. Some letters concerned themselves with the relationships of the court to gods such as Dagan and Baal and involved risk assessment issues such as the estimation of success of going on a hazardous journey. Others discussed risk management issues such as the propitiation of a particular god to prevent a particular adverse consequence.

Given the long history of risk assessment and management, it is not surprising that they have undergone a good deal of evolution. Recently, an important aspect of that evolution has been the introduction of information from molecular biology, biomarkers of toxicity, pharmacokinetics, and structure-activity relationships (SAR) into the process. In order to make the best judgments on risk, one must use the best estimations of risk. To make the best estimate of risk, one must use the best science available. This conference is trying to highlight that science and how it is being applied.

To provide a framework for the work presented in this conference, this discussion will begin with a short historical section on why cancer risk assessment is of public concern, followed by a brief analysis of how this concern has been manifested. We will conclude with a short overview of some of the tasks that risk assessors will have to face in order to improve the process.

Why U.S. Society Is Concerned

Public interest in the long-term effects of environmental agents arose first from the atom bomb tests in the 1950s. These tests resulted in worldwide radioactive fallout, thereby making a weapons test performed near Irkutsk of intense interest to someone in Minneapolis. Public interest was compounded by colorful media characterizations which depicted the production of monstrous insects and the insidious nature of radiation. Models of radiation action emerged, one of the most popular being the "single-hit" model, in which a single DNA damage site would result in mutation and cancer. With these models, and the database generated from the increasing number of people

Banbury Report 31: Carcinogen Risk Assessment: New Directions in the Qualitative and Quantitative Aspects © Cold Spring Harbor Laboratory. 0-87969-231-6/88. $1.00 + .00

exposed to radiation, statisticians attempted to calculate the population risk for cancer. This effort has continued and has recently resulted in compensation tables for people exposed to certain levels and types of radiation. Parenthetically, the public perception of relative health risk from radiation, e.g., from nuclear power plants, is still much greater than that estimated by public health experts.

Public concern about radiation set the stage for a broader concern about the role of chemicals in and on the environment. These matters were intermingled and amplified when evidence emerged that some of the effects of chemicals were mediated, similar to radiation, by effects on DNA. This led to the use of similar models and similar concepts for predicting the long-term effects of both agents. Although it was known from before 1920 that chemical treatments could induce cancer, in the context of public health this concept was fairly new. An example of the concepts brought over from radiation biology was the single-hit model of chemical carcinogenesis and subsequently pronouncements that indicted a single molecule of chemical in the production of a cancer. This was despite the long-standing tradition in toxicology of using modalities such as safety factors in extrapolating effects across species.

The public implications of pronouncements such as these on risks from chemicals, coupled with the seemingly ubiquitous presence of unseen environmental chemicals, were enormous. This was especially true because, as a postindustrialized nation in this century, the United States was in a position which made it very sensitive. After the conquest of tuberculosis and polio, the focus for public health had shifted from acute, infectious diseases to the chronic ones, such as cancer. Only very recently has acquired immunodeficiency syndrome (AIDS) turned public attention back to infectious diseases. One of the reasons for this shift was the large increase in average lifespan over the last century, mainly as a result of public sanitation, clean food, and better health care. This increased lifespan allowed people to live long enough to get cancer, Alzheimer's Disease, and so forth. The inevitable and terrible consequences of chronic diseases to people who had become unaccustomed to the ravages of diseases such as influenza and polio, coupled with their increasing incidence and familiarity, made them the major sources of public concern.

The Response to This Concern

As a result of the public concern, Congress responded first by amending previous laws concerning food safety. These were originally enacted to keep the food supply free of obvious poisons, such as antifreeze, and to preserve good sanitation. These laws were altered to include oversight of any substance that could result in a long-term effect (e.g., the Delaney Amendment to the Food, Drug, and Cosmetic Act). Similar concerns spread to occupational health as well as environmental health, abetted by statements by some scientists that a large portion of the annual cancer incidence in the United States resulted from exposure to environmental agents. This again resulted in new legislation. These concerns have, if anything, intensified over the last number of years. One result is the laws passed over the last three decades, some of which are shown in Table 1. As alluded to above, some of these laws led regulatory agencies to acquire a new set of responsibilities in addressing chronic endpoints. Others led to the creation of entirely new agencies, such as the Environmental Protection Agency, the Consumer Products Safety Commission, the Agency on Toxic Substances and Disease Registry, and so forth. Also present, although not on the list, is the increasing sensitivity to environmental and health concerns in all aspects of government. For example, the Department of Defense now considers environmental and health effects when it conducts projects that could effect the environment.

THE PROBLEM

To take on the responsibilities demanded by the public is not a simple task, even if we consider only chemicals. Presently, there are about 50,000–60,000 "manmade" chemicals in everyday commerce in significant production (over 1 ton/annum). Newly classified chemicals are being increased by 10% per year. There may be 50,000 dump sites with hazardous chemicals, with significant amounts of these substances being found at almost 2000 dump sites. As staggering as this is, there is a growing appreciation that our foodstuffs contain the majority, both in number of chemicals and quantity, of the chemicals to which people are exposed (Doll and Peto 1981; Ames 1983). Biologically active substances, sometimes with toxicity comparable to manmade chemicals, are ingested in milligram and gram quantities in food, as opposed to exposure to micrograms or less in the environment.

Ironically, the task of addressing the risks from exposure to chemicals, especially the goal of risk assessment, which is to estimate these risks under practical conditions of use and exposure, has been complicated, not simplified, by many of the mechanistic discoveries of the last number of years. For example, in assessing the risk of carcinogenesis, the simple picture of the 1950s has been replaced with multistage models involving different stages, some with reversible steps. It has been found that the same chemical can promote or inhibit carcinogenesis depending on the circumstances of exposure. Essential nutrients and hormones can be carcinogenic. Thoughts about the relationship of mutation and cancer have undergone considerable revision in the last few years as the significance of promotion and progression have been better appreciated. The idea of a simple cheap test to predict car-

Table 1
Federal Laws Related to Exposures to Toxic Substances

Legislation	Agency	Area of concern
Food, Drug, and Cosmetics Act (1906, 1932, amended 1958, 1960, 1962, 1968, 1976 1962, 1968, 1976)	FDA	food, drugs, cosmetics, food additives, color additives, new drugs, animal and feed additives, and medical devices
Federal Insecticide, Fungicide, and Rodenticide Act (1948, amended 1972, 1975, 1978)	EPA	pesticides
Dangerous Cargo Act (1954)	DOT USCG	water shipment of toxic materials
Atomic Energy Act (1954)	NRC	radioactive substances
Federal Hazardous Substances Act (1960, amended 1981)	CPSC	toxic household products
Federal Meat Inspection Act (1987) Poultry Products Inspection Act (1968)	USDA	food, feed, color additives, and pesticide residues
Federal Meat Inspection Act (1967) Poultry Products Inspection Act (1968) Egg Products Inspection Act (1970)	USDA	food, feed, color additives, and pesticide residues
Occupational Safety and Health Act (1970)	OSHA NIOSH	workplace toxic chemicals
Poison Prevention Packaging Act (1970, amended 1981)	CPSC	packaging of hazardous household products

Law	Agency	Regulates
Clean Air Act (1970), amended (1974, 1977)	EPA	air pollutants
Hazardous Materials Transportation Act (1972)	DOT	transport of hazardous materials
Clear Water Act (formerly Federal Water Control Act) (1972, amended 1977, 1978)	EPA	water pollutants
Marine Protection, Research, and Sanctuaries Act (1972)	EPA	ocean dumping
Consumer Product Safety Act (1972, amended 1981)	CPSC	hazardous consumer products
Lead-based Paint Poison Prevention Act (1973, amended 1976)	CPSC, HEW (HHS) HUD	use of lead paint in federally assisted housing
Safe Drinking Water Act (1974, amended 1977)	EPA	drinking water contaminants
Resource Conservation and Recovery Act (1976)	EPA	solid waste, including hazardous wastes
Toxic Substances Control Act (1976)	EPA	hazardous chemicals not covered by other laws, includes premarket review
Federal Mine Safety and Health Act (1977)	DOL, NIOSH	toxic substances in coal and other mines
Comprehensive Environmental Response, Compensation, and Liability Act (1981)	EPA	hazardous substances, pollutants, and contaminants contaminants

Abbreviations: (EPA) Environmental Protection Agency; (FDA) Food and Drug Administration; (CPSC) Consumer Products Safety Commission; (DOL) Department of Labor; (DOT) Department of Transportation; (HEW) (HHS) Department of Health, Education, and Welfare (many functions assumed by HHS Department of Health and Human Services); (HUD) Department of Housing and Urban Development; (NIOSH) National Institute of Occupational Safety and Health; (NRC) Nuclear Regulatory Commission; (USCG) United States Coast Guard; (OSHA) Occupational Safety and Health Administration; (USDA) United States Department of Agriculture.

A sampling of the laws enacted up to 1982 concerning public health and environmental agents. (Adapted from Office of Science and Technology Policy 1986.)

cinogenesis has foundered when the multitude of possible carcinogenic mechanisms are appreciated. Even the bedrock of modern testing programs, i.e., the ability of a compound to induce carcinogenesis in inbred rodent strains to predict effects in humans, has been brought into serious question as a quantitative tool, especially as there has been an increasing understanding about the effects of modulators of toxicity such as diet, strain, physiological state, and so forth.

Against this complicated background, regulators must make decisions every day concerning the safety of food additives, action levels for contaminants, levels of pesticide residues, limits in the workplace to chemical exposure, and whether a fence should be placed around a toxic waste dump and where it should be placed. These decisions are of intense interest to the society at large and can effect all sectors of the society. Of special importance to this conference is how science can be used to help resolve problems identified by the process of risk assessment.

ANALYSIS OF RISK ASSESSMENT

Introduction

As discussed in a number of documents in risk assessment (National Academy of Sciences 1983; CCEHRP 1985; Office of Science and Technology Policy 1986), risk assessment is based on a series of assumptions. In actuality, these assumptions are frequently default assumptions used to span the gaps in scientific knowledge and current understanding. They result in a good deal of uncertainty in the final evaluations derived from the risk assessment process. Indeed, based upon the assumptions used, the final level established may vary by more than six orders of magnitude. In order to appreciate how the assumptions are used and to place in context how certain aspects may be improved, it is useful to have a schema of how risk assessment is done.

Process

There are generally four parts to a risk assessment, as identified by the Office of Science and Technology Policy (1986): (1) hazard identification, (2) exposure assessment, (3) dose-response assessment, and (4) risk characterization (Table 2).

Hazard Identification. Hazard identification entails a qualitative evaluation of both the data bearing on an agent's ability to produce deleterious effects and the relevance of this information to humans. Three sources of information can contribute to identifying hazards: (1) epidemiological studies, (2) long-term animal bioassays, and (3) other tests. In understanding the use of

Table 2
Four Steps in Quantitative Carcinogenic Risk Assessment

Hazard identification (carcinogenic to humans?)
Exposure assessment (number of people exposed, length and route of exposure)
Hazard or dose-response assessment (animal effects and maximum effect as projected by mathematical models)
Risk evaluation

assumptions to identify hazards, one can group the assumptions into three different extrapolations. One is extrapolation across conditions, i.e., where data from a test under some particular conditions are used to make some characterization about a population. These are relevant to all types of data used. Another is extrapolation over species, and a third is extrapolation across end points, where an end point, such as mutation, is used to represent another, such as carcinogenesis. A number of assumptions are used in this process.

Use of Data from Epidemiological Studies

Extrapolation across conditions
1. Genetic factors are not confounding for extrapolation to total population.
2. Sex is not confounding for toxic effect.
3. Different physiological states, e.g., age, hormonal status, stress, disease, etc. are not confounding.
4. When routes of exposure are different in populations of potential risk, this is not confounding.

Use of Data from Animal Assays
Many of the same assumptions used for epidemiology are also used for this, plus

Extrapolation across conditions
1. Average dose is equivalent to dose varying in duration, frequency, and rate.
2. Agent is delivered in a form which is similar to that present in the environment.
3. Total body dose can be calculated for one route of exposure from other routes of exposure, generally by assuming equal absorption by different routes.
4. Diseases act independently, especially tumors.
5. Adverse biological effects increase with increasing chemical dose (monotonicity).
6. Target site dose is directly proportional to administered dose.

Extrapolation across species
7. Similarity in animal and human metabolism.
8. Exposure for a fraction of a lifetime of an animal (raised to some power, usually between two and eight) is equivalent to human exposure for the same fraction of a lifespan.

Use of Data from Short-term Tests

1. Extrapolation across conditions—test tube conditions can adequately model doses varying in duration, pattern, and rate.
2. For extrapolation across species—human response can be adequately modeled in Chinese hamster ovary cells and in bacteria.
3. For extrapolation across end point—mutagenesis and chromosomal aberrations adequately model carcinogenesis.

Work such as consideration of SARs directly tries to estimate hazard to humans from structure. As such it synthesizes much of the information in the extrapolation across end points and species using numerical analysis. It is especially important to cope with the magnitude of the problem, as set forth above, since it is not practical to even do long-term assays on a great number of chemicals not to mention epidemiological studies. Some paradigms are attempting to incorporate biological information to further improve the process. Recent attempts to replace long-term assays by short-term tests such as the Ames assay have not been successful, and the more analytical approach used in SAR may be successful. This will be covered in Section 1.

Much of the work in molecular biological parameters is also relevant to hazard identification. If a reliable biomarker for toxicity can be found, this would significantly shorten the time to determine hazard and improve extrapolation across conditions. If a biomarker can be found, one could, in theory, measure the effects of conditions on the biomarker and determine how the marker is being modulated. This would be a key step in determining risk under practical conditions of use and exposure.

A similar analysis can be made for the work in pharmacokinetics. Determining a dose closer to the effective dose has the probability of removing a good deal of uncertainty in evaluating the effects of many modulators. This will be covered in Section 2.

Exposure Assessment. Exposure assessment estimates the number of individuals who are likely to be exposed along with the types, magnitudes, and durations of their anticipated exposures. Without human exposure, there is no risk to the human population, regardless of the potency of an agent under consideration. Thus, exposure evaluation is a critical component of the risk assessment process. Some important assumptions are:

1. Certain spatial distributions of compounds, e.g., point estimates or distributions can model real-life distributions.
2. Time variations of distributions, dependent on physical factors are known.
3. Dietary habits are irrelevant.
4. Different units of dose can be compared in combining studies.

In addition to its relevance to hazard identification, the work in molecular biology and biomarkers as well as the efforts in pharmacokinetics and absorption, are relevant to exposure assessment. Success in defining an integrated measure of human exposure, e.g., blood adducts of a compound, could ultimately make many of the current problems in exposure assessment moot. In clarifying the relationship of administered and proximal dose, pharmacokinetics has the potential to address many of the same problems as a molecular biological marker for those agents for which it is difficult to define a biomarker. Both areas of research also have the potential to add significantly to the mechanistic understanding of carcinogenesis by helping to define an effective dose since definition of a marker for an effective dose will demand a better understanding of the crucial steps in the carcinogenic process. Much of these data will be covered in both Section 2 and Section 3.

Hazard or Dose-response Assessment. Hazard or dose-response assessment uses the information on toxic effects from the hazard identification phase together with techniques to estimate the magnitude or an upper bound on the magnitude of the toxic end point at any given dose level, usually at levels below the observable range. There are three different approaches used in extrapolation: (1) low-dose extrapolation, (2) no observed effect level, and (3) margin-of-safety. Low-dose extrapolation is usually used in carcinogenesis, with the multistage model currently the preferred model for low-dose extrapolation. Some of the assumptions used include:

Epidemiological Data

1. The model of extrapolation to low-dose is known.
2. Short follow-up time is not confounding for dose response.
3. Different temporal exposures are not dealt with, e.g., a dose in old age similar to a dose in childhood.
4. Different physiological factors in different populations are not factored in.

Animal Data

1. Interspecies conversion of dose.
2. Data available for more than one strain are combined using ad hoc techniques.
3. Method of high- to low-dose extrapolation.

4. Method of extrapolation from animal species to humans (in a broad sense, this category includes most of the factors considered in hazard identification, but, the narrow sense used here limits the term to mathematical prediction of tumor incidence in one species from results in another).
5. Use of standardized dosage scales (e.g., mg/kg body weight, concentration).
6. Considerations of biochemical target site and factors influencing the interaction of agent and site.

Research directions in this area are included in Section 4 and somewhat in Section 5 of this volume. Defining the uncertainty in species extrapolation and developing new models for low-dose extrapolation, e.g., recent ones which incorporate biological data such as information on proliferation, are pointing out important areas to pursue.

Risk Characterization. The final step in the risk assessment process, risk characterization, usually involves a total evaluation of the qualitative evidence, the exposure information, and the quantitative results. The final product of this evaluation is, typically, the generation of a quantitative estimate of the human cancer risk associated with the projected exposure profile. There has been a valuable effort to evaluate qualitative evidence by a weight-of-the-evidence approach where the uncertainties in the data are rationalized using best scientific judgment. There is also an effort to express the results of a risk assessment so there is a clear distinction drawn between what is scientific consensus and what is policy. Finally, there is an important effort to characterize the uncertainty in the assessment and where the cause of the uncertainty lies. These points and others will arise when the policy considerations of the new directions in risk assessment are evaluated predominantly in Section 5, as well as throughout the volume.

CONCLUSION

Risk assessment has an important role in risk management. By emphasizing research areas and directions that improve the ability of risk managers to make decisions, research in risk assessment will not only improve risk estimates but will also result in a more complete and comprehensive understanding of the basic processes involved in evaluating risk and understanding the biology of the organism of interest, man.

REFERENCES

Ames, B.N. 1983. Dietary carcinogens and anticarcinogens. *Science* **221:** 1256.
Doll, R. and R. Peto. 1981. The causes of cancer: Quantitative estimates of avoidable risks of cancer in the United States. *J. Natl. Cancer Inst.* **66:** 1193.

Executive Committee of the Coordinating Council on Environmental Health and Related Programs (CCEHRP). 1985. *Risk assessment and risk management in the Department of Health and Human Services.* Department of Health and Human Services, Washington, D.C.

National Academy of Sciences. 1983. *Managing the process: Risk assessment in the Federal Government.* National Academy of Sciences Press, Washington, D.C.

Office of Science and Technology Policy. 1986. Chemical carcinogens: A review of the science and associated principles. *Environ. Health Perspect.* **67**: 201.

Structure-Activity
Relationship Data

Structure-Activity Relations among Nitrogen-containing Alkylating Carcinogens

WILLIAM LIJINSKY
Laboratory of Chemical and Physical Carcinogenesis
BRI-Basic Research Program
NCI-Frederick Cancer Research Facility
Frederick, Maryland 21701

OVERVIEW

Most N-nitroso compounds and related nitrogen-containing aliphatic carcinogens are alkylating agents. A large proportion are methylating or ethylating agents, which alkylate DNA and other macromolecules as would be predicted from their chemical structures. Qualitatively and quantitatively the alkylation patterns in rats or in hamsters are similar, whether the carcinogen is directly acting or requires metabolic activation. However, the tumors induced by the methylating agents are often very different between compounds, as they are between ethylating agents. The differences are particularly great between nitrosamines and nitrosoalkylureas, which induce respectively a particular set of tumors in rats (or in hamsters) but few tumors in common. The types of tumor induced by nitrosamines in some cases differ greatly between different dose rates, even though the route of administration and total dose delivered are the same. The results suggest that alkylation of DNA by these carcinogens might be an important event in carcinogenesis but that other properties of the carcinogen determine whether or not tumors arise in a particular organ.

INTRODUCTION

It is 30 years since the alkylating agents, such as the carcinogenic nitrogen mustards, were proposed to act through alkylation of DNA. Since then, a very large number of simple nitrogen compounds have been shown to be carcinogenic; subsequent, biochemical studies of many of these compounds showed them to alkylate DNA in vivo. These carcinogens belonged to several chemical groups, including N-nitroso compounds, hydrazines, triazenes, azoxy compounds, and azo compounds. Most of these compounds have induced tumors in the liver of rodents, and it is alkylation in the liver that has been most studied. The largest of these groups of carcinogens has been the N-nitroso compounds; a large subdivision of this group, nitrosoalkylureas,

Banbury Report 31: Carcinogen Risk Assessment: New Directions in the Qualitative and Quantitative Aspects © Cold Spring Harbor Laboratory. 0-87969-231-6/88. $1.00 + .00

usually induces tumors of many organs but not in the liver. The reason for this is not known, but it is one of the important questions for which answers are needed. The reason for the failure of liver enzymes to activate a number of liver carcinogens to bacterial mutagens, although alkylation of liver DNA by these compounds has usually been demonstrated, is also unknown.

In the early years of work with *N*-nitroso compounds begun by Magee and Barnes, and greatly expanded by Druckrey, Preussmann and their associates, much attention was given to the structures that could and could not give rise to an alkylating agent. For example, the finding that nitrosomethyl-tertiary-butylamine was not carcinogenic and did not alkylate DNA (Magee and Lee 1964) lent strong support to the concept of DNA alkylation as a principal mechanism of carcinogenesis. During the structure-activity studies of Druckrey and Preussmann (Druckrey et al. 1967), a discrepancy was found in the form of nitrosomethylaniline, which does not alkylate DNA (and is not mutagenic) but is carcinogenic, inducing only tumors of the esophagus in rats, however. Since then, several other compounds with activities that do not fit have been discovered, and these have suggested that some modification of the earlier simple hypothesis is in order. An examination of the relation between chemical structure and carcinogenic activity among these compounds gives indications of the routes of metabolism, by which the compounds are activated, and offers hope that the number of different mechanisms by which they induce such a variety of tumors in different species might be small. Nevertheless, there is sufficient complexity to suggest that simplified systems, such as preparations of microsomes from organs containing several types of cell, will not duplicate the metabolism of those nitrosamines that leads to tumor induction in vivo. This is most likely why many carcinogenic alkylating compounds are not active in the bacterial mutagenesis assays. For example, the potently carcinogenic azoxyalkanes are not mutagenic in the Ames assay (Lijinsky et al. 1985), although they are as effective alkylating agents in vivo as the nitrosamines with which they are isomeric.

RESULTS AND DISCUSSION

Carcinogenesis by Methylating Agents

A large variety of carcinogenic nitrogen compounds are agents that lead to methylation of DNA in vivo. The formation of a methylating agent is often obvious, as from nitrosodimethylamine, nitrosomethylurea, azoxymethane, and nitrosomethylurethane. It is almost equally obvious that nitroso-methylethylamine, nitrosomethyl-*n*-propylamine, and the homologs with longer or more complex alkyl chains should be methylating agents. It has been recently shown (von Hofe et al. 1987) that many of these compounds give rise to methylation of DNA in the rat esophagus, which is a common target organ, in addition to the liver in some cases. There is a rough correlation of the extent of DNA methylation in the esophagus with the potency of the compound as an esophageal carcinogen, but nitrosomethyl-n-hexylamine is a more potent esophageal carcinogen than would be indicated by its methylation of esophageal DNA.

When considering the activity of asymmetric nitrosamines, it is obvious that two different positions of α-oxidation exist and that two different alkylating agents (presumably alkyldiazonium ions) can be formed; in vitro studies have shown the formation of both possible aldehydes by the action of microsomal enzymes (Farrelly and Stewart 1982). However, even in the case of nitrosomethylethylamine, ethylation of liver DNA is two orders of magnitude smaller than methylation (von Hofe et al. 1986). The role of the longer alkyl group in carcinogenesis by, for example, the homologous series of nitrosomethyl-n-alkylamines appears to be small, since the homologs from n-propyl (C-3) to n-hexyl (C-6) induce mainly esophageal tumors in rats with similar potency, and methylation of esophageal DNA is prominent. The nitrosomethyl-n-alkylamines with longer carbon chains induce tumors of the liver, lung, and bladder, but not tumors of the esophagus in rats (Table 1). This suggests a role for the long alkyl group in organ-specific carcinogenesis, which has been shown to include chain shortening by β-oxidation to form a series of nitrosamino acids (Singer et al. 1981). In the case of those compounds with alkyl chains having an even number of carbon atoms, one end product is nitrosomethyl-3-carboxypropylamine, giving rise to nitrosomethyl-2-oxo-propylamine that appears to be the proximate bladder carcinogen and is present in the urine of rats given nitrosomethylalkylamines with even-carbon chains that induce bladder tumors in rats (Lijinsky et al. 1981). These nitrosamines also induce bladder tumors in hamsters (but not in guinea pigs), suggesting that the same metabolic pathways are followed, and most of these nitrosamines also induce liver tumors in hamsters. Nitrosomethyl-2-oxo-propylamine, the proximate carcinogen in the bladder, is a comparably effective methylating agent to nitrosodimethylamine, but the mechanism of formation of the methylating agent is not known.

The complexity of many carcinogenic nitrosamines suggests that there are quite different alkylating agents formed from them. However, nitroso-2,6-dimethyl-morpholine and the β-oxygenated propyl-nitrosamines that are formed metabolically from it (Gingell et al. 1976) are primarily methylating agents in vivo. Although several of these compounds have one or more common target organs in rats or hamsters, they also differ in some other types of tumor they induce. It appears that formation of a common methylating agent (e.g., a methyldiazonium ion) is not the only reaction of importance, since they all methylate DNA in many organs but do not induce tumors in all

Table 1
Carcinogenesis by NO-Me-Alkylamines in Male F344 Rats

NO-Me-	Relative potency	Dose (mmole) 2 × week (gavage)	$t_{1/2}$	% Animals with tumors					Other
				liver	esophagus	lung	bladder		
Methylamine	+++	0.025	50	50	0	80	0		kidney 50, nasal 20
Ethylamine	++++	0.025	38	94	0	44	0		nasal 50
n-Butylamine	++++	0.021	26	12	100	0	0		nasal 50
n-Hexylamine	++++	0.04	31	95	95	45	5		nasal 5
n-Heptylamine	++	0.11	27	70	0	40	0		trachea 60, nasal 10
n-Octylamine	++	0.11	35	85	0	60	70		nasal 85, trachea 25
n-Nonylamine	++	0.11	43	90	0	60	0		nasal 40, trachea 5
n-Decylamine	+	0.11	81	10	0	40	85		nasal 5
n-Undecylamine	++	0.11	48	90	10	80	0		
n-Dodecylamine	+	0.05	101	15	0	25	95		forestomach 35
n-Tetradecylamine	+	0.11	84	0	0	15	100		kidney 10

organs. It is possible that other forms of alkylation are responsible for the differences. The role of a particular alkylating agent in carcinogenesis by N-nitroso compounds (and probably by other nitrogen-containing carcinogens) might be hard to predict merely from looking at its chemical structure.

Ethylating Compounds

Most ethylating compounds seem to have the rat esophagus as a target, including nitrosodiethylamine and azoxyethane, but neither these nor any other compound induces tumors in the esophagus of the syrian hamster or the guinea pig. These structural requirements of an alkylating agent for induction of tumors in the rat esophagus suggest the presence in the rat esophagus, but not in the hamster esophagus, of a specific receptor. Nitrosamines, azoxyalkanes, and triazenes with appropriate structures induce tumors of the esophagus in rats. However, nitrosoalkylureas and nitrosoalkylcarbamates do not induce esophageal tumors in rats, although they are powerful, directly acting alkylating agents. This suggests that the carbamyl structure lacks affinity for the esophageal receptor, and perhaps that metabolism is required in the esophagus for the alkylating agent to induce tumors in that organ. A similar suggestion can be made about the nasal mucosa of the rat or hamster, in which no nitrosoalkylurea or nitrosoalkylcarbamate has induced tumors, although a large number of nitrosamines and azoxyalkanes have.

Nitrosamines and Nitrosoalkylureas

There is a large contrast between the carcinogenic effect of a nitrosoalkylurea, which generates a particular alkylating diazonium ion, and that of a nitrosamine which can generate the same alkyldiazonium ion. For example, nitrosomethylurea induces nervous system tumors in rats and tumors of the forestomach, whereas nitrosodimethylamine induces tumors of liver, kidney, lung, and nasal mucosa; excepting brain, both compounds give rise to almost identical patterns of methylation in those organs following administration of equimolar doses. The same is true of nitrosoethylurea and nitrosodiethylamine, although a different spectrum of tumors is induced by the ethylating agents. A series of nitrosoalkylureas has been examined in rats, and the effects of administration of approximately equimolar doses to rats are shown in Tables 2 and 3. Although there are some differences in potency and in the frequency of various types of tumors induced, the carcinogenic effects of the nitrosoalkylureas are quite similar. However, they differ considerably from the effects of the nitrosamines containing the same alkyl groups, which would be expected metabolically to give rise to the same alkylating agent (Table 4). It is probable that the alkyl groups of the nitrosamines are oxidized or

Table 2
Carcinogenesis by Nitrosoalkylureas in Male Rats (Gavage)

1-Nitrosourea		Mutagenicity (rev/µmole)	Total dose (mmole)	$t_{1/2}$ (weeks)	Tumors induced					
1	3				lung	nervous system	forestomach	intestine	mesothelioma	zymbal gland
Methyl	H	1700	0.8	35		++	++			
Methyl	methyl	73	1.2	81		++			++	
Methyl	ethyl	86	1.2	28	+	++				+
Ethyl	H	31	1.1	30	+	+	++	+	+	+
Ethyl	ethyl	34	1.2	33	++			++	+	+
Ethyl	methyl	34	1.2	34	++			+	+	+
Ethyl	hydroxyethyl	180	1.4	56	++	+		+	++	+

Table 3
Carcinogenesis by Nitrosoalkylureas in Female Rats (Gavage)

1-Nitrosourea		Mutagenicity (rev/µmole)	Total dose (mmoles)	$t_{1/2}$ (weeks)	Tumors induced						
1	3				lung	mammary gland	uterus	nervous system	forestomach	intestine	zymbal gland
Methyl	H	1700	0.4	33				++	++		
Methyl	methyl	73	1.2	40	+			++			
Methyl	ethyl	86	0.6	34				++			
Ethyl	H	31	0.4	40	+	+	+	+	++	+	
Ethyl	ethyl	34	0.6	29		++	++				
Ethyl	methyl	34	0.6	37	+	++	++	+		+	+

Table 4
Carcinogenesis by Nitrosoalkylamines and Analogous Nitrosoalkylureas: Tumors Induced in Rats by Oral Administration (Gavage)

Alkyl group	Dialkylnitrosamine	Alkylmethylnitrosamine	Alkylnitrosourea
Methyl	liver, lung, kidney	—	nervous system, forestomach
Ethyl	liver, esophagus, nasal	liver, lung, nasal	lung, forestomach, intestines, mammary gland, zymbal gland
n-Propyl	liver, esophagus, lung, nasal	esophagus, forestomach	duodenum, intestine, zymbal gland
n-Butyl	liver, lung, bladder, forestomach	esophagus, forestomach, nasal	lung, forestomach, mammary gland, colon, uterus
n-Amyl	liver	esophagus	lung, forestomach, uterus, mammary gland, zymbal gland, intestine
n-Hexyl	—	esophagus, liver, lung	lung, forestomach, uterus, colon, mammary gland
n-Octyl	0	esophagus, liver, bladder, lung	—
Allyl	0	esophagus, kidney, nasal	mammary gland, forestomach, uterus, colon, zymbal gland, thymus
2-Hydroxyethyl	liver, esophagus, nasal	liver, nasal	thyroid, lung, duodenum, forestomach, colon, zymbal gland, bladder
2-Hydroxypropyl	esophagus, lung, thyroid, liver, nasal	esophagus, lung, nasal	thymus, forestomach

otherwise metabolized, particularly if the alkyl groups are large, whereas it is less likely that the alkyl groups of nitrosoalkylureas are metabolized before these rather unstable compounds break down to the alkyldiazonium ion. Therefore, it is remarkable that there is so great a similarity in the tumors that nitrosoalkylureas of various structures induce in rats and an even greater similarity in hamsters.

Nitrosoalkylureas

The much more stable nitrosodialkylureas and nitrosotrialkylureas appear to form the same alkylating agent as the corresponding nitrosomonoalkylurea, and the nitrosodialkylureas are similarly mutagenic to bacteria (Lijinsky et al. 1987a). In hamsters, they all induce hemangiosarcomas of the spleen, whatever their structure, but in rats the tumors induced by nitrosodialkylureas are sometimes similar but often different from those induced by the corresponding nitrosomonoalkylurea (Tables 2 and 3).

Nitrosodimethylurea is a much weaker mutagen and a weaker carcinogen than nitrosomethylurea, although it induces the same tumors (of the nervous system) as nitrosomethylurea in rats (Lijinsky 1987). However, nitroso-1-methyl-3-ethylurea has similar mutagenic potency to nitrosodimethylurea, but similar carcinogenic potency to nitrosomethylurea, also inducing tumors of the nervous system. Methylation of rat liver DNA by all three compounds is similar; however, none of them induced tumors of the liver in rats after chronic oral administration. Methylation of DNA by these nitrosomethylureas appears to depend, predictably, on the simple chemical formation of the same alkylating agent, probably a methyldiazonium ion. Tumor induction might depend on other properties of the compounds.

Liver Carcinogens

The focus of much interest has been on those compounds that induce tumors in the liver, and this organ is the site of induction of tumors by many of the compounds considered here, in rats and in hamsters. Although induction of liver tumors by the directly acting nitrosoalkylureas is not unknown, the overwhelming majority of these compounds that induce tumors in the liver require metabolic activation. Microsomal oxidases seem to be involved in many cases, but not in all since microsomal enzymes do not appear to activate azoxyalkanes (Lijinsky et al. 1985), for example, or a number of nitrosamines that bear an oxygen function on the 2-carbon, such as nitrosodiethanolamine (Farrelly et al. 1984). These compounds are not oxidized by microsomal preparations in vitro, nor are they converted to bacterial mutagens by these enzymes. Nevertheless, there must be enzymes in the liver that convert them to active intermediates.

One of the notable difficulties in understanding liver carcinogenesis by the alkylating agents we are considering is the dependence of the effectiveness of the carcinogen on the dose rate and the route of administration. Even when the route is the same, for example by mouth, there is often a large difference in the incidence of liver tumors and of other tumors in rats between administration in drinking water and by gavage, as well as a difference between different doses. As examples, high doses of nitrosodiethylamine in drinking water induce a high incidence of liver tumors in rats; lower doses induce mainly esophageal tumors and few liver tumors (Table 5). Nitrosodimethylamine in drinking water induces liver tumors in rats at all dose rates, but no other tumors, but similar doses by gavage induce fewer liver tumors and high incidences of tumors of the lung, kidneys, and nasal mucosa. The isomeric azoxymethane in drinking water induces liver tumors in rats together with tumors of the colon, but similar doses by gavage induce only tumors of the colon and kidneys but no liver tumors (Table 6). These results are difficult to explain in light of the more extensive, but similar in pattern, methylation of liver DNA by azoxymethane, compared with the effects of the same dose of nitrosodimethylamine. Pharmacological factors related to the dose seem to play a role in determining whether tumors ensue, quite apart from the extent of alkylation of DNA produced, which is obviously adequate to initiate tumors even after administration of low drinking water doses to the rats.

Alkylation of liver DNA in hamsters by ethylating agents and by methylating agents seems to be similar to that in rats, and the extent of ethylation is much smaller than the extent of methylation by an equimolar dose of a methylating agent. Yet, in rats a given dose of nitrosodiethylamine or azoxyethane is much more effective in inducing tumors than the same dose of nitrosodimethylamine or azoxymethane. In contrast, the relative effects in hamsters are reversed, so that nitrosodimethylamine and azoxymethane are much more effective than nitrosodiethylamine and azoxyethane; all except the latter induce mainly liver tumors in hamsters, but the animals treated with the ethyl compounds survived much longer (Lijinsky et al. 1987b). In hamsters nitrosomethylethylamine resembled nitrosodiethylamine rather than nitrosodimethylamine in carcinogenic effects. However, in both rats and hamsters the methylating properties of nitrosomethylethylamine resembled those of nitrosodimethylamine, and in ethylating properties nitrosomethylethylamine resembled nitrosodiethylamine. This suggests that the alkylating activities of these compounds in rats and hamsters are parallel and predictable from the chemistry of the compounds, but that the carcinogenic activities in the two species does not follow the same rules.

Table 5
Tumors Induced by Ethylating Carcinogens in Rats and Hamsters

Compound	Route of administration	Rat	Hamster
Nitrosodiethylamine	water	esophagus, liver	—
	gavage	liver, esophagus, nasal	liver, nasal
Azoxyethane	water	esophagus, liver, nasal	—
	gavage	nasal, liver	nasal (liver)
Nitrosomethylethylamine	water	liver, esophagus	—
	gavage	liver, lung, nasal	liver, nasal
Nitrosoethylurea	gavage	lung, forestomach, colon, nervous system, zymbal gland, mesothelioma	spleen, forestomach
Nitrosodiethylurea	water	lung, zymbal gland, mesothelioma	—
	gavage	lung, colon, zymbal gland, mesothelioma	spleen

Table 6
Tumors Induced by Methylating Carcinogens in Rats and Hamsters

Compound	Route of Administration	Rat	Hamster
Nitrosodimethylamine	water	liver	—
	gavage	liver, lung, kidney	liver
Azoxymethane	water	liver, colon	—
	gavage	colon, kidney, zymbal gland	liver, colon
Nitrosomethylethylamine	water	liver, esophagus	—
gavage	liver, lung, nasal	liver, nasal	
Nitrosomethylurea	gavage	nervous system, forestomach	spleen, forestomach
Nitrosodimethylurea	water	nervous system	—
	gavage	nervous system, thyroid, mesothelioma	spleen
Nitrosobis-(2-oxopropyl)-amine	water	lung, thyroid	—
	gavage	lung, thyroid, bladder	liver, pancreas

Hydroxyethylating Compounds

If we examine the effects of hydroxyethylating agents as carcinogens, there are considerable differences from the effects of ethylating agents, at least in rats. For example, nitrosohydroxyethylurea induced tumors of the thyroid, glandular stomach, and bone, but few mammary tumors and no mesotheliomas, whereas the converse was true of nitrosoethylurea. Nitrosodiethanolamine was a less effective alkylating agent of many orders of magnitude than nitrosodiethylamine, and the former was a weaker carcinogen, although the types of tumors induced by the two nitrosoamines were similar. Nitrosooxazolidone is a potent carcinogen and gives rise to the same alkylating intermediate, a hydroxyethyl donor, as nitrosohydroxyethylurea and nitrosodiethanolamine, but nitrosooxazolidone induces only forestomach tumors in rats or in hamsters. The hybrid nitrosodialkylurea, nitroso-1-hydroxyethyl-3-ethylurea, which is comparably effective as an hydroxyethylating agent in vivo to nitrosohydroxyethylurea, induces all of the tumors in rats that are induced by the latter, but in addition a high incidence of tumors of the nervous system and of the liver, which nitrosohydroxyethylurea does not induce at all (Table 7). Nitroso-1-hydroxyethyl-3-chloroethylurea, in contrast, induced only tumors of the liver and kidney in rats. On the other hand, nitrosodiethylurea or nitroso-1-ethyl-3-methylurea induce the same spectrum of tumors as nitrosoethylurea, that is, few tumors of the nervous system and none of the liver. These differences suggest that the alkylation these compounds produce in tissues are only part of the process of tumor induction and other properties of the carcinogen determine whether tumors ensue. On the other hand, organs in which for reasons of metabolism or of the lack of access, the carcinogen does not produce alkylation of DNA, are unlikely to give rise to tumors. The example can be cited of nitrosodiethanolamine, which is carcinogenic but not detectably mutagenic in any system, yet alkylates rat liver DNA, albeit at a very low level.

CONCLUSION

There are sharp differences between nitrosamines and nitrosoalkylureas in the types of tumor they induce as a class in rats and in hamsters (Table 8). It is an enigma that nitrosoalkylureas given to rats in drinking water do not induce tumors of the esophagus, although so many nitrosodialkylamines forming the same alkylating diazonium compound have the rat esophagus as their primary target.

It seems that, although alkylation of target cell DNA by the nitrogen-containing alkylating carcinogens might be necessary (except in the case of cyclic nitrosamines, which have not been shown to alkylate DNA), it is not

Table 7
Carcinogenesis by Hydroxyalkylnitrosoureas in Male Rats (Gavage)

1-Nitroso-		Mutagenicity (rev/μmole)	Total dose (mmoles)	$t_{1/2}$ (weeks)	Tumors induced						
1	3				lung	liver	kidney	intestine	thymus	mesothelioma	nervous system
Ethyl	H	31	1.1	30	+			+		+	+
Hydroxyethyl	H	2400	0.8	45	++			++			
Hydroxyethyl	ethyl	2900	1.4	65	+	++		+		++	++
Hydroxyethyl	chloroethyl	1900	1.3	78	++	++	++				
3-Hydroxypropyl	H	220	1.3	70	+	+					
2-Hydroxypropyl	H	3100	1.3	32	+				++		
2-Hydroxypropyl	chloroethyl	3700	1.3	90	+	++			+	+	

Table 8
Tumor Types Not Induced

By nitrosamines or azoxyalkanes	By nitrosamides
(a) *Rats*	(a) *Rats*
Mesothelioma	Esophagus
Nervous system	Nasal mucosa
Mammary gland	Trachea
Uterus	Pancreas
Zymbal gland	
Intestine	(b) *Hamsters*
Glandular stomach	Mesothelioma
Pancreas	Esophagus
	Nervous system
(b) *Hamsters*	Lung
Mesothelioma	Trachea
Esophagus	Bladder
Nervous system	Mammary gland
Mammary gland	Nasal mucosa
Lymphoma	Lymphoma
Kidney	Thyroid
Thyroid	Colon
Intestine	Intestine
	Kidney

sufficient to determine the induction of tumors. For this, other properties of the carcinogen, presently not understood, come into play.

ACKNOWLEDGMENTS

Research sponsored by the National Cancer Institute, Department of Health and Human Services, under contract no. NO1-CO-74101 with Bionetics Research, Inc. The contents of this publication do not necessarily reflect the reviews or policies of the Department of Health and Human Services, nor does mention of trade names, commercial products, or organizations imply endorsement by the U.S. Government. By acceptance of this article, the publisher or recipient acknowledges the right of the U.S. Government to retain a nonexclusive, royalty-free license in and to any copyright covering the article.

REFERENCES

Druckrey, H., R. Preussmann, S. Ivancovic, and D. Schmähl. 1967. Organotrope carcinogene Wirkungen bei 65 verschiedenen N-Nitroso-Verbindungen an BD-Ratten. *Z. Krebsforsch.* **69**: 103.

Farrelly, J.G. and M. Stewart. 1982. The metabolism of a series of methylalkylni-trosamines. *Carcinogenesis* **3**: 1299.

Farrelly, J.G., M.L. Stewart, and W. Lijinsky. 1984. The metabolism of nitrosodi-n-propylamine, nitrosodiallylamine and nitrosodiethanolamine. *Carcinogenesis* **5**: 1015.

Gingell, R., L. Wallcave, D. Nagel, R. Kupper, and P. Pour. 1976. Common metabo-lites of N-nitroso-2,6-dimethylmorpholine and N-nitrosobis-(2-oxopropyl)amine in the Syrian hamster. *Cancer Lett.* **2**: 47.

Lijinsky, W. 1987. Structure-activity relations in carcinogenesis by N-nitroso com-pounds. *Cancer Metastasis Rev.* **6**: 301.

Lijinsky, W., R.K. Elespuru, and A.W. Andrews. 1987a. Relative mutagenic and prophage-inducing effects of mono- and di-alkylnitrosoureas. *Mutat. Res.* **178**: 157.

Lijinsky, W., R.M. Kovatch, and C.W. Riggs. 1987b. Carcinogenesis by nitrosodial-kylamines and azoxyalkanes given by gavage to rats and hamsters. *Cancer Res.* **47**: 3968.

Lijinsky, W., J.E. Saavedra, and M.D. Reuber. 1981. Induction of carcinogenesis in Fischer rats by methylalkylnitrosamines. *Cancer Res.* **41**: 1288.

Lijinsky, W., A.W. Andrews, R.K. Elespuru, and J.G. Farrelly. 1985. Lack of genetic and *in vitro* metabolic activity of potently carcinogenic azoxyalkanes. *Mutat. Res.* **157**: 23.

Magee, P.N. and K.Y. Lee. 1964. Cellular injury and carcinogenesis. *Biochem. J.* **91**: 35.

Singer, G.M., W. Lijinsky, L. Buettner, and G.A. McClusky. 1981. Relationship of rat urinary metabolites of N-nitrosomethyl-N-alkylamine to bladder carcinogenesis. *Cancer Res.* **41**: 4942.

von Hofe, E., J. Schmerold, W. Lijinsky, and P. Kleihues. 1987. DNA methylation in rat tissues by a series of homologous aliphatic nitrosamines ranging from N-nitrosodimethylamine to N-nitrosomethyl-dodecylamine. *Carcinogenesis* **8**: 1337.

von Hofe, E., F. Grahmann, L.K. Keefer, W. Lijinsky, V. Nelson, and P. Kleihues. 1986. Methylation versus ethylation of DNA in target and non-target tissues of Fischer 344 rats treated with *N*-nitroso-methylethylamine. *Cancer Res.* **46**: 1038.

COMMENTS

Weisburger: Now we have time for one or two questions.

Hart: In work that was done by Mel Newman, Tom Slaga, and myself, we used 7,12-dimethylbenzanthracene, and we did one full substitution around the ring, similar to the benzo[a]pyrene substitution work that you have yet to discuss. Tom looked at mutagenicity and carcinogenici-ty, I looked at adduct formation and removal, and Mel Newman did most of the synthesis.

When we started to look at rat strains, although we thought, as you do, that unlike the bacterial system, the initial cell culture system was predictive. We found, however, that it was not as predictive as we originally assumed. The primary difference appears due to an element that hasn't yet been mentioned by anyone. Kleihus, Koestner, and myself did similar work with the alkylating agents, regarding the differences in proliferation of tissues. For example, cellular proliferation tends to have an equal, if not greater, impact than any of the chemical or metabolic changes that we noted, based upon whether the damage is actually going through DNA replication. It's interesting that now some models in the area of risk assessment are attempting to take proliferation into account. So, in addition to the parameters listed earlier, I think a biological parameter that must be considered, one which varies between tissues and even between strains of the same tissue, is the proliferation rate within those tissues.

Weisburger: Yes. Anytime you test a chemical, you have to think about both the chemical and the animal in which you are going to test it.

Wilson: Regarding the increasingly sophisticated and exquisite sensitivity of activity to the details of the structure of the compound, I've become more and more interested in the question of whether binding to the DNA macromolecule is even relevant to the carcinogenic process. In this case, it has begun to look to me more like a case of something involved in a receptor-type mechanism. The tetraol, the diol epoxide, or something perhaps derived from them is reacting with some undiscovered element in the cell. The result is either proliferation and the increasing of the proportion of background initiation that is captured as a mutated cell or the indirect increase of the relative fitness of the transformed cells that already exist. Has anyone done, or is it even possible to do, a definitive experiment that shows that, in fact, only reaction of these compounds or derivatives of these compounds with DNA leads to tumors?

Thakker: I don't know of an experiment that can really show that. My comment is that we have obviously reached an impasse. We know over the past few years that binding to DNA probably is an important event. I think most people have tried to show that these compounds tend to have more adducts or are more carcinogenic. When you don't have an answer, the simplest explanation that fits the data should be the one that is posed. In my opinion, the simplest explanation that one can come up with is that the biological differences that are seen, despite the formation of similar adducts from a number of different derivatives, may lie in the selectivity of the sequence that is involved.

That really is testable. For example, we know that four optically active benzo[a]pyrene diol epoxides all react with DNA, but they have tremendously different biological activity. Looking at the sequences around the codon of the adducts could be one place to start.

Singer: If you measure gross binding of an alkylating agent to DNA, you will find that poor carcinogens, such as dimethylsulfate, can give you the highest amount of binding in vitro and in vivo. So, a long time ago, people began to give up the idea that gross measurement had anything to do with carcinogenesis. I, of course, would like Willy's (Lijinsky) comments on that. I also will speak about specific kinds of adducts.

There is another factor, and that is that there is much more to the equation than DNA. We have proteins and we have RNA, neither of which we can ignore. Most of the types of carcinogens with which Willy and I work bind better to protein than they do to DNA. In this case, of course, you could be losing an essential function.

Lijinsky: That idea of controlling protein interaction goes back to Jim Miller and Betsy (Weisburger). About the alkylation, we have not measured the gross binding. We have measured the "pattern of O^6 alkylation" as well as the extent, which has been known for 20 years or more.

Michejda: That comment needs a reply. I think that is a crucial point of the conference.

Weisburger: We'll bring it up again.

Use of Structure-Activity Relationships in Assessing the Risks of New Chemicals

CHARLES M. AUER
Office of Toxic Substances
U.S. Environmental Protection Agency
Washington, D.C. 20460

OVERVIEW

Under Section 5 of the Toxic Substances Control Act (TSCA), manufacturers and importers of "new" chemicals (those not on an inventory of "existing" chemicals) must submit a Premanufacture Notification (PMN) to the U.S. Environmental Protection Agency (EPA) 90 days before they intend to commence manufacture or import. Whereas the notification must include information such as chemical identity, use, production volume, etc., there is no requirement that the notifier conduct health or environmental testing on the new chemical prior to submission. Since 1979, EPA has received notifications on over 9000 new chemicals; of these, fewer than 50% contained health or environmental test data. The task before EPA under TSCA Section 5 is to determine, despite the limited available test data, whether the new chemical presents an "unreasonable risk" of injury to health or the environment. This paper describes EPA's approach to assessing new chemicals with particular emphasis on the Agency's use of structure-activity relationships (SAR) analysis.

INTRODUCTION

TSCA was enacted in 1976 and provided certain authorities to EPA. The stated purpose of TSCA is to "protect human health and the environment by requiring testing and necessary use restrictions on certain chemical substances." The term "chemical substance" includes any organic or inorganic substance occurring in nature or as a result of chemical reaction; the term

This article has been reviewed by the Office of Toxic Substances, U.S. Environmental Protection Agency, and approved for publication. Approval does not signify that the contents necessarily reflect the views and policies of the Agency nor does mention of trade names or commercial products constitute endorsement or recommendation for use.

References in the previous discussion to the use of structure-activity relationships to address the greater number of chemicals EPA is required to delineate in the premanufacturing notice procedures are detailed in this paper.

does not include drugs, pesticides, foods, food additives, cosmetics, and certain other chemicals that are controlled by other statutes.

TSCA makes a clear distinction between so-called new and existing chemical substances. The latter have been enumerated in the TSCA Inventory of existing chemicals which contains over 60,000 entries. New chemicals, that is those not appearing on the TSCA Inventory, are subject to premanufacture reporting requirements under Section 5 of TSCA. Under these requirements, the manufacturer or importer of a new chemical must submit a PMN to EPA 90 days before it intends to commence manufacture or importation. This 90-day period, extendable with cause to 180 total days, is available to EPA for assessing the new chemical. Since publication of the initial TSCA Inventory in July 1979 through the end of 1987, the Agency has received PMNs on over 9000 new chemicals (Table 1). Of these, approximately 40% were polymeric substances, whereas the remaining PMNs were discrete chemicals or complex reaction products (EPA 1987).

The task before EPA under TSCA Section 5 is to distinguish between new chemicals that present reasonable risk versus those presenting unreasonable risk and to control the latter to minimize the risk (as used in TSCA, risk is a function of hazard [i.e., toxicity] and exposure). Determinations of unreasonable risk also involve consideration of economic and relative risk factors (these can include, for example, the cost or performance-based benefits of the new chemical, the economic impact of testing or regulation on the submitting company, and the relative hazards of the PMN chemical vis-á-vis those of substitutes). If it is determined that a PMN chemical may or will present unreasonable risk, the Agency can take action to control the risk.

Table 1
Annual Receipt of PMNs

Fiscal year[a]	Number
1979	9
1980	281
1981	580
1982	839
1983	1196[b]
1984	1192
1985	1462
1986	1693
1987	1761
Total	9012

[a]Corresponds to the period October 1 of the previous year through September 30 of the indicated year.
[b]106 synfuel chemicals are counted as one PMN (EPA 1987).

TSCA Section 5 requires that certain information be provided in the PMN, including: (1) a description of the new chemical substance, including by-products and impurities; (2) estimated annual production volume; (3) proposed uses; (4) estimates of the number of individuals expected to be exposed and the expected duration of exposure; and (5) any test data in the possession or control of the notifier that are related to the health or environmental effects of the substance. Thus, TSCA Section 5 does not require that submitters conduct toxicity testing prior to submission of a PMN, although they must supply any health or environmental test data that are available to them at the time of submission.

Currently, EPA receives test data on less than 50% of all PMN chemicals submitted. In general, health test data are more commonly provided than are environmental fate or effects data. The most commonly received health test data are the results of various acute tests (acute toxicity and irritation studies), whereas mutagenicity, repeated dose toxicity, reproductive effects testing, and so on, are submitted less frequently. Despite the paucity (often absence) of submitted test data, the Agency must determine whether PMN chemicals, under their projected conditions of manufacturing, processing, or use, may pose an unreasonable risk of injury to health or the environment.

In performing this risk determination, EPA must consider the potential hazards presented by the new chemical within the context of the projected human and environmental exposures. Descriptions of EPA's risk assessment process can be found elsewhere (DiCarlo et al. 1985; EPA 1986; Auer and Gould 1987). Because of the limitations in the available test data on PMN chemicals, EPA has had to develop an approach to assessing potential hazards in the presence of limited test data. This approach is known generically as SAR analysis and will be discussed in the section that follows.

In the event that the Agency, after completing its risk assessment, determines that a new chemical may present an unreasonable risk, it can under TSCA Section 5e prohibit or limit manufacture, processing, use, or disposal of a new chemical pending development of test data sufficient to permit a reasoned evaluation of the risk posed by the chemical. When the Agency can support the finding that a new chemical will present an unreasonable risk, it can take action under TSCA Section 5f to control the new chemical without requiring the development of additional test data. Through 1986 (EPA 1987), EPA has issued TSCA Section 5e orders on 216 PMN chemicals (counting a set of 106 synfuel chemicals received in FY83 as one PMN and one Section 5e action) and Section 5f rules on four PMN chemicals. An additional 150 PMN chemicals have been the subject of voluntary actions, agreed to by EPA and the submitter, involving testing, exposure controls, or other voluntary measures. A total of 313 PMN chemicals have been voluntarily withdrawn by the submitter in the face of a likely TSCA Section 5e (154 PMNs) or 5f (14 PMNs) action, or for other reasons (145 PMNs).

If EPA chooses not to take action to control a PMN chemical, the submitter is free to manufacture or import the chemical following expiration of the review period. Chemicals that are subject to voluntary or formal control action can also commence manufacture subject to the requirements of the specific action. Upon commencement of manufacture or importation, the submitter is required to provide written notification of such activity to EPA, after which the chemical will be added to the TSCA Inventory. To date, a notice of commencement of manufacture or importation has been received on approximately 56% of all PMNs submitted to the Agency through FY85 (EPA 1987).

DISCUSSION

As indicated earlier, TSCA Section 5 does not require the generation of test data prior to the submission of a PMN. Submitters must, however, provide any test data that are available to them at the time of submission. Table 2 presents summary statistics on test data submitted with PMNs. As can be seen, fewer than half of all PMNs contain test data. The situation is somewhat better for nonpolymeric PMN chemicals, of which approximately 60% contain some test data, whereas only 30% of the polymeric PMNs contain test data. Nonetheless, when test data are submitted they most commonly report the results of various acute tests (acute oral and dermal lethality studies [LD_{50} determinations] and skin and eye irritation studies). Mutagenicity or sensitization studies are received with less than one in six PMNs, whereas repeated-dose toxicity studies, developmental toxicity tests, reproductive toxicity assays, and other tests are received with less than 1% of all PMNs. (For additional discussion, the reader is referred to earlier evaluations of the test data provided in PMNs [Office of Technology Assessment 1983; Auer and Gould 1987].)

Given the qualitative and quantitative limitations of the test data provided with PMNs, EPA was confronted with the difficulty of assessing chemicals in the presence of limited test data. From this experience evolved EPA's reliance on SAR analysis as a tool for identifying and assessing the potential hazards presented by PMN chemicals. The major components of EPA's approach to hazard assessment in the presence of limited test data include the following: (1) critical review of available test data on the PMN chemical; (2) identification and selection of potential analogs and/or prediction of key PMN metabolites or environmental degradation products, followed by critical review of test data available on these chemicals; (3) use of quantitative structure-activity relationships (QSAR) methods when available and applicable; and (4) the experience and judgment of scientific assessors in interpreting, weighing, and integrating the often limited information developed per the above components.

Table 2
Submission of Test Data on PMN Chemicals

Test data type	All (% PMNs)	Nonpolymer (% PMNs)	Polymer (% PMNs)
(a) *Health data*			
Acute oral	38	50	22
Acute dermal	23	29	14
Acute inhalation	11	14	7
Eye irritation	36	47	21
Skin irritation	38	50	22
Mutagenicity	15	23	6
Sensitization	11	17	5
Other[a]	11	16	4
(b) *Environmental effects data*			
Acute lethal vertebrate	6	9	3
Acute lethal invertebrate	3	3	2
(c) *Environmental fate data*			
Biodegradation	6	8	2
Log P	4	5	1
No submitted test data	51	38	68

Based on the PMNs received through September 1985 (EPA 1987).
[a]The "other" health data category includes acute toxicity studies by other routes (ip, iv, etc.), repeated-dose toxicity studies, teratogenicity assays, phototoxicity, neurotoxicity, and a variety of other toxicity tests.

As discussed above, little or no test data are generally submitted with PMNs, and, furthermore, in EPA's experience only rarely are data on the PMN chemical found in the published literature. Thus, in many instances, this component contributes little to the overall assessment of the PMN chemical.

The second component, the identification and selection of analogs and the prediction of potential metabolites or degradation products, represents one of the unique aspects of EPA's approach. In order for an analog to be useful to EPA, it must resemble the PMN chemical in one or more critical aspects (e.g., structurally, substructurally, physicochemically, etc.) and also have pertinent toxicological data available in the literature. An analysis by the National Research Council (NRC) (1984) reported that available test data are limited for most chemicals, but especially so for TSCA chemicals (the analysis examined pharmaceuticals, pesticides, food additives, and industrial [TSCA] chemicals). The NRC estimated that no toxicity information was available in the published literature for over 75% of the chemicals on the TSCA Inventory. This factor imposes major limitations on the usefulness of many potential analogs.

EPA relies on two principal means to identify chemical analogs. These consist of analog recommendations offered by technical staff and structural analogs retrieved from several publicly available, automated chemical substructure and nomenclature search systems. (Examples of publicly available automated substructure and nomenclature search systems include: SANSS [Structure and Nomenclature Search System] in the Chemical Information System, available from CIS, Inc.; CAS-ONLINE, available from Chemical Abstracts Service; and DARC, available from Questel, Inc.) Analogs recommended by technical staff often provide a wealth of pertinent information that can be applied to the assessment effort. These individuals also provide guidance in developing the strategy for the automated analog searches. This guidance consists of the identification, based on chemistry, metabolism, mechanisms of toxicity, etc., of key features (e.g., potential toxicophores) within the PMN chemical's structure, which may be associated with some potential toxicity or the mitigation of toxicity. Potential analogs resembling the PMN chemical in the structure or function of these key features are then identified using one of the automated substructure search capabilities. When selecting analogs for literature search and subsequent assessment purposes, similarity in the structure or function of the potential toxicophore(s) is an essential element. The physicochemical properties of the PMN chemical are also considered in selecting potential analogs; ideally, analogs resemble the PMN chemical both physicochemically and in the structure or function of the potential toxicophore(s). The physicochemical and other factors considered in comparing the PMN chemical with potential analogs can include relative differences in molecular weight, molecular topology, log P, water solubility, pKa, presence and position of reactive or potentially reactive groups, and possible steric or electronic effects. Once potential analogs have been selected, they are subjected to an automated literature search using a variety of readily available bibliographic systems and data bases to determine the availability of pertinent toxicity information. Only those analogs that yield test data are carried forward in the assessment process.

A second major aspect of the effort to identify test data on "related" chemicals involves the identification of potential metabolites and environmental degradation products of the PMN chemical. Metabolism studies that are directly applicable to the PMN chemical are rarely available, thus, the effort focuses on the metabolic potential of the new chemical (DiCarlo et al. 1986a). Key potential metabolites are identified by applying established principles of xenobiotic metabolism (taken, for example, from Williams 1959; Parke 1968; Jacoby 1980; Jacoby et al. 1982; Caldwell and Jacoby 1983; Anders 1985) and by considering metabolism studies on chemical analogs.

The emphasis in this analysis, which uses a "weight of the evidence" approach, is to establish likely activation and deactivation pathways for the PMN chemical with the objective of identifying potential reactive metabolites. For example, if a postulated metabolite is projected to be formed only by an unusual reaction or to require a series of biotransformation steps for its formation, these points will be considered in reaching the overall assessment conclusions. In much the same general way, EPA attempts to identify environmental degradation products that might result from release of the PMN chemical. Potential metabolites or environmental degradation products identified per the above are then subjected to analog search and literature search as was described earlier.

The use of the third component, QSAR methods, is currently limited to the estimation of certain physicochemical properties or environmental fate parameters (such as water solubility, vapor pressure [Lyman et al. 1982], log P [Chou and Jurs 1979]), environmental effects (prediction of acute LC_{50}s in aquatic organisms; see, for example, Konemann 1981; Hermans 1983; Lipnick and Dunn 1983; Veith et al. 1983, Lipnick et al. 1985), and bioconcentration factors (Veith et al. 1979).

The last of the components, the experience and judgment of the scientific assessors in interpreting and integrating the available information, is the most critical. This is especially so in the case of information developed on analogs, metabolites, or degradation products that must be weighted as a function of their similarity to the target chemical or, in the case of metabolites and degradation products, the likelihood and significance of their formation. In performing an evaluation of potential analogs, assessors consider a variety of factors as they apply to the PMN chemical and then, using these factors, compare the PMN chemical with the proposed analogs. The factors can include molecular shape and size, physicochemical properties, the presence and positions of potentially activating or deactivating functional groups, potential for oral, dermal, and inhalation absorption, biotransformation pathways, distribution and excretion, possible mechanisms of toxicity, possible idiosyncratic toxicity of analogs, etc. (Arcos 1983; DiCarlo et al. 1985, 1986a,b; Auer and Gould 1987).

Thus, in the presence of limited test data on PMN chemicals, an SAR-based approach is used by EPA to evaluate the potential hazards of new chemicals. The conclusions of the hazard analysis are combined with the determinations developed by exposure assessors and economists to yield an overall risk conclusion for the PMN chemical. In making projections about the risks of most PMN chemicals, EPA is handicapped by the limited test data that are available on the new chemical and its analogs. For this reason, EPA's hazard predictions tend to take the form of conservative, worst-case analyses that reflect the uncertainties inherent in a process using limited test data. The

TSCA Section 5e "may present" language recognizes the uncertainties that are likely to confront EPA in assessing the risks of PMN chemicals under these circumstances. Accordingly, TSCA Section 5e permits EPA to meet a less stringent regulatory finding in requiring the development of needed test data on those new chemicals that may have the potential for presenting unreasonable risks.

ACKNOWLEDGMENT

The author gratefully acknowledges the assistance of Juanita Herman in typing the manuscript.

REFERENCES

Anders, M.W., ed. 1985. *Bioactivation of foreign compounds.* Academic Press, New York.

Arcos, J.C. 1983. Comparative requirements for premarketing/premanufacture notification in the EC countries and the USA, with special reference to risk assessment in the framework of the U.S. Toxic Substances Control Act. *J. Am. Coll. Toxicol.* **2**: 131.

Auer, C.M. and D.H. Gould. 1987. Carcinogenicity assessment and the role of structure activity relationships (SAR) analysis under TSCA Section 5. *Environ. Carcinogen. Rev.* **C5(1)**: 29.

Caldwell, J. and W.B. Jacoby, eds. 1983. *Biological basis of detoxication.* Academic Press, New York.

Chou, J.T. and P.C. Jurs. 1979. Computer assisted computation of partition coefficients from molecular structures using fragment constants. *J. Chem. Inf. Comput. Sci.* **19**: 172.

DiCarlo, F.J., P. Bickart, and C.M. Auer. 1985. Role of the Structure Activity Team in the premanufacture notification process. In *QSAR in toxicology and xenobiochemistry* (ed. M. Tichy), p. 433. Elsevier, Amsterdam.

———. 1986a. Structure-metabolism relationships (SMR) for the prediction of health hazards by the Environmental Protection Agency. I. Background for the practice of predictive toxicology. *Drug. Metab. Rev.* **17**: 171.

———. 1986b. Structure metabolism relationships (SMR) for the prediction of health hazards by the Environmental Protection Agency. II. Application to teratogenicity and other toxic effects caused by aliphatic acids. *Drug. Metab. Rev.* **17**: 187.

EPA. 1986. *New chemical review process manual* (EPA 560/3-86-002). Office of Toxic Substances, Washington, D.C.

———. 1987. Data printouts retrieved from MITS or PENTA, EPA in-house PMN information systems. Office of Toxic Substances, Washington, D.C.

Hermans, J. 1983. The use of QSAR in toxicity studies with aquatic organisms. Correlation of toxicity of different classes of organic chemicals with Poct, pKa and chemical reactivity. In *Quantitative approaches to drug design* (ed. J.C. Dearden), p. 263. Elsevier, Amsterdam.

Jacoby, W.B., ed. 1980. *Enzymatic basis of detoxication,* vols. I and II. Academic Press, New York.

Jacoby, W.B., J.R. Bend, and J. Caldwell, eds. 1982. *Metabolic basis of detoxication.* Academic Press, New York.

Konemann, H. 1981. Quantitative structure-activity relationships in fish toxicity studies. I. Relationship for 50 industrial pollutants. *Toxicology* **19:** 223.

Lipnick, R.L. and W.J. Dunn III. 1983. An MLAB study of aquatic structure toxicity relationships. In *Quantitative approaches to drug design* (ed. J.C. Dearden), p. 265. Elsevier, Amsterdam.

Lipnick, R.L., D.E. Johnson, J.H. Gilford, C.K. Bickings, and L.D. Newsome. 1985. Comparison of fish toxicity screening data for 55 alcohols with the QSAR predictions of minimum toxicity for nonreactive nonelectrolyte organic compounds. *Environ. Toxicol. Chem.* **4:** 281.

Lyman, W.J., W.F. Reehle, and D.H. Rosenblatt. 1982. *Handbook of chemical property estimation methods.* McGraw-Hill, New York.

National Research Council. 1984. *Toxicity testing: Strategies to determine needs and priorites.* National Academy Press, Washington, D.C.

Office of Technology Assessment. 1983. The Information Content of Premanufacture Notices—Background Paper, OTA-BP-H-17 Washington, D.C.

Parke, D.V. 1968. *The biochemistry of foreign compounds.* Pergamon Press, Oxford.

Toxic Substances Control Act (TSCA). 1976. Public Law 94-469, 90 Stat. 2003, October 11, 1976.

Veith, G.D., D.J. Call, and L.T. Brooke. 1983. Structure-toxicity relationships for the fathead minnow, *Pimephales promelas:* Narcotic industrial chemicals. *Can. J. Fish. Aquat. Sci.* **40:** 743.

Veith, G.D., D.L. De Foe, and B.V. Bergstedt. 1979. Measuring and estimating the bioconcentration factor of chemicals in fish. *J. Fish Res. Board Can.* **36:** 1040.

Williams, R.T. 1959. *Detoxication mechanisms.* Wiley, New York.

Commentary

WILLIAM FARLAND
U.S. Environmental Protection Agency
Washington, D.C. 20460

Farland: Earlier, we discussed the various attributes of chemicals that concern us when we talk about structure activity. As we proceed, we will discuss the ability to alkylate, confirmation, stereochemistry, substituents, and how these chemical properties can be applied to risk assessment process.

One of the things that is important to understand is that in federal government risk assessment, we sit in a central position because we provide one component of information for risk managers who have to make decisions and who have to deal with the economics and the politics of risk management decisions, along with many other things. We also are able to deal with the research and data collection that goes on outside. Also, ours is the ability to influence data collection and research, in the sense that risk assessment ends up stimulating as many questions as it answers.

I like to look at risk assessment as a process that is made up of hazard identification, dose/response assessment, and exposure assessment. That leads us to risk characterization and to the idea that risk characterization is the product of this process and that it has a central role in risk management. Frequently, we don't have the answers that people want to hear when they ask questions about uncertainties. That will be my viewpoint.

Despite the admonition from Dr. Lijinsky regarding not using stucture-activity relationships, we at the EPA do use them. Let me put that in perspective. In 1986, EPA published some guidelines for doing risk assessment, carcinogenicity in particular. Our idea was to improve the technical quality of our risk assessment, so that we would have something consistent against which to work. Clearly, there was a mandate to clarify scientific assumptions and to get them into these group discussions, in order to provide flexibility in the way we work. Thereby, we provided both our internal groups and the public with a road map of how we conduct business.

In terms of these guidelines, we looked at hazard identification and the weight of evidence analysis, which Ron (Hart) discussed, as an important component in the risk assessment process. For carcinogenicity, we directed attention to various subjects of hazard identification: (1)

clearly, review and analyses of all of the data available on a particular chemical is important; (2) questioning whether a particular end point could be ascribed to that chemical and what data base support was available is critical; and (3) finally questions are asked whether data on animal modeling pertain to that same event occurring from other routes with other species.

That is generally the list used when we study the kinds of information for our hazard identification step in carcinogenicity risk assessment. Aside from the animal studies and epidemiology, which certainly form a very strong base for the analyses that we do, there are many things that need to be studied. Earlier, questions were raised dealing with the issues of chemical and physical properties, the structure-activity issue, and metabolism and pharmacokinetics. All of these things add weight to the evidence that a chemical may be carcinogenic.

Generally, with risk assessments that I do at the Office of Research and Development, structure activity is used as supportive information. We have data from long-term bioassays or epidemiology regarding a chemical's carcinogenicity to humans. We say that structure activity provides important supportive information that a chemical belongs to a class of carcinogenic chemicals or that the chemical may be metabolized to a particular chemical structure that we know, from long-term bioassays, is carcinogenic.

So far I have reviewed chemicals for which there is long-term bioassay data under the Toxic Substances Control Act. However, EPA must also deal with new chemical substances that are coming into the marketplace. In fact, since 1979, EPA has reviewed about 9000 substances that have been proposed to the market. Those 9000 substances, primarily industrial chemicals, are evaluated with the understanding that this is preliminary testing. If there is a need, based on the evidence that is available to us at the time, for additional testing, that is the time that we ask for more testing to be done. If there is a need to control exposure in some particular way, that is the time to get it on the books.

The Congress was generous in giving us 90 days to do such assessments and to suggest that we really didn't need a base set of testing in order to make determinations. Last year, there were some 1760 chemicals tested at the office with which Charlie Auer and I used to be associated. Of those, 60% were discrete chemicals and about 40% were polymers. Clearly, different issues are associated with these two classes, and this distinction needs to be considered.

As I indicated, the law says that there is no necessary base set of information, but that we must be supplied with available information on the new chemical when it is proposed for manufacture. As soon as there is a small amount of the chemical available, as soon as there is something known about the physicochemical properties, and as soon as there is an acute test, submission is made. In fact, we get test data, any test data, on less than 50% of the chemicals that are sent through. We may know what the structure is and a little bit about the purity but that's about it. We get acute testing data on about 40% of the chemicals, so that is a test that the industry does very early and supplies to us very early on, so that we have something to go on in terms of acute toxicity. Just for your information, we get some mutagenicity data and some sensitization data on less than 15% of the chemicals, and we get repeated dose studies on less than 1% of all of those chemicals that come to us.

What I have tried to explain is the task that we are faced with and the fact that, despite the admonition that we heard earlier, we have to use structure-activity relationships. The only thing we have to go on, in terms of particular chemicals, is what we know from the available data base and how we can use structures that we have reviewed in the past. The decisions that we make at that point are not about regulation but about determining whether additional testing should be done.

That is an important distinction, because we need to determine if there is enough suspicion based on informed, scientific judgment to require testing. In terms of requiring the testing, we place a burden of evidence that the chemical will support or will not support. Then a decision is made as to whether the chemical will go into the marketplace and potentially effect the public. That's the second way that we use structure-activity relationships.

Lijinsky: Does the use of the chemical have any effect on how you evaluate it?

Farland: Absolutely. Certainly it does, in terms of the exposure component. Basically, we evaluate the chemical's test data as a hazard identification step. As I said, we very rarely have much information from that standpoint. We then look at analogs or potential metabolites. Again, that is an issue for expert judgment, not quantitative structure-activity relationships. Studies of quantitative structure-activity relationships, from our perspective, have not developed to the point that they are particularly useful for health end effects. They are used fairly routinely for some ecological environmental effects. There is a much larger data base, that is quite useful in that regard.

Basically, we try to conclude the likelihood of hazard if there is exposure to this chemical and what types of testing would be needed to characterize that hazard. Probably one of the most important issues is how we will get that information. Will we be getting that information while the chemical is in production and under use with certain protective equipment required, or will it be basically a ban on the chemical until information is available?

We have a committee of about 40% of our senior scientists that essentially spends all of its time dealing with dossiers on these chemicals. The initial decision comes out of the structure-activity team, goes through a review by a division-level board, and then it goes through an additional review. There are at least three studies by people with slightly different perspectives on the issues of potential hazard, the exposure that might be seen on the new chemical, and the use of the structure activity in a strong way to determine the need for additional test data on that chemical.

One thing struck me earlier. Ron (Hart) mentioned that there is an attempt now to use additional biological information in terms of modeling risks. That is information to which we hope that the basic research community will help to contribute and that our statisticians will help us use.

Dr. Lijinsky's point about site concordance of tumors becomes very important. What we are going to end up with is a situation where our models are going to reflect cell proliferation rates and to reflect various types of handling of chemicals in specific organs in rodents. Then, we have to ask the question of how we translate that to a human model. Are we going to say that any organ that functions similarly is going to potentially show a carcinogenic response? Or, are we going to say that there may be a human organ that functions in the same way? Thereby, we can begin to predict risks using that type of a response.

This gives us a little bit of a lead-in to some of our discussions on quantitation and modeling and how we can use structure activity to get to the issue of site concordance. That one is an issue that has swung like a pendulum. There was a time when we felt that there was not a need to worry about site concordance. We were concerned that if you had the potential to produce a tumor in an animal, you had the potential to produce a tumor in a human at some site. Now, there is a data base building and there is more information there that should be studied in terms of the site concordance. Dave Rall has recently published an analysis of the data base indicating that, although there are exceptions, site concordance may be stronger than we suspect for some chemicals. That is really just an introduction to some of the topics that are particularly important to us in the regulatory community.

Weisburger: Thank you, Bill. I think Dr. Farland has done an excellent summary of how the EPA uses this data. I really hadn't known all the details myself, other than that the structure-activity relationships were used a great deal.

Panel Discussion

CHRISTOPHER J. MICHEJDA
NCI-Frederick Cancer Research Facility, Maryland

DONALD E. STEVENSON
Shell Oil Company, Texas

KURT ENSLEIN
Health Designs, Inc., New York

Weisburger: Now we will have the panel period. First is Dr. Christopher Michejda, from the NCI-Frederick Cancer Research Facility.

Michejda: There are several points and questions that I would like to raise. Willy (Lijinsky) mentioned N-nitrosomethylaniline. The reason we are interested is that, unlike most nitrosamines, which are metabolized to a highly reactive alkyldiazonium ions, this one is metabolized to a rather less reactive benzenediazonium ion plus formaldehyde. Yet, it is quite a good carcinogen, and the carcinogenic effect is exclusively in the esophagus in the rat.

   Although the proof is still lacking in vivo, we have recently found that in in vitro systems there is a binding to DNA that is quasitransient. That raises an interesting issue. These so-called nonbinders may bind for a brief period of time. If the tissue is suitable, such as in the esophagus, which sloughs off cells continually and, therefore, actively undergoes DNA synthesis and replication, then perhaps, a transient binding can be imprinted as an error. Without going into the chemistry, the product that is formed in a test tube is stable; however, when it's formed in a physiological situation, it is unstable or quasitransient. Dr. Hart mentioned this subject.

   The correlation between alkylation and carcinogenicity is, in some cases, extremely good. One might mention the tobacco-specific nitrosamines, in particular, that the people at the American Health Foundation have been studying: Steve Hecht, Dietrich Hoffmann, John Weisburger, and others. In their studies, the degree of methylation by these carcinogens in target tissue and carcinogenicity is very good. The carcinogens are compounds such as 4-N-nitrosomethylamino-1-(3-pyridyl)-1-butanone, for example.

   Very recently, we examined the DNA alkylation by N-nitrosomethyl-(2-hydroxethyl)amine, which is a liver carcinogen in rats but is particularly potent in female rats rather than male rats. What we found is that the amount of alkylation, integrated over a period of time, is greater in females than it is in males. This doesn't prove that alkylation is the thing, but, clearly, the data tend to support alkylation as being a critical

Banbury Report 31: Carcinogen Risk Assessment: New Directions in the Qualitative and Quantitative Aspects © Cold Spring Harbor Laboratory. 0-87969-231-6/88. $1.00 + .00   **47**

factor in initiation of cancer. We measured specific adducts, we measured dose responses in these adducts, and we also measured the persistence of the adducts. I mention this because there are data regarding nitrosamines and other types of carcinogens where there is a good correlation between adduct formation and cancer initiation.

Dr. Thakker said something about polycyclic aromatic hydrocarbons. He talked about benzo[a]pyrene. One of our colleagues at FCRF, Tony Dipple, has been looking at adducts produced by many polycyclic aromatic hydrocarbons, particularly dimethylbenzanthracene, and more recently, benzo[c]phenanthrene and 5-methylchrysene. One of the most interesting findings in his work is the excellent correlation between carcinogenic potency of a given metabolite and the ability to bind to the amino group of adenine.

Focusing on adducts at the 2-amino group of guanosine may be appropriate since the correlation appears to be better with adducts to adenine, according to Dr. Dipple and his coworkers. Their numbers provide one of the strongest indications that PAH binding to DNA is one of the necessary, but clearly not sufficient, factors in cancer initiation.

Lastly, Dr. Farland talked about the structure-activity relations. These are viewed by many chemists as the way to bring about order from chaos. One would like to be able to reduce everything to a very simple equation. What I would like to point out is that structure-activity relations are a valid concept. Structure-activity relations are an extension of the "linear free-energy relationship" theory that was initiated by Bronsted and Louis Hammett. However, a long time ago chemists found that one has to be careful in applying linear free-energy relationships. One must apply them to a strictly defined data set. As long as you are studying the right things, you are probably correct in applying structure-activity relationships. However, as Willy (Lijinsky) explained, given the amazing amount of data, it is very difficult to pick out the correct things to compare.

Weisburger: Thank you, Chris, for giving us these points to consider and to keep in mind. Our next discussant is Dr. Donald Stevenson, from Shell Oil Company.

*   *   *

Stevenson: The Science Committee of the American Industrial Health Council, of which I am the Chair, recently had an informal meeting with Charlie Auer of EPA and some of his staff to review structure activity. What Charlie told us is almost exactly what Bill (Farland) described at this meeting.

For that meeting, we had been supplied with about a dozen structures by EPA which asked us to assess them for carcinogenic activity. I gave the structures to two biochemists, one being Bob Neal and the other was a student of Bob Neal's who works for Shell. When the structures were discussed, it was found that our agreement with the EPA assessment was almost complete. In other words, competent biochemists or chemists sitting in a group discussing structural activity can achieve a great deal in determining what is the likely outcome.

One further suggestion did come out of that meeting. As Bill mentioned, the EPA looks at what is significant in the practical context, and one area where we both have found difficulty in making predictions is in the estimation of dermal absorption, which in the industrial context is often the major route of exposure. We did debate the possibility of following up by getting additional information, and so forth. Certainly in our company, in doing our risk assessments, we find it difficult to determine the amount of the substance that will get into the body over a given timespan.

We have also submitted a group of 12 compounds to the two structure-activity methods discussed by the two next speakers. Our results there were not so promising. In one case, of the 12, 4 were in fact misdiagnosed, 3 false positives and 1 false negative. In the other case, all the results were indeterminant, i.e., no definite predictions were possible. So, I think that one has to be careful when you use these systems in isolation.

Our current feeling is that structure-activity systems do have their use when balanced by good judgment, but they are not reliable on their own. The judgment factor is still very important.

The implication of what Bill mentioned was that there were a lot of new chemicals coming into commerce. One has to be very careful with that word "chemical," because it applies to substances rather than to chemicals, per se.

In our own case, many of the things that we submit are minor structural variants of substances already marketed. As an example, we market detergent alcohols. A new substance, according to the TSCA definition, might have only a slightly different range of molecular sizes. So, in fact, we might market a range that is 12–15 carbons in the chain length. A customer may not want that particular mixture, but he may want a 13–14, or just a 12, or just an 11 length. If these lengths are not marketed and included in the TSCA Inventory, then they automatically become a new substance under the definition of the Act. Those are such minor variants that one wouldn't necessarily test them.

Another example would be in the resins area, where again one modifies a chain length to a certain degree by adding another phenol group or something similar. Again, one probably would not be changing the risk by any significant degree. Therefore, I think the numbers can be misleading, if you don't understand the context in which substances are produced.

The other thing, of course, is that, as an oil company, we often sell products on physical or performance specifications rather than on chemical specifications. That presents a different kind of problem altogether, because we are dealing with complex mixtures.

In the case of oils, there has been a tremendous amount of testing done in the generic sense. You have to understand, with oils, that an oil obtained from different oil wells may vary in composition even from others in the same field. Oil from the same oil well over a period of time may vary, also. So, in that situation, you can't test every different new product. We do have a large amount of generic information on, for example, refinery streams. Much of that information has been correlated with individual short-term tests now and allows risk determinations to be made with reasonable certainty on individual streams.

Various companies have different approaches. Mobil, for instance, has developed a modified Ames test, which is based on testing a DMSO extract, and they are utilizing this to make a prediction of carcinogenicity. We, in fact, have a somewhat similar test, except it is based on a DMSO extract that is looked at in terms of the polycyclic content, and it is on that basis that we make a judgment. There are also other test systems that have been developed that relate to short-term effects directly on, for example, mouse skin. There is a range of useful tests that have now been developed on which you can make predictions of potential carcinogenic activity.

I would also like to get back to Ron's (Hart) original point, because I think what he said is a cliche in the suggestion that there are X thousands of compounds out there, and that if we could test those and find which are carcinogenic, we could solve the cancer problem. I think an uninformed person sitting in this audience might well have come to that conclusion, and we have to be very careful not to give that impression.

The numbers quoted may be based on the TSCA Inventory, although I have learned that some companies have a data base that has information on that large a number of compounds. However, I suspect that we are dealing with the old 80/20 rule, that perhaps 20% of the number of chemicals represent 80% of the total tonnage or exposure. Certainly, when you look down the list of those materials that are around, it is surprising that many of the "golden oldies" are still at the top of the list, things like sulfuric acid, sodium hydroxide, the inorganics, and so forth.

Therefore, I think that more work is required to investigate what really is the profile of exposure. Certainly, if you take it to be that large and test a few compounds a year, take those out of the total, and then add a few more, you are really not going to have any effect on the overall problem. If we are really concerned about cancer, I think that our approach should be capable of producing a definable benefit in terms of reducing incidence. Some of the legislation actually requires that an agency demonstrates that whatever it does has a defined benefit.

Going back to the structure activity topic for a moment, I have discussed mixtures. Another thing about which we have to be very careful is minor contaminants. I once spent ten years on a particular investigation because we didn't realize that there was a minor contaminant in a particular product. That was not a carcinogenic end point, it was another end point. We picked up the mode of action very quickly, but we couldn't explain it on a chemical basis. It literally took us ten years to solve that particular problem. It wasn't until we finally learned the details of the actual manufacturing route that we realized everything would just fall into place.

When a compound is tested, very often we don't know exactly what is examined, and so I am rather reluctant to accept a result from a bioassay unless I know what actually was tested. I think in many cases we just don't have that kind of information.

We have already touched on the concept that a carcinogen is not just a carcinogen. We also have to consider the context in which it may work. Last week, I had two extensive conversations with somebody who called me about a good, new test for carcinogenic activity. If I supplied a material, they could tell me whether it was a carcinogen or not. This led to a long debate, since they wouldn't disclose the system because it was going to be patented. All I discovered was the fact that it was a range of test systems, which from what I gleaned was a rational approach. However, unless I knew what I was letting myself in for, in terms of the system, I would be very reluctant to use it. Is it very useful, for instance, to know whether a certain effluent or substance is carcinogenic, but that is only half the answer. The questions really are important. How carcinogenic is the substance? Is this test going to provide you with a certain cutoff? The questions imply that we do have to develop an approach that is quantitative, we have to have an approach that tells us how we can estimate and manage risk on a rational basis, rather than simply listing hazards.

We must get back to the first lesson we ever received in toxicology in the 16th century, when Paracelsus said, "Everything is harmful, everything is safe; it all depends on the dose." Really, we shouldn't be talking about toxic chemicals, because in fact everything is toxic. We really have to discover how we can limit risk and not simply do this by eliminating those things that appear to be superficially attractive on the surface.

Weisburger: Thank you. I always like to tell people that Dr. Stevenson has said everything is toxic, that even water is toxic, and that there was a case where somebody drank 17 liters within a short time and died from it. So remember, water is a very toxic chemical.

Dr. Kurt Enslein, from Health Designs in Rochester, New York, is with us, and he is one of our panelists. Dr. Enslein.

*   *   *

Enslein: For the past several years we have been engaged in applying principles of structure-activity relationships (SAR) to the modeling of toxic end points. By the use of these SAR equations, it is possible to estimate the probability of a particular toxic response for untested chemicals. These estimates are useful for setting testing and developmental priorities, and thus also in the risk assessment process. The current equations do not estimate potency, but they identify those compounds that may present risks, in this case, carcinogenic risk. These equations have been implemented in the TOPKAT program, which operates on a number of advanced personal computers.

The equation for the prediction of the probability of carcinogenicity is based on three categories of data: (1) NCI/NTP 2-year bioassays, as evaluated by Dr. Richard Griesemer, now at Oak Ridge National Laboratory; (2) compounds identified as human carcinogens listed in the 1985 Annual Report on Carcinogens, not already included in the NCI/NTP assays; and (3) food additives used for substantial periods of time, sometimes in quantity, and putatively noncarcinogenic, selected from those listed in Code of Federal Regulations (CFR) 21. Table 1 shows which chemical groups are represented in the data base.

Each chemical is described by parameters that are then used to develop SAR equations. These parameters consist of substructural keys and molecular connectivity indexes. The equations are developed by means of discriminant analysis procedures. The parameters that are found to be statistically important in distinguishing carcinogens from noncarcinogens are listed in Table 2, together with the signs of the discriminant coefficients for each parameter. A positive sign indicates that the parameter adds to the probability of carcinogenicity, and a negative sign reduces that probability. We have not listed the coefficients for the sake of simplicity.

Using the resubstitution method for evaluating the performance of the equation, we have the results shown in Table 3. These results show that taking into account seven chemicals for which decisions cannot be made, i.e., their predicted probabilities are too near 0.5, 97% of the other chemicals are assigned to their correct carcinogenesis categories.

Due to the high accuracy of the SAR equation it is then possible to estimate

Table 1

Heterogeneous Data Set Classification by Chemical Groups

	Number of compounds	
Group	positives	negatives
Aryl (amines, azo-amines, amides, nitro)	34	13
acridine/quinoline	0	2
one ring	19	3
two or more rings	15	8
Aryl azo (not amine)	2	3
N-nitrosoamines	2	0
Di-or-polyhalogenated alkanes and cycloalkanes	16	0
Halogenated alkenes	4	1
Aryl and heteroaryl halogens	11	1
Hydrazines and hydrazides	4	0
Aliphatic azo, azoxy, and diazo	0	1
Strained rings (not otherwise classified)	2	0
Lactones, lactams, anhydrides	1	3
PAHs and hetero analogs (fused rings only)	7	4
Triazenes	1	1
Purines, pyridines, pyrimidines	3	4
Thio analogs	4	7
Carbamates and unsaturated carbonyl compounds	3	3
Benzylic alcohols	1	31
Aliphatic alcohols	0	35
Aliphatic and alicyclic esters	1	17
Aromatic esters	2	26
Aliphatic and alicyclic carboxyls and nonring lactones	1	7
Aromatic carboxyls	1	3
Aldehydes (any and all)	0	34
Ketones (any and all)	0	25
Furans	0	4
Thiazoles	2	0
Carbazoles	1	0
Alkyl benzenes (i.e., toluene, styrene, and derivatives)	0	4
Aliphatic amines	1	1
Aliphatic (nitrosos, alkanes, alkenes)	1	1
Cyanates and isocyanates	2	0
Phosphates	6	0
Benzene	1	—
Total	114	229

the probability of an untested compound producing a positive result if a 2-year NCI/NTP assay were performed with it. Using these estimates, it is possible to rank a series of chemicals with these probabilities to determine priorities for testing and other investigations. It is important to realize that

Table 2
NCI/NIP Bioassay Model Final Equation Keys and Coefficients

Key	Name	Sign
K11000	Longest atom chain in nonring molecule (scaled)	+
K11100	Longest atom chain in ring molecule (scaled)	−
K16200	Hydrazine	+
K16700	Bromide fragment	+
K17024	Aryl nitro	+
K17208	Azo fragment (β-phenyl)	+
K2000	Longest aliphatic carbon chain in molecule	−
K2140	Di-acyl ethyl fragment	−
K26001	Aliphatic alcohol or salt of alcohol	−
K26007	Aryl alcohol or salt of aryl alcohol	−
K26008	Nonaromatic ring alcohol or salt of alcohol	−
K26559	Aliphatic carboxylic acid or salt of acid	−
K26654	1,1,1-Trichloro fragment (non-β-phenyl) (carc.)	+
K3010	2-Methyl-2-butene fragment	−
K36220	Aliphatic amide	+
K36435	Carbonyl substituted aryl ester	−
K36445	Oxygen substituted aryl ester	−
K36605	Aliphatic aldehyde	−
K36610	Aliphatic ketone	−
K36640	Aliphatic halogen	+
K36671	Nonaromatic ring chloride	+
K37629	Aryl sulfonic acid or salt	−
K38228	Ethane/ethylene fragment (see documentation)	+
K38338	Propane/propylene fragment (see documentation)	+
K38607	Di-acyl fragment	−
K4099	Longest perimeter in a ring	+
K4501	Oxirane	+
K6105	Aryl NH$_2$	+
K6156	Aryl 3-branched nitrogen (nonamide)	+
K6603	Aryl aldehyde	−
K6653	1,1-dichloro (non-β-phenyl)	+
K6670	Aryl chloride	+
K72RNH	NH or N subst., with electron releasing groups only	−
K76100	Aliphatic NH$_2$ or NH or 3-branched nitrogen (nonamide)	+
K76425	Alkyl or nonaromatic ring ester	−
K7WRNW	N with 1 elec. rel. and 2 with draw. grps. or 3 with draw. grps.	+
DIFPATO	Difference path MCI order 0	+
KR1245	1, 2, 4, 5 substituted benzene	+
SIMPC4	Simple path/cluster MCI order 4	+
VALPAT4	Valence adjusted path MCI order 4	+
KWRNH	NH subst., with 1 elec. rel. grp. and 1 elec. with draw. grp.	+

the SAR equation produces an estimate of the probability of a compound being a carcinogen, not its carcinogenic potency.

Table 3
Discriminant Analysis Classification

Actual class	Negative	Indeterminate	Positive
Negative	217	4	7
Positive	3	3	101

% Indeterminate: $7/335 = 2.1\%$; % false positives: $7/328 = 2.1\%$; % false negatives: $3/328 = 0.9\%$; Overall accuracy: $325/335 = 97.0\%$.
$F = 25.6$ with 41 and 293 D.F.

The TOPKAT program includes facilities for entering structures, displaying these, determining the parameters that influence a particular estimate, and validating the estimate by calling up those compounds in the data base which contributed to the substructural keys used for the estimate in question. A typical sequence is shown in the following figures. Figure 1 shows the estimate for tolbutamide with the parameters used for that estimate. Several keys were generated as warnings: the tautomeric fragment to warn of the possibility of the alternate form, and the sulfonamide bound to benzene as a key that has produced misclassifications in some instances. Figure 2 shows the substructures used in the estimate. The substructures are outlined by balloons. Figure 3 is part of the search for compounds in the data base with structures related to tolbutamide and a display of their carcinogenicity information. These compounds contain the structure (2 electron-withdrawing groups bound to NH) most responsible for the noncarcinogenicity estimate for tolbutamide (Fig. 1B). One notes that most of these compounds are not carcinogens and have structures quite well-related to tolbutamide, thus at least partially confirming that estimate. It is desirable to repeat this process for all the parameters used in the estimate, but this detail is now shown here to conserve space.

Not all compounds for which assay data are available are used in the development of the model. Figure 4 shows four compounds which were not included in the calculations. Trifluralin (Fig. 4A) always turned out to be a severe outlier, for reasons that we did not understand, so we had no choice but not to use it. Pentachloronitrobenzene (Fig. 4B) would be expected to be a carcinogen on the basis of its substructures, but is not carcinogenic in the NCI/NTP bioassay. The last two compounds in Figure 4 contain rare substructures, i.e., features that exist but infrequently in the data base. These features thus cannot be used in the SAR equation, and therefore these compounds cannot be included as they would be inadequately described. As the data base grows in the future, it may well be possible to include these compounds again. In conclusion, SAR models of carcinogenicity perform at a high level of accuracy and can be used for the identification of chemicals that may present a carcinogenic risk. SAR models can be used as part of the armamentarium of carcinogenic risk estimation.

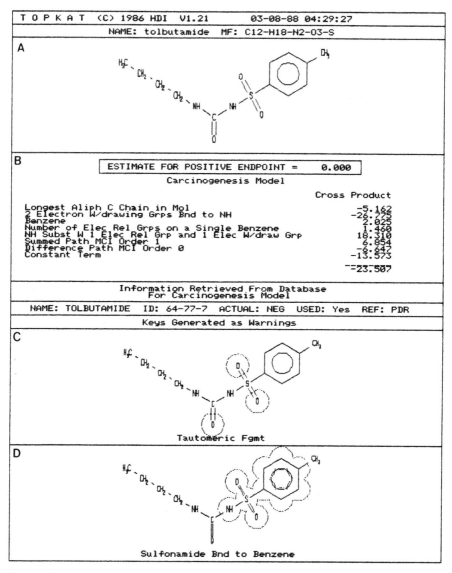

Figure 1

(*A*) Structure of tolbutamide. (*B*) Parameters used for the estimate of carcinogenicity of tolbutamide. Each parameter has a value which is multiplied by the coefficient for that parameter in the discriminant equation, resulting in a cross-product. A positive cross-product adds to the probability of the compound being a carcinogen, a negative cross-product reduces that probability. MCI is the molecular connectivity index. (*C* and *D*) Substructural keys generated as warnings (see text).

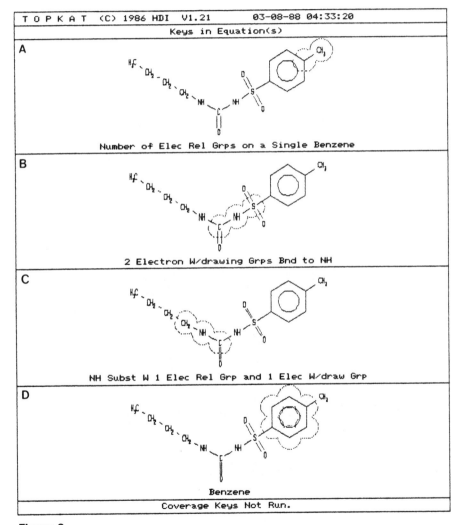

Figure 2
(*A–D*) Substructures identified in tolbutamide that are also present in the discriminant equation.
These substructures are used in the calculation of the estimate.

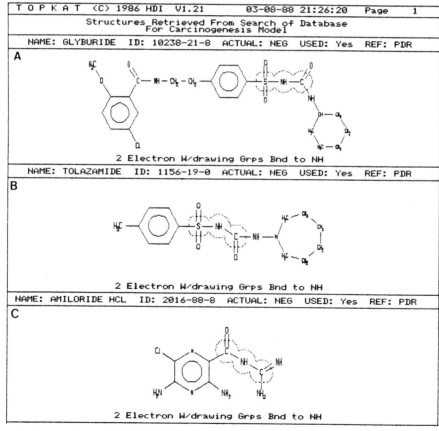

Figure 3 (*See facing page for legend.*)

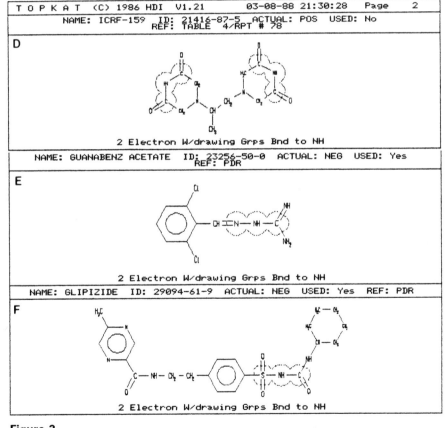

Figure 3

(*A–F*) Chemical structures retrieved from the data base associated with a substructure used for the calculation of the estimate for tolbutamide (see text).

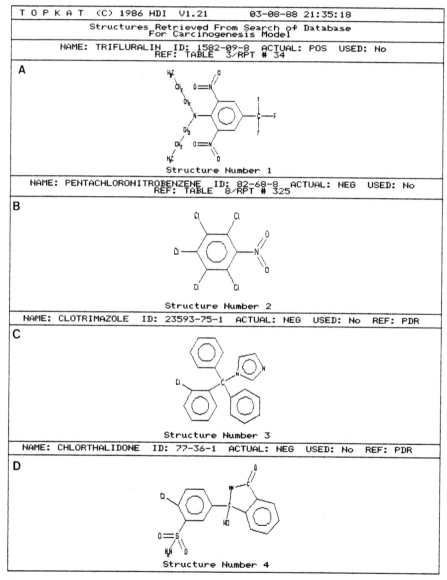

Figure 4

Structures of some chemicals not used in the development of the SAR model.

Open Discussion

Weisburger: Since I am the Chair, I am going to ask my question first. Dr. Farland, of those 9000 or so chemicals that EPA has looked at in the PMN, how many of them actually got out there into the world?

Farland: We don't know. That's a complex question because many of these chemicals are used as chemical intermediates as well, and so they are not going to get out into the world at any time, even if they are in use. They are captured intermediates in processes. We take that into consideration when we talk about a need for testing or controls. There are also a large number that are not commercialized. In other words, even though they have been approved, we never see a notice of intent to manufacture. So, I can't answer the question at this point.

Weisburger: Maybe the marketplace fizzled.

Farland: Could be.

Michejda: I would just like to add one thing that I think is very important, and something that Dr. Enslein said jogged my memory. Lots of the carcinogenicity tests—in fact, by far the majority of them—have been carried out on pure substances. Yet, we do know that combination treatments of various kinds frequently produce not just additive but synergistic effects. This is a real can of worms that simply has not been addressed very properly in many studies.

Farland: Just a quick follow-up on that. Joe Arcos's volumes have come out every few years. This next one is actually looking at the interaction literature, and it's complete now. The manuscript is in place, and I hope that it will be out very shortly. It has been a tremendous study. There is actually a fairly complex data base that starts to look at interactions. It should be a real contribution to the scientific community at large.

Hart: I'd like to go back to the original charge of the conference. One of the reasons why this session was called was because we are using structure-activity relations (SAR) in some of the regulatory agencies. We have also heard from Willy (Lijinsky) and others this morning that there are limitations, and there's no doubt about that. Also, our total dependency upon the animal bioassay data can sometimes lead us astray. Is it appropriate to use SAR, are we using SAR in a proper fashion, and are there ways we can use SAR more effectively to answer regulatory questions? That was the reason to build a bridge between the basic science and the regulatory aspects now. That question has not really been addressed so far. Are we doing the best we can with what we have,

Banbury Report 31: Carcinogen Risk Assessment: New Directions in the Qualitative and Quantitative Aspects © Cold Spring Harbor Laboratory. 0-87969-231-6/88. $1.00 + .00   **61**

or can we do it better? Has there been anything out of the basic science that can help us in modifying what we are doing now?

Clayson: Dr. Lijinsky and several other speakers have emphasized that DNA adduct formation isn't the end-all and be-all of carcinogenesis, and I don't think anybody in the room would disagree with that. However, this raises a question with me. Is it not the end-all and be-all of carcinogenesis because the chemical has some other action on some other part of the cellular mechanism, or is it not the end-all because different species react in different ways to this insult?

My reading, and it's no more than that, suggests very strongly that the species differences are important, because recent work has shown that DNA binding in cells seems to be specific to certain bases within the whole gamut of the bases of that nature. Also, looking at the oncogenes, it appears that they must attack specific sites to be effective. It seems to me that we should be looking very hard at the differences between species. I think it makes a tremendous difference to risk assessment because, if we are looking at two different chemical attacks on a cellular level, then we will get a very different pattern of dose/response curves to those that we will get if we are looking at a difference in the host response.

Singer: I am going to bring up a subject which I don't think anybody intends to talk about, and that is called repair. I know it wasn't the charge of the speakers, but it turns out that, in talking about species differences, organ differences, and so on, you impinge directly upon repair. Data coming from other laboratories, and particularly Tony Pegg's lab, find that the human liver has approximately 10^3 times as much of the repair enzyme, O^6-methylguanine methyltransferase, as does the hamster. That is only one factor that can account for species differences. In all animals that have been tested so far, the brain has the lowest capacity, the liver has the greatest capacity, and that is probably true of a lot of other enzymes. In various types of human disease, again, variations in repair capacity for exactly the same kind of damage is such that one person will have the disease and others will not.

Weisburger: We're glad you brought it up.

Lijinsky: The importance of the quantitative structure-activity relations is the quality of the data that are used. A lot of the data goes into the data base mechanically, without thought, without knowledge, without criticism, and that is a problem. Dr. Enslein's example of trifluralin is a perfect example. I think in many cases no biochemist ever sees the data.

Something else, I want to agree that there are enormous differences between species in response to carcinogens, and this might involve responses to the same lesion in the DNA. However, other properties of the carcinogen are things that we miss considering. There are certainly carcinogens that do not interact with DNA but produce exactly the same tumor, and they do not seem to be promoting agents. If there is another mechanism for producing tumors, by an indirect effect on the genome, then a lot of chemicals are actually genotoxic and employ that mechanism in addition. That implies that there are other properties of carcinogens involved, and those are the things to which we should be paying some attention.

Enslein: In response to your comments, there is no data base that is ever perfect. Regarding Ron's question, how could one use these tools in the regulatory process? I don't think they should be used at all as the sole decision point. I think it's another way of getting another piece of information, of gaining perhaps some insight, for raising questions regarding important parameters for that particular chemical. You might ask what else we know about such chemicals, what is in the data base about such chemicals, in order to set priorities, to make you think further, but by no means to act as a replacement for human judgment. No assay is a replacement for human judgment either. When you do a two-year carcinogenesis bioassay, you've done it once. That just represents the results of one assay, as evaluated by one or several people.

Guengerich: I go back to the issue of the DNA binding. For instance, if you look at Lutz's work in terms of covalent binding index, and you look at all the carcinogens versus DNA binding, you find a pretty reasonable correlation when you do the covalent binding properly in vivo. Along with that, there have been experiments with oncogenes, where it is actually shown that if you modify a piece of DNA with an ultimate carcinogen, do a transfection into 3T3 cells, and then inject those cells, you can actually produce real tumors in nude rodents under conditions where you have had a single modification. That doesn't mean that every tumor is due to this mechanism, but it shows what you can experimentally produce.

In terms of the matter of DNA adducts, Chris (Michejda) brought out that sometimes we pass things off as no DNA damage just because we aren't properly looking for them. Chris mentioned a diazonium arylating agent. Another example that comes to mind, though, comes from our own experience with acrylonitrile. When we started working on acrylonitrile, which avidly binds to protein, everybody said that it was nongenotoxic and there was some kind of an epigenetic mechanism. After a few years, we found low levels of some DNA adducts. Now, Jim Swenberg, using different experimental conditions, is finding horrendous levels of DNA adducts in the tumor tissues. So, we have gone almost completely from an epigenetic mechanism to a hard-core genetic mechanism.

Weisburger: The techniques are always very important.

Hart: There is one point about which you have to be very careful. DNA damage is very important, and repair is even more important. However, when you look at the binding index, the coefficients of binding, versus carcinogenicity, you've got to be very careful how you use those data. Many of the compounds that are selected for carcinogenicity studies, whole animal bioassays, and so on, are selected because they damage DNA, induce mutagenesis, or cause adduct formation. So, you are selecting for those compounds that damage DNA.

Guengerich: There will also be a lot of fluctuations along that, as well. One other thing, which has not really been addressed much in the literature, is that many of the alkylating agents actually rely on their alkylating properties in acting as promoters. There are only a few examples. One comes from some recent work from the Millers' laboratory with 1-hydroxyestragole. For instance, using brachymorphic mice and pentachlorophenol and sulfation, they found that you could actually affect the properties of the 1-hydroxyestragole as a promoter of diethylnitrosamine-initiated tumors. In searching the literature, I didn't find much about this. We don't know if this represents a second hit on DNA or a modification of something else, but it is a factor we have to consider, especially in terms of some of these complete carinogenesis protocols.

Mason: My question about the function of alkylated DNA has been answered. Once that molecule is alkylated, does it have its normal function? Can it produce its normal enzyme?

Wilson: It alkylates or dealkylates all the time.

Mason: I know that, but while it's alkylated does it have any function? Does it function normally, or does the problem occur in the next generation when the chromosomes reproduce?

Guengerich: Then you're putting in mutations, and the subject is where they are and what is the process.

Mason: What I'm asking is do we have to have a mutated gene before the molecule functions, or does the alkylated DNA function?

Poirier: In terms of the *ras* activation story, the codon 12 or the codon 61 mutations are enough to activate the *ras* gene. Then what you get is an altered protein that somehow acts as an intermediary for tumorigenesis.

Guengerich: You have to have some kind of reading, either DNA or RNA.

Ahmed: I'd like to ask a question about the polycyclic aromatics. You mentioned the two diol-epoxide molecules, and you mentioned that P-450 selected ones that are more mutagenic. Have you any idea about the relative thermodynamic stability of the two compounds, 1 and 2? In one case I noticed that the epoxide group and the hydroxyl group were *trans* to each other and the hydroxyl group was *trans* to the other hydroxyl group. However, in the first one you find them on the same side or *cis* to each other? In the nonenzymic production of these epoxides in vitro, do you see any difference in the actual relative amounts formed?

Thakker: There is considerable selectivity when benzo-ring dihydrodiols are epoxidized with peroxyacid. Facial selectivity of the oxidation is determined by the conformation of the hydroxyl groups.

Ahmed: So the P-450 selects?

Thakker: The way P-450 selects has more to do with the way they sit at the binding site.

Beland: But that's just one specific isozyme, P-450c, isn't it?

Thakker: No other homogeneous isozymes have yet been studied adequately.

Guengerich: Marnett has shown that if you go to prostaglandin-synthetase, you actually get a stereochemically different adduct.

Thakker: Which is more like a chemical peroxidation.

Fu: I want to get back to Dr. Hart's original question, whether or not SAR is good for assessment of the human health risk. Personally, with reservations, I think this is a very good approach. For bioassay, usually we select the strains that are very sensitive to the carcinogens and produce a high incidence of tumors. The question is whether human beings are genetically similar to those strains. To utilize the experimental animal data for risk assessment, the first thing is to search for the rodents that have similar polymorphism as human beings. SAR, based on the data from these rodents, would be much more reliable.

Weisburger: Also, the regulatory agencies have to think of the whole population, not just the tough people who are out there but also the sensitive people as well. In starting the bioassay, we did not take the most sensitive animal models. We took some that seemed to be reasonable and that had been used where there was some experience. We could have used the Sencar mouse and maybe even had 100% response.

Farland: Just to comment, when the National Academy went through its evaluation of risk assessment in the federal government, it looked at that issue specifically. It comes under this heading of inference, the idea that you have to make a decision in the absence of data, and that you are asked to look at the information and say which is the species that is most relevant to humans. If you have an answer to that question, you use that species. If you don't have an answer, then the recommendation is that you see the most sensitive responder, with the likelihood that either the human population is similar or there are individuals in the human population that may be similar to that most sensitive responder. That is an inference that can be tested, but in the absence of the data we have only one route.

Hart: Have we ever used strains other than the ones that we always use? We have never found one that was relevant.

Farland: No, but as an example, if we look at liver carcinogenicity, many times we get an argument regarding response in a high-background strain. I look at the complete database, and I find that I have liver tumors in a low-background strain in the females. Doesn't that provide me with some additional support for the fact that perhaps there is a response that I ought to consider relevant. That is a case where you are not simply focusing on the most sensitive strains to provide support.

Pfitzer: I think some of the discussion and comments made here have been too demanding on what they expect out of SAR. The regulatory agencies use SAR as supportive evidence, and we all agree that's appropriate. What I have been missing here is a better and a more precise definition of the activity part of structure-activity relationship. There is a big difference between talking about a cancer in a tissue in a bioassay and looking at a DNA adduct. There are many things that occur: all of the binding, the interactions, the transformation, and the repair. Making decisions about a structure-activity relationship on such a complex activity as the end result of a tumor in an animal may be far too much to expect from the system. It's important information, but all the studies on mechanisms that have been done are extremely important to understanding the activity. The SAR should not be condemned because of uncertainties, when we are dealing with so complex a system.

Wilson: The use of structure-activity relationships, in both industry and in the government, is not in the assessment phase and not in the characterization phase, but in the hazard identification step, where nonquantitative inferences are drawn about what information is useful.

In that case, it is quite feasible and proper to look at very gross estimates of activity, saying that cancer as an end point is a very gross estimate of activity, and then correlating that with structure. However, no one that I know of takes additional steps within that assessment scheme, as Ron (Hart) and Bill (Farland) described, without additional information.

Hart: Precisely.

Pharmacokinetic and
Metabolic Activity Data

Interindividual Metabolic Variation in Humans: Mechanisms, Methods of Assessment, and Consequences

F. PETER GUENGERICH
Department of Biochemistry and Center in Molecular Toxicology
Vanderbilt University School of Medicine
Nashville, Tennessee 37232

OVERVIEW

Evidence has been obtained in animal models that differences in the metabolism of procarcinogens and protoxicants can influence the susceptibility to risk. In recent years, the biochemical understanding of these animal systems has been developed considerably and extended to humans. However, little direct evidence has yet been obtained to support the view that these metabolic differences are important in humans. Several lines of future investigation are suggested to address the working hypothesis that major metabolic differences exist in humans and are important in the risk of individuals to chemical carcinogenesis.

INTRODUCTION

The subject of risk assessment deals not only with evaluation of risks of the general population to specific chemicals but also with prediction of risks of chemicals to specific individuals. This latter area is often considered under the heading of "host factors." In this chapter, evidence for variation in rates of metabolism of foreign chemicals as a factor in risk from protoxicants and procarcinogens will be reviewed. Points to be considered will be evidence for variation in metabolism in humans, the relevance of studies in animal models, the significance of variation in metabolism as a host factor for risk in humans, and current and future strategies for assessing human populations and obtaining more information.

RESULTS AND DISCUSSION

Basic Concepts and the Role of Animal Studies

Today we know much about many of the enzymes involved in the metabolism of xenobiotics, although key pieces of basic information remain elusive. Most of these enzymes have been purified from animal tissues. However, many of

Banbury Report 31: Carcinogen Risk Assessment: New Directions in the Qualitative and Quantitative Aspects © Cold Spring Harbor Laboratory. 0-87969-231-6/88. $1.00 + .00

these proteins exist as parts of multigene or supergene families. For instance, about 20 different distinct cytochrome P-450 proteins have now been purified from rat liver microsomes, and all appear to have some common elements of structural similarity.

Even in single-gene systems such as nicotinamide adenine dinucleotide phosphate (NADPH)-cytochrome P-450 reductase and microsomal epoxide hydrolase, a complete description of the regulation is lacking, even though regulatory elements of genes coding for several proteins involved in xenobiotic metabolism have been identified. When multigene families exist, individual proteins in each family may differ in their catalytic as well as regulatory properties. Many of the enzymes are induced and suppressed by drugs and chemicals in the environment. Usually one finds that individual gene products (enzymes) have at least some specificity for carrying out individual reactions; in some cases, this can be quite striking. Another matter that has only been dealt with briefly is the effect of amino acid substitutions (in proteins) upon catalytic function.

We see that the complement of enzymes that metabolize xenobiotics might be expected to be influenced by both genetic and environmental factors. As discussed under the subject of aryl hydrocarbon hydroxylase inducibility, genetic and environmental factors can also interact in determining the balance of enzyme activity. Can changes in the balance of enzymes alter the metabolism of chemicals? A number of examples are known. For instance, genetic strains of mice that vary in their expression of cytochrome P-450 enzymes show altered abilities to metabolize a number of drugs and other chemicals. Such differences can influence toxicity and susceptibility to carcinogenesis. An example in this latter aspect is brachymorphic mice, which lack sulfotransferase activity and do not develop tumors when administered certain carcinogens. The same protection can be achieved in normal mice by inhibiting the enzyme with the chemical pentachlorophenol (Boberg et al. 1983). Thus, we see that the enzyme balance can influence risk as well as metabolism. Although the questions that have been asked in this regard are relatively restricted to date, experiments of this type can be extended.

What can we learn from studies on such enzymes in animals? In general, experience has shown that the animals are fairly reasonable models. The availability of sequencing methods has revealed clear structural homology of the proteins in the cases of cytochrome P-450, alcohol dehydrogenase, glutathione S-transferase, and epoxide hydrolase. In general, primary sequence similarity is reflected in catalytic specificity. However, numerous exceptions do exist, particularly in some of the more complex gene families. For instance, human S-mephenytoin 4-hydroxylation P-450 and rabbit P-450 1 cDNA sequences are more than 80% identical, yet the proteins differ radically in substrate specificity (Umbenhauer et al. 1987). Although regulatory patterns tend to be similar, some caution is also needed. Rodents greatly overemphasize sex differences in metabolism, and such dimorphism is not very striking in humans. Rabbits also demonstrate some peculiarities as well. Much can be gained from studying animal models, however, and at the least they provide probes for analyzing human systems.

Evidence for Differences in Xenobiotic Metabolism in Humans

Considerable evidence exists for variation in the rates of metabolism of drugs and other xenobiotics in humans. It is common to observe a difference of an order of magnitude in any in vitro or in vivo parameter related to the metabolism of a drug; indeed, it is uncommon to observe a smaller difference. Actually, the differences attributable to sex and age are far less than the idiotypic variation. Examples of variation can be seen with nifedipine area under the curve (Kleinbloesem et al. 1984), debrisoquine 4-hydroxylation metabolic ratio (Magoub et al. 1977), and mephenytoin 4-hydroxylation (Wedlund et al. 1984; Shimada et al. 1986). Examples for variation in rates of metabolism of nontherapeutic xenobiotics are not as extensive. However, Autrup et al. (1984) found considerable variation in rates of the metabolism of several procarcinogens by human tissue explants and variations in rates of microsomal metabolism of compounds such as benzo[a]pyrene and trichloroethylene have been reported (Miller and Guengerich 1983; Beaune et al. 1986).

In some cases evidence has been presented that a true genetic polymorphism exists in the variation of drug metabolism. The best documented cases involve debrisoquine 4-hydroxylation and S-mephenytoin 4-hydroxylation (Magoub et al. 1977; Küpfer and Preisig 1983; Wedlund et al. 1984). In some cases genetic polymorphism has been proposed but the evidence is not so clear, i.e., antipyrine (Vessell and Page 1968), tolbutamide (Scott and Poffenbarger 1979), nifedipine (Kleinbloesem et al. 1984). Yet, in other cases the variation is probably distributed in a unimodal manner, although it should be pointed out that patterns can be misleading and the type of parameter utilized may influence the apparent modality.

Current Biochemical Information in Humans

In recent years considerable attention has been directed towards understanding the enzymes that metabolize drugs and carcinogens in human tissues. This effort has been fueled by technical developments and the increasing availability of tissue samples. Considerable progress has been made with both the so-called phase I (oxidizing) and phase II (conjugating) enzymes.

At least eight forms of human cytochrome P-450, five forms of glutathione S-transferase, two forms of uridine diphosphate (UDP)-glucuronosyl transferase, one form of epoxide hydrolase, and NADPH-cytochrome P-450 reductase have now been purified from human liver. In addition, cDNA and genomic clones related to many of these enzymes have also been obtained and sequenced. The field is moving rapidly. Although a detailed review of the entire field is not possible in the space available, current work suggests that variations in enzymatic function occur at several levels:

"Isozymic" Differences. In short, different proteins exist within each enzyme class. These are not really appropriately termed isozymes, for the individual proteins often have distinct functions. The proteins can be grouped into families on the basis of their primary structures, and the different proteins generally have distinct catalytic specificities towards xenobiotic substrates.

Variation in Amounts of Enzyme. In some cases, the level of a catalytic activity in different individuals is highly correlated to the amount of detectable enzyme protein. Examples include cytochrome P-450 nifedipine oxidase ($P450_{NF}$) and phenacetin O-deethylase. The basis of the variation may be at the level of transcription, although results involving mRNA quantitation are not yet as clear in human tissues as in rats. These variations may be influenced by environmental factors that regulate putative *trans*-acting factors affecting transcription, as well as genetic variations in these regulatory factors. Gonzalez et al. (1988) have recently indicated that at least some of the variation in levels of cytochrome P-450 debrisoquine 4-hydroxylase may be due to DNA mutations that give rise to abnormal mRNA splicing and mRNAs that are not converted into stable proteins.

Mutations in Structural Genes That Affect Catalytic Activity. Distinct examples of such alterations in human systems have not been identified, although a prime candidate is the genetic polymorphism in mephenytoin 4-hydroxylase activity, where a restriction fragment length polymorphism (RFLP) in genomic DNA has been tentatively identified (Guengerich et al. 1988) and several other lines of evidence are consistent with such a mechanism.

Do Individual Humans Vary in Risk as a Result of Metabolic Differences?

Although this hypothesis has often been assumed, a dearth of supporting information is actually available. The evidence for the influence of environmental factors on the incidence of certain diseases and cancer is well-documented. For instance, twin studies show differences in the incidence of Parkinson's Disease, implicating nongenetic factors, and the incidence of particular cancers is influenced by dietary lifestyle. Do differences in metabolism actually influence risk, however?

One case that has been studied is the influence of N-acetylation phenotype on cancers of the bladder and other tissues. The results are not completely clear but do suggest that slow metabolizers may be at increased risk, at least in the case of bladder cancer. Kellerman et al. (1973) examined levels of lymphocyte aryl hydrocarbon hydroxylase activity and concluded that cigarette smokers with a high degree of inducibility were more likely to develop lung cancer. The status of this hypothesis is still unclear, however. More recently Ayesh et al. (1984) reported that cigarette smokers having squamous cell lung cancer were more likely to be unusually rapid phenotypic hydroxylators of debrisoquine.

It should be pointed out, however, that in none of the above cases has a metabolic basis been established. Even if a high degree of correlation can be found, nonmetabolic explanations such as gene linkage can be invoked. More direct evidence is needed.

Future Directions

Although much has already been learned in recent years about differences in the way that humans metabolize xenobiotic chemicals, more can be learned by applying several approaches. The suggestion made here is to use and test the working hypothesis that metabolic differences exist and are important in individual risk assessment. Evaluation of the hypothesis can be done through several lines of investigation.

Development of More Information. Many of these enzymes exist in multigene families with closely-related forms that catalyze different reactions and pose problems in the development of specific molecular probes and the assessment of catalytic specificity (i.e., cytochrome P-450, glutathione S-transferase, UDP glucuronosyl transferase). Fortunately, new methods in the application of high-resolution chromatography, use of oligonucleotide probes and monoclonal antibodies, and protein expression have been developed and can be applied to these problems. The definition of catalytic specificity is a particular problem in the multigene enzyme systems, for the separation of closely related proteins can be difficult and elucidating catalytic specificities of related proteins is difficult when immunochemical cross-reactivity is a consideration.

Searches for New Variants. Drugs can be extremely valuable in the identification of metabolic variations in human populations. They are administered in quantities large enough to produce physiological effects and levels of exposure and metabolite production can be documented. In general, approved drugs can be administered without major ethical considerations. Some chemotherapeutic agents give rise to the formation of DNA adducts.

The appearance of quantitatively unusual patterns of drug action is often a clue to abnormally slow or rapid metabolism of drugs, as manifested by adverse side effects or lack of drug efficacy. These observations can be followed up at the level of clinical pharmacology to establish whether pharmacokinetic or pharmacodynamic variations are involved. If alterations in metabolism are implicated, then the logical course of investigation involves characterization of the enzyme(s), elucidation of the mechanism for the defect, and identification of other chemicals that are handled primarily by the same system.

At this time only a few polymorphisms have actually been identified. It would be of use to find more and, subsequently, to characterize them. Furthermore, a need also exists for the development of better methods for phenotyping individuals after polymorphisms have been identified. There are two major approaches in this area. The first involves selection of better drugs that can be used in metabolic analysis. For instance, dextromethorphan is a useful substitute for phenotyping individuals for debrisoquine 4-hydroxylase activity because of its lack of major physiological activity and its clearance for use in many countries. In a similar way, several recent studies suggest that theophylline metabolism may be useful in the phenotyping for phenacetin O-deethylase activity (Birkett et al. 1988). The identification of P-450$_{NF}$ as the major cortisol 6β-hydroxylase permits inferences to be made about enzyme status from the amount of urinary excretion of 6β-hydroxycortisol (Ged et al. 1988).

The other approach of phenotyping involves the use of RFLP analysis, which is based upon changes in electrophoretic patterns of genomic DNA after digestion with endonucleases. Such an approach, of course, requires not only the isolation and characterization of DNA related to the protein under consideration but also the existence of mutations in the genes that are responsible for altered catalytic activity. Such changes have been identified, for instance, in human alcohol and aldehyde dehydrogenases (Jörnvall et al. 1984). Ultimately, RFLP offers many advantages (once the basis is established), for many analyses can be done with DNA obtained from a single, small (15 ml) blood sample.

Development of In Vitro/In Vivo Relationships. In vitro assays can be used to predict which other compounds may be handled by abnormal metabolizers in such a way as to place them at increased risk. Methods for the establishment of catalytic specificity in vitro include copurification of activity, enzyme reconstitution, immunochemical inhibition, diagnostic and competitive inhibition, and correlation of activities (Beaune and Guengerich 1988). Again, the importance of utilizing drugs should be emphasized, for they can be used to establish in vitro/in vivo relationships, which are important, as exemplified in the case of tolbutamide (Knodell et al. 1987).

Another point to be considered is that in vivo information can be obtained about the metabolisim of certain industrial chemicals when they are ingested at levels below allowed daily levels. Such situations permit the testing of hypotheses made from in vitro observations at the in vivo level. In vivo relationships can be examined in situations where accidents or oversights have exposed selected groups of individuals to unusually high levels of chemicals under consideration for risk assessment. Societal habits such as smoking can also be considered in terms of establishment of relationships, although major difficulties exist in dealing with complex mixtures of materials. The point about mixtures must also be considered with industrial chemicals and drugs as well, however.

Development of In Vivo Models That Utilize In Vitro Data. Under this heading we consider studies on species extrapolation. An example is provided from studies on the metabolism of methylene chloride, which is under consideration for its carcinogenic risk. In vivo data were collected on the disposition of methylene chloride in rats and used in the development of a pharmacokinetic model. In vitro data on the rates of oxidative and conjugative metabolism were obtained in rat and human liver samples, with the assumption (based upon the literature) that the former pathway involves detoxication and the latter route represents an activation pathway. The in vitro kinetic constants were then utilized in the in vivo model to predict levels of various metabolic products in individual compartments and assess the relative risk of methylene chloride in man relative to test animal species (Andersen et al. 1987). Many other problems are probably amenable to such analysis and these extrapolations should be experimentally testable (Table 1).

Table 1

Interspecies Comparisons of First Order Rate Constants Estimated In Vivo and In Vitro for Glutathione S-Transferase-catalyzed Reaction of Glutathione and Methylene Chloride

Species	In vivo[a] (h^{-1})	In vitro[b] $(ml\ min^{-1}\ [mg\ protein]^{-1})$
Mouse	4.3	0.75
Rat	2.2	0.12
Hamster	1.5	0.03
Human	0.5	0.09

[a]Data from Andersen et al. (1987).
[b]Data from Reitz et al. (1988).

ACKNOWLEDGMENTS

Research related to this article due in the author's laboratory was supported by United States Public Health Service Awards ES 00267, CA 30907, and CA 44353.

REFERENCES

Andersen, M.E., H.J. Clewell III, M.L. Gargas, F.A. Smith, and R.H. Reitz. 1987. Physiologically based pharmacokinetics and the risk assessment process for methylene chloride. *Toxicol. Appl. Pharmacol.* **87**: 185.

Autrup, H., C.C. Harris, S.-M. Wu, L.Y. Bao, X.-F. Pei, S. Lu, T.-T. Sun, and C.-C. Hsia. 1984. Activation of chemical carcinogens by cultured human fetal liver, esophagus, and stomach. *Chem. Biol. Interact.* **50**: 15.

Ayesh, R., J.R. Idle, J.C. Ritchie, M.J. Crothers, and M.R. Hetzel. 1984. Metabolic oxidation phenotypes as markers for susceptibility to lung cancer. *Nature* **312**: 169.

Beaune, P.H. and F.P. Guengerich. 1988. Human liver drug metabolism *in vitro*. *Pharmacol. Ther.* (in press).

Beaune, P., P. Kremers, L.S. Kaminsky, J. DeGraeve, and F.P. Guengerich. 1986. Comparison of monooxygenase activities and cytochrome P-450 isozyme concentrations in human liver microsomes. *Drug Metab. Dispos.* **14**: 437.

Birkett, D.J., J.O. Miners, M.E. McManus, I. Stupans, and R.A. Robson. 1988. The methylxanthines and tolbutamide as model substrates for cytochrome P-450 isozymes in animal and man. In *Microsomes and drug oxidations* (ed. D.J. Birkett et al.). Taylor and Francis, London. (In press.)

Boberg, E., E.C. Miller, J.A. Miller, A. Poland, and A. Liem. 1983. Strong evidence from studies with brachymorphic mice and pentachlorophenol that 1'-sulfooxysafrole is the major ultimate electrophilic and carcinogenic metabolite of 1'-hydroxysafrole in mouse liver. *Cancer Res.* **43**: 5163.

Ged, C., P. Maurel, I. Dalet-Beluche, and P. Beaune. 1988. Cortisol 6β-hydroxylase in human liver microsomes: Implication of cytochrome P-450-5(NF). *Biochem. Pharmacol.* (in press).

Gonzalez, F.J., J.P. Hardwick, M. Umemo, R.C. Skoda, E. Matsunaga, T. Matsunaga, B.J. Song, S. Kimura, D.W. Nebert, H.V. Gelboin, and U.A. Meyer. 1988. Human and rat debrisoquine hydroxylase and ethanol inducible cytochrome P-450 gene families: Structure, regulation and polymorphisms. In *Microsomes and drug oxidations* (ed. D.J. Birkett et al.). Taylor and Francis, London. (In press.)

Guengerich, F.P., D.R. Umbenhauer, P.H. Beaune, M.V. Martin, C. Ged, T. Muto, R.W. Bork, R.G. Knodell, and R.S. Lloyd. 1988. Characterization and functional significance of forms of human cytochrome P-450. *Proc. Int. Congr. Pharmacol.* **10**: (in press).

Jörnvall, H., J. Hempel, B.L. Vallee, W.F. Bosron, and T.-K. Li. 1984. Human liver alcohol dehydrogenase: Amino acid substitution in the $\beta_2\beta_2$ Oriental isozyme explains functional properties, establishes an active site structure, and parallels mutational exchange in the yeast enzyme. *Proc. Natl. Acad. Sci.* **81**: 3024.

Kellerman, G., C.R. Shaw, and M. Luyten-Kellerman. 1973. Aryl hydrocarbon hydroxylase inducibility and bronchiogenic carcinoma. *New Engl. J. Med.* **289:** 934.

Kleinbloesem, C.H., P. van Brummelen, H. Faber, M. Danhof, N.P.E. Vermuelen, and D.D. Breimer. 1984. Variability in nifedipine pharmacokinetics and dynamics: A new oxidation polymorphism in man. *Biochem. Pharmacol.* **33:** 3721.

Knodell, R.G., S.D. Hall, G.R. Wilkinson, and F.P. Guengerich. 1987. Hepatic metabolism of tolbutamide: *In vitro* characterization of the form of cytochrome P-450 involved in methyl hydroxylation and relationship to *in vivo* disposition. *J. Pharmacol. Exp. Ther.* **241:** 1112.

Küpfer, A. and R. Preisig. 1983. Inherited defects of drug metabolism. *Semin. Liver Dis.* **3:** 341.

Magoub, A., L.G. Dring, J.R. Idle, R. Lancaster, and R.L. Smith. 1977. Polymorphic hydroxylation of debrisoquine in man. *Lancet* **II:** 584.

Miller, R.L. and F.P. Guengerich. 1983. Metabolism of trichloroethylene in isolated hepatocytes, microsomes, and reconstituted enzyme systems containing purified cytochromes P-450. *Cancer Res.* **43:** 1145.

Reitz, R.H., A.L. Mendrala, and F.P. Guengerich. 1988. *In vitro* studies of methylene chloride metabolism in human and animal tissues: Use in physiologically-based pharmacokinetic models. *Toxicologist* **8:** 156.

Scott, J. and P.L. Poffenbarger. 1979. Pharmacogenetics of tolbutamide metabolism in humans. *Diabetes* **28:** 41.

Shimada, T., K.S. Misono, and F.P. Guengerich. 1986. Human liver microsomal cytochrome P-450 mephenytoin 4-hydroxylase, a prototype of genetic polymorphism in oxidative drug metabolism: Purification and characterization of two similar forms involved in the reaction. *J. Biol. Chem.* **261:** 909.

Umbenhauer, D.R., M.V. Martin, R.S. Lloyd, and F.P.Guengerich. 1987. Cloning and sequence determination of a complementary DNA related to human liver microsomal cytochrome P-450 S-mephenytoin 4-hydroxylase. *Biochemistry* **26:** 1094.

Vessell, E.S. and J.G. Page. 1968. Genetic control of drug levels in man: Antipyrine. *Science* **161:** 72.

Wedlund, P.J., W.S. Aslanian, E. Jacqz, C.B. McAllister, G.R. Wilkinson, and R.A. Branch. 1984. Mephenytoin hydroxylation deficiency in Caucasians: Frequency of a new oxidative drug metabolism polymorphism. *Clin. Pharmacol. Ther.* **36:** 773.

Acetylation Pharmacogenetics: Acetylator Phenotype and Susceptibility to Arylamine Carcinogenesis

WENDELL W. WEBER, SUSAN S. MATTANO, AND GERALD N. LEVY
Department of Pharmacology and
Department of Toxicology
University of Michigan
Ann Arbor, Michigan 48109

OVERVIEW

Epidemiological studies show that the acetylator phenotype is a determinant of susceptibility to arylamide-induced cancer. There is a statistically significant association of the slow acetylator phenotype to urinary bladder cancer, whereas the rapid phenotype is associated with colorectal cancer and breast cancer of women. Investigations in rapid and slow inbred mouse strains show that three acetylation activities are involved in the bioactivation of arylamines to carcinogens, and that all three activities are identified with a single, homogeneous 31,500 dalton protein. ^{32}P-postlabeling of DNA adducts has been adapted to high-performance liquid chromatography (HPLC) analysis for rapid assessment of DNA damage, and carcinogen-nucleotide adducts formed in the DNA of liver and skin of mice exposed to arylamines and other aromatic carcinogens have been resolved by this technique.

INTRODUCTION

Beginning with Rehn's report almost 100 years ago (1895) of urinary bladder cancer among aniline dyestuff workers, this disorder has become almost synonymous with that of "industrial" bladder cancer (Parkes and Evans 1984). Case et al. (1954) showed further that aniline dyestuff workers were about 30 times more likely to contract bladder cancer than the general population. Since then, occupational exposure to arylamines has become widely regarded as the major cause of this disorder.

Shortly before Rehn's report on bladder cancer, acetylation was identified by the German organic chemist, Cohn (1893), as one of the nine major synthetic (conjugation) reactions that humans and animals use to dispose of drugs and other chemicals. Biological acetylation is a common reaction of primary amine groups such as occur in the aromatic amine drugs and car-

Banbury Report 31: Carcinogen Risk Assessment: New Directions in the Qualitative and Quantitative Aspects © Cold Spring Harbor Laboratory. 0-87969-231-6/88. $1.00 + .00

cinogens. The acetyl group, supplied by acetyl coenzyme-A, is transferred to these substances enzymatically during conjugation.

About the time of Case's report on industrial bladder cancer in aniline dye workers in 1954, reports of genetic differences in acetylating capacity first appeared in the German and American literature (for review, see Weber 1987). The human acetylation polymorphism has since been shown to be an autosomal, monogenic, Mendelian trait that enables persons to be identified as rapid (RR or Rr) or slow (rr) acetylators of aromatic amines and hydrazines. The acetylator genes specify qualitatively distinct isozymic variants of the drug acetylating enzymes of liver, intestinal mucosa, and other tissues that differ in their activities toward these chemicals. They also modify the response of persons to these chemicals and are associated with aromatic amine-induced cancer and other sporadic human disorders (Table 1).

Currently, our assessment of the importance of the acetylator genes as determinants of individual susceptibility to aromatic amine-induced cancer is based chiefly on two lines of investigation: genetic epidemiology studies of human populations and the experimental study of animals that express a genetic acetylation polymorphism.

RESULTS AND DISCUSSION

Genetic Epidemiology of Aromatic Amine-induced Cancer

The importance of human acetylator genes to cancer has been reported for the urinary bladder, the colorectum, and the breast of women. Urinary

Table 1
The Relative Risk of the Rapid (R) and Slow (S) Acetylator Phenotypes to Various Sporadic Disorders in Human Subjects

Sporadic disorder	Number of studies	Relative risk	Chi-square
Isoniazid hepatitis	6	S/R = 2.21	14.50 ($p < 0.001$)
Bladder cancer			
all studies	11	S/R = 1.36	10.45 ($p < 0.01$)
high risk of			
exposure	3	S/R = 1.70	7.82 ($p < 0.01$)
Colorectal cancer	2	R/S = 3.03	11.90 ($p < 0.001$)
Breast cancer	2	R/S = 2.05	8.99 ($p < 0.01$)
Type I diabetes			
(Europeans)	4	R/S = 1.62	21.82 ($p < 0.001$)

Relative risks computed by Haldane's modification (1956) of Woolf's method (1955). Summarized from Weber (1987).

bladder cancer in persons exposed to aromatic amines such as benzidine has been most intensively studied. A significant excess of slow acetylators occurs among those affected (Table 1). The difference is most pronounced in the slowest of the slow acetylators, among smokers as compared to nonsmokers and among workers at high risk of exposure to aromatic amines (Table 1; Mommsen and Aagaard 1986). In addition, there is a significant association of tumor aggressiveness to the acetylator phenotype (Cartwright et al. 1982). Slow acetylators are more susceptible to bladder cancer because they maintain higher concentrations of these amines and transport more of them to the bladder, as shown for benzidine (Dewan et al. 1986), where they are activated to DNA-reactive metabolites that initiate the malignancy.

In contrast to the association of slow acetylation with bladder cancer, two studies (Lang et al. 1986; Ilett et al. 1987) find a relative mean excess of 3.03 rapid acetylators to slow acetylators associated with colorectal cancer in men and women (Table 1). Studies of human tissues by Flammang and his colleagues indicate that high levels of acetyltransferase activity are present in human colonic mucosa and that the mucosa catalyzes the O-acetylation of the N-hydroxy metabolites to DNA-reactive metabolites (Flammang et al. 1985; Flammang and Kadlubar 1985, 1986) that could initiate cancer of the large bowel. Additional evidence indicates that several aromatic amines identified as pyrolysis products formed during food cooking (Sugimura and Sato 1983; Stormer et al. 1987) are highly mutagenic and carcinogenic in experimental animals (Takayama et al. 1984a,b). Polymorphic acetylation of some of these pyrolsate products has been reported by Shinohara et al. (1985). Therefore, the genesis of human colorectal cancer may involve aromatic amine carcinogens and rapid acetylator genes may favor the susceptibility of individuals to this disorder.

Evans (1986) reports a significantly greater relative risk ratio of 2.05 of rapid acetylators compared to slow acetylators in two breast cancer studies of Caucasian women (Table 1). The reason for this association is not clear, but because Shore et al. (1979) have shown a strong relationship between use of arylamine-containing hair dyes in women over age 50, but not in younger women, and because these substances are mutagenic (Searle et al. 1975) and carcinogenic in rats (Rojanapo et al. 1986), acetylation may be implicated in this disorder.

The Acetylator Genes and Bioactivation of Carcinogenic Aromatic Amines

The link between acetylator-phenotype- and arylamine-induced cancer involves three acetylation reactions (Fig. 1) (Weber et al. 1987; S. Mattano et al., in prep.). In humans, benzidine and 2-naphthylamine provide much of the

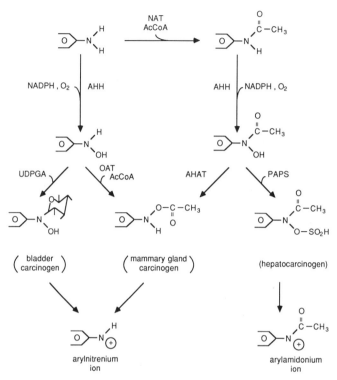

Figure 1

Bioactivation pathways of arylamine carcinogens.

epidemiological evidence for arylamine cancer. These chemicals are poly-morphically acetylated by human and rabbit liver N-acetyltransferase (N-AT) preparations suggesting not only that N-acetylation is an early step in arylamine bioactivation, as Poirier originally proposed (1963), but also that a difference in tumorigenic response to these substances in rapid and slow acetylators might be expected (Glowinski et al. 1978). The intramolecular transfer of the acetyl group from N to O to form an N-acetyoxyarylamine mediated by arylhydroxamic acid acyltransferase (N-O-AT) is another acetyl transfer step in bioactivation. The N-AT and N-O-AT are both cytosolic proteins. The N-AT and N-O-AT reactions are both catalyzed through an ordered ping-pong mechanism by a single enzyme or closely linked enzymes that are genetically polymorphic in rabbit liver (Glowinski et al. 1980). The O-acetyltransferase (O-AT) activity of liver has been identified as the third acetyl transfer step in bioactivation of arylamines. O-AT catalyzes the activa-tion of N-hydroxylated arylamines such as N-OH-2-aminofluorene (N-OH-

AF) and N-OH-3,2'-dimethyl-4-aminobiphenyl (N-OH-DMABP) by direct O-acetylation to form the acetoxyarylamine (Flammang and Kadlubar 1986). The acetoxyarylamines are highly reactive intermediates that react rapidly and spontaneously to form adducts of the amine with macromolecules including DNA (Westra et al. 1985).

We have investigated the bioactivation of arylamines in A/J (A, slow acetylator) and C57BL/6J (B6, rapid acetylator) inbred mouse strains (Weber 1987). The arylamine N-AT enzymes of these mouse strains differ qualitatively since there are differences in their apparent affinities for 2-aminofluorene, and their degree of inhibition by DMSO (Glowinski and Weber 1982b; Mattano and Weber 1987).

To isolate the difference due to the N-AT genes from differences due to other polymorphic background genes in A and B6 strains, we have constructed congenic rapid (A.B6-Nat^r) and slow (B6.A-Nat^s) acetylator mouse strains from these parental strains (S. Mattano et al., in prep.) The A.B6-Nat^r line has the Nat^r/Nat^r genotype on the A background, whereas the B6.A-Nat^s line has the Nat^s/Nat^s genotype on the B6 background. The arylamine N-AT activities with p-aminobenzoic acid, 2-aminofluorene, and 4-aminobiphenyl in mouse liver cytosols of B6, A, AC57F1, and in the congenic lines are shown in Table 2. The differences in activity between the B6 and the A strains is about 2-fold, which agrees reasonably well with the 2.5–3-fold differences that we reported previously (Mattano and Weber 1987). The A.B6-Nat^r activities are about two times greater than the B6 activities, and the B6.A-Nat^s activities are about half those of the A activities. Although somewhat surprising, these findings are, however, consistent with previous observations of the strain distribution patterns for liver and blood arylamine N-AT from recombinant inbred strains derived from A and B6 mice (Glowinski and Weber 1982a), and they provide further support for the existence of mouse genes that modify the expression of arylamine N-AT activity.

Table 2
Mean Acetyltransferase Activity in Inbred Mouse Liver Cytosols

Mouse strain	Acetylator genotype[a]	N	N-AT activity			O-AT activity
			PABA	AF	ABP	N-OH-DMABP
C57BL/6J	rr	5	7.35	2.80	1.01	0.96
AC57F1	rs	5	4.18	1.79	0.75	1.30
A/J	ss	5	3.88	1.45	0.65	1.58
A.B6	rr	9	14.5	4.09	2.25	0.50
B6.A	ss	5	2.00	0.61	0.36	1.82

Summarized from D. Hein et al. (in prep.).
[a]rr, rs, and ss = rapid heterozygous and slow mouse genotypes.

The acetyl coenzyme-A-dependent binding of N-OH-DMABP was also examined in the liver cytosols of these five mouse strains (Table 2). N-OH-DMABP was chosen because its metabolic activation occurs solely through direct O-acetylation and not via N-O-AT-mediated intramolecular acetyl transfer (Flammang et al. 1985). Similar levels of N-OH-DMABP O-AT activity were found in these mouse strains as Flammang and Kadlubar reported (1985). In addition, we found similar levels of O-AT activity in the AC57F1 and in both congenic acetylator strains.

We have copurified arylamine 2-aminofluorene N-AT, N-OH-2-acetyl-aminofluorene N-O-AT, and N-OH-DMABP O-AT to homogeneity from B6 mouse liver. The enzyme has a molecular weight of 31,500 on poly-acrylamide gel electrophoresis. The relative amounts of N-AT/O-AT/N-O-AT in this protein band were in the ratio of 1000-2000/3-4/1. All three acetyltransferase activities are thus catalyzed by a single protein or very similar proteins (S. Mattano et al., in prep.).

Since acetyl transfer is a ping-pong reaction, the N-AT, O-AT, and N-O-AT reactions probably involve a common acetylated enzyme intermediate. Once formed, this intermediate may catalyze the N-acetylation of the acrylamine or the conversion of N-OH-amine by O-AT or N-O-AT to the acetoxyarylamine. The extent to which any of these reactions occurs is substrate-dependent. It also depends on the pharmacokinetics of the arylamine in tissues of the individual and on the genetic capacity of different tissues for bioactivation.

HPLC Analysis of ^{32}P-postlabeled DNA Adducts

The formation of a covalent adduct between the carcinogen/mutagen and a DNA nucleotide is generally believed to be a crucial step in a common mechanism of carcinogenesis/mutagenesis. The technique of ^{32}P-postlabeling of DNA carcinogen adducts and their separation by thin-layer chromatography is proving to be advantageous for detecting such adducts and quantitating DNA damage (Randerath et al. 1981; Gupta et al. 1982). We have adapted this method to the HPLC analysis of DNA adducts of several classes of aromatic carcinogens (G. Levy and W. Weber, in prep.). Following DNA isolation, hydrolysis, and postlabeling, the ^{32}P-postlabeled nucleotides are resolved by reversed-phase ion-pair HPLC. The HPLC technique rapidly resolves DNA-carcinogen adducts from 1 μg or less of mouse liver DNA after as little as three hours of exposure to the carcinogen.

Our initial studies indicate that the method resolves the acetylated and nonacetylated adducts from liver of mice treated with 2-aminofluorene (Fig. 2B). 4-Aminobiphenyl and 2-naphthylamine each showed an adduct peak with a retention time similar to the nonacetylated 2-aminofluorene adduct,

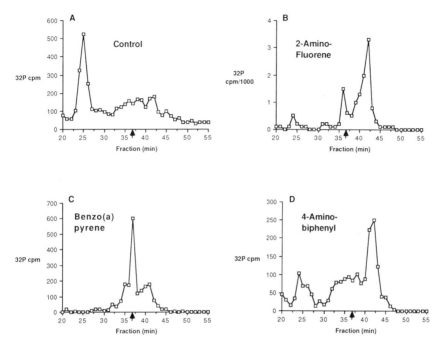

Figure 2

HPLC analysis of ^{32}P-postlabeled adducted nucleotides: (*A*) from a control mouse; (*B*) from a 2-aminofluorene-treated mouse, less control; (*C*) from benzo[a]-pyrene-treated mouse skin, less control; and (*D*) from a 4-aminobiphenyl-treated mouse, less control.

whereas benzidine gave a major adduct that eluted earlier as would be expected from an acetylated adduct (data not shown). DNA adducts from mice treated with alkenylbenzenes such as safrole and methyleugenol and from mouse skin painted with benzo[a]pyrene were also detected and resolved by this technique.

We think that HPLC ^{32}P-postlabeling of DNA will be useful for the assessment of the extent of DNA damage caused by aromatic amines and other aromatic carcinogens to target and nontarget organs. We are currently applying this technique to the assessment of DNA damage induced by exposure to arylamine carcinogens of the inbred mouse strains mentioned above (Table 2) and the "double congenic" mouse strain (B6.A-Nat^s.D2-Ah^d) that we have recently constructed. The latter mouse strain has the slow acetylator genotype and the low inducible Ah (dd) genotype on the B6 genetic background. Pairwise comparisons of these mouse strains should enable us to evaluate the effects of the acetylator and Ah-inducible hydroxylator genes in different combinations (rapid acetylator-high inducible, rapid acetylator-low inducible, slow acetylator-high inducible, slow acetylator-low inducible) in the absence of other polymorphic background genes and, thus, obtain greater insight into the bioactivation of arylamine carcinogens.

Human epidemiological studies indicate remarkable differences in the susceptibility of individuals to arylamine-induced cancer that are attributable to the acetylator trait. The safe levels of exposure to these chemicals will thus vary from one person to another. However, the toxicity of any environmental chemical is a complex event whose expression usually depends on more than a single hereditary factor, and on extrinsic influences too. Even so, we would not lose sight of the fact that susceptibility to the environmental chemical may be largely determined in certain instances by one or two specific genetic traits, and that a number of these traits can now be identified in the individual.

ACKNOWLEDGMENT

These investigations were partially supported by Public Health Service grants CA-39018 and GM-27028.

REFERENCES

Cartwright, R.A., R.W. Glashan, H.J. Rogers, R.A. Ahmad, D.B. Hall, E. Higgins, and M.A. Kahn. 1982. The role of N-acetyltransferase phenotypes in bladder carcinogenesis. A pharmacogenetics epidemiological approach to bladder cancer. *Lancet* **II**: 842.

Case, R.A.M., M.E. Hosker, D.B. McDonald, and J.T. Pearson. 1954. Tumours of the urinary bladder in workmen engaged in the manufacture and use of certain dyestuff intermediates in the British chemical industry. *Br. J. Ind. Med.* **11**: 75.

Cohn, R. 1893. Ueber das Auftreten acetylirter Verbindungen nach Darreichung von Aldehyden. *Z. Physiol. Chem.* **17**: 274.

Dewan, A., J.P. Jani, D.S. Shah, and S.K. Kashyap. 1986. Urinary excretion of benzidine in relation to the acetylator status of occupationally exposed subjects. *Hum. Toxicol.* **5**: 95.

Evans, D.A.P. 1986. Acetylation. In *Ethnic differences in reactions to drugs and xenobiotics* (ed. W. Kalow et al.), vol. 214, p. 209. Alan R. Liss, New York.

Flammang, T.J. and F.F. Kadlubar. 1985. Acetyl CoA-dependent, cytosol-catalyzed binding of carcinogenic N-hydroxy-arylamines to DNA. In *Microsomes and drug oxidations* (ed. A.R. Boobis et al.), p. 190. Taylor and Francis, London.

———. 1986. Acetylcoenzyme A-dependent metabolic activation of N-hydroxy-3,2'-dimethyl-4-aminobiphenyl and several carcinogenic N-hydroxy arylamines in relation to tissues and species differences, other acyl donors, and arylhydroxamic acid-dependent acyltransferases. *Carcinogenesis* **7**: 919.

Flammang, T.J., J.G. Westra, F.F. Kadlubar, and F.A. Beland. 1985. DNA adducts formed from the probable proximate carcinogen, N-hydroxy-3,2'-dimethyl-4-

aminobiphenyl, by acid catalysis or S-acetyl coenzyme A-dependent enzymatic esterification. *Carcinogenesis* **6:** 251.

Glowinski, I.B. and W.W. Weber. 1982a. Genetic regulation of aromatic amine N-acetylation in inbred mice. *J. Biol. Chem.* **257:**1424.

————. 1982b. Biochemical characterization of genetically variant aromatic amine N-acetyltransferases in A/J and C57BL/6J mice. *J. Biol. Chem.* **257:** 1431.

Glowinski, I.B., H.E. Radtke, and W.W. Weber. 1978. Genetic variation in N-acetylation of carcinogenic arylamines by human rabbit liver. *Mol. Pharmacol.* **14:** 940.

Glowinski, I.B., W.W. Weber, J.M. Fysh, J.B. Vaught, and C.M. King. 1980. Evidence that arylhydroxamic acid N,O-acyltransferase and the genetically polymorphic N-acetyltransferase are properties of the same enzyme in rabbit liver. *J. Biol. Chem.* **255:** 7883.

Gupta, R.D., M.V. Reddy, and K. Randerath. 1982. ^{32}P-postlabeling analysis of non-radioactive aromatic carcinogen-DNA adducts. *Carcinogenesis* **3:** 1081.

Haldane, J.B.S. 1956. The estimation and significance of the logarithm of a ratio of frequencies. *Ann. Hum. Genet.* **20:** 309.

Ilett, K.F., B.M. David, P. Detchon, W.M. Castleden, and R. Kwa. 1987. Acetylation phenotype in colorectal carcinoma. *Cancer Res.* **47:** 1466.

Lang, N.P., D.Z.J. Chu, C.F. Hunter, D.C. Kendall, T.J. Flammang, and F.F. Kadlubar. 1986. Role of aromatic amine acetyltransferase in human colorectal cancer. *Arch. Surg.* **121:** 1259.

Mattano, S.M. and W.W. Weber. 1987. Kinetics of arylamine N-acetyltransferase in tissues from rapid and slow acetylator mice. *Carcinogenesis* **8:** 139.

Mommsen, S. and J. Aagaard. 1986. Susceptibility in urinary bladder cancer: Acetyltransferase phenotypes and related risk factors. *Cancer Lett.* **32:** 199.

Parkes, H.G. and A.E.G. Evans. 1984. The epidemiology of the aromatic amine cancers. In *Chemical carcinogens* (ed. C.E. Searle), vol. 1, p.277. American Chemical Society, Washington, D.C.

Poirier, L.A., J.A. Miller, and E.C. Miller. 1963. The N and ring hydroxylation of 2-acetylaminofluorene and the failure to detect N-acetylation of 2-aminofluorene in the dog. *Cancer Res.* **23:** 790.

Randerath, K., M.V. Reddy, and R.C. Gupta. 1981. ^{32}P-postlabeling test for DNA damage. *Proc. Natl. Acad. Sci.* **78:** 6126.

Rehn, L. 1895. Bladder tumors in fuchsin workers (from German). 1963. *Arch. Klin. Chirurgie* **50:** 588.

Rojanapo, W., P. Kupradinun, A. Tepsuwan, S. Chutimataewin, and M. Tanyakaset. 1986. Carcinogenicity of an oxidation product of phenylenediamine. *Carcinogenesis* **7:** 1997.

Searle, C.E., D.G. Harnden, S. Veniott, and O.H.B. Gyde. 1975. Carcinogenicity and mutagenicity tests of some hair colourants and constituents. *Nature* **255:** 506.

Shinohara, A., K. Saito, Y. Yamazoe, T. Kamataki, and R. Kato. 1985. DNA binding of N-hydroxy-Trp-2 and N-hydroxy-Glu-P-1 by acetyl-CoA dependent enzyme in mammalian liver cytosol. *Carcinogenesis* **6:** 303.

Shore, R.E., B.S. Pasternack, E.U. Thiessen, M. Sadow, R. Forbes, and R.E.

Albert. 1979. A case-control study of hair dye use and breast cancer. *J. Natl. Cancer Inst.* **62**: 277.

Stormer, F.C., J. Alexander, and G. Becher. 1987. Fluorometric detection of 2-amino-3-methylimidazo[4,5-f]quinoline,2-amino-3,4-dimethylimidazo[4,5-f]quinoline and their N-acetylated metabolites excreted by the rat. *Carcinogenesis* **8**: 1277.

Sugimura, T. and S. Sato. 1983. Mutagens-carcinogens in foods. *Cancer Res.* **43**: 2415s.

Takayama, S., M. Masuda, M. Mogami, H. Ohgaki, S. Sato, and T. Sugimura. 1984a. Induction of cancers in the intestine, liver and various other organs of rats by feeding mutagens from glutamic acid pyrolsate. *Gann* **75**: 207.

Takayama, S., Y. Nakatsuru, M. Masuda, H. Ohgaki, S. Sato, and T. Sugimura. 1984b. Demonstration of carcinogenicity in F344 rats of 2-amino-3-methylimidazo-[4,5f]quinoline from broiled sardine, fried beef and beef extract. *Gann* **75**: 467.

Weber, W. 1987. *The acetylator genes and drug response.* Oxford University Press, New York.

Weber, W., S.S. Mattano, and G.N. Levy. 1987. Acetylation pharmacogenetics and aromatic amine-induced cancer. In *Carcinogenic and mutagenic N-substituted aryl compounds* (ed. C. King et al.), p. 20. Elsevier Science Publishers, New York.

Westra, J.C., T.J. Flammang, N.F. Fullerton, F.A. Beland, C.C. Weis, and F.F. Kadlubar. 1985. Formation of DNA adducts in vivo in rat liver and intestinal epithelium after administration of the carcinogen 3,2'-dimethyl-4-aminobiphenyl and its hydroxamic acid. *Carcinogenesis* **6**: 37.

Woolf, B. 1955. On estimating the relation between blood group and disease. *Ann. Hum. Genet.* **19**: 251.

COMMENTS

Pfitzer: Is there any sex or age variation among these different acetylators?

Weber: In the most recent studies that we have done with the congenics, we have started to measure the acetylator effects and DNA binding in males versus females. It appears there is a sex effect, but one we don't understand. The females seem to have severalfold higher DNA binding than the males, but there is a lot of variability in the data. That is why we are only happy right now with the qualitative detection, using this method that we are developing. There are some problems to be worked out with the quantitation side of it. I'm not sure of what we have yet, but it appears there is more DNA binding in the female congenic line that has the rapid acetylator gene on the slow background (A.B6-Nat^r).

Estabrook: Wendell, is there any relationship to the activities one sees for the acetylation of o-hydroxy fatty acids or prostaglandins?

Weber: That's an interesting question because the *O*-acetylation story has only just begun to develop. It would be interesting to look at some reactions other than the *N*-acetylation reactions to see if there is anything similar going on.

Estabrook: What about the 3-hydroxy group of some steroids?

Weber: The answer to that isn't known.

Estabrook: Dehydroisoandrosterone (DHA) is very easily acetylated. Of course, DHA is an interesting agent to many people at the moment.

Weber: Investigations by Rosenkranz in the U.S. and by Saito and associates in Japan opened up the *O*-acetylation story within the last five or six years, and others have contributed after them.

Michejda: What is the evidence that colorectal cancer is produced by anything that can be acetylated?

Weber: Sugimura and Sato have found some tryptophan pyrolysates in cooked food, and Shinohara, another Japanese investigator, has found that in rapid and slow acetylator rabbit liver preparations those compounds are polymorphically acetylated. That is, the rapid phenotype acetylates them more rapidly than the slow, suggesting there could be an important connection to acetylation. Another important subject is whether there is a difference in the acetylation of those compounds by rapid and slow acetylator individuals.

Michejda: There is the story of the picopentanes, which are polyhydroxy polyenes. I wonder whether they might be acetylated.

Beland: With regard to the protein pyrolysates, Sugimura, in *Environmental Health Perspectives* just last year, concluded that there probably was not enough in the diet to make a significant difference.

Weber: I'm always suspicious when I come to the quantitative aspect. I'd rather reserve judgment on whether there is enough produced or not.

Weisburger: They are present to the extent of about 0.1 part per billion.

Weber: But how much does it take?

Weisburger: You need it about 60 or 70 years.

Perera: I have a question for Dr. Guengerich. You didn't mention the fairly sizable body of human data on the relationship between AAH inducibility and lung cancer risk.

Guengerich: You're talking about the Shaw and Kellerman studies. Those have been controversial. Those started about 1973, as I understand it.

At that time, there were mainly three populations identified in terms of cancer risk and there was some relationship to the inducibility of AAH levels. A number of laboratories have trouble really repeating that. There were a lot of problems and a lot of people left the business. The latest I read was a couple of years ago. I think Khouri had some information that there still seemed to be a correlation between the basal activity with lung cancer.

Weber: They studied a distribution of about 30 people. Most of the cancer patients were at the high-inducible end of that.

Guengerich: Here again, we're discussing the basal levels, so there may still be something to that.

Wilson: It's a very tough assay.

Guengerich: It's a tough assay, and some people can go quite a way on something that's not really clear.

Perera: How do you distinguish the effect of genetic factors from environmental factors on AAH activity? How can you say this is a truly genetic phenomenon that we're seeing?

Guengerich: That's difficult. The other problem is, with something like AAH, what you are actually measuring is genetic effects on the inducibility, as well. At least, that's what the animal studies say.

Weber: You probably remember Beverly Paigen's paper in the *New England Journal* (1977), in which she looked at families of people who had a member with cancer. They didn't see the same effects in white cells of the family members that they saw in the cancer patients, so the conclusion was there could not have been a genetic effect because the family members didn't show it. I think that's the answer to your question.

Estabrook: I believe that current results suggest that there are at least five regulatory elements involved in the expression of the AAH system. When these regulatory elements become understood and established, it may be appropriate to go back and reexamine some of that data using more modern probes.

Guengerich: Yes. Studies have recently looked at the correlation between mRNA levels and AAH. I think you see a good relationship there, as I recall, but I think that's as far as it goes. I still am a little uneasy about the relationship to lung cancer.

Commentary

MURRAY S. COHN
U.S. Consumer Product Safety Commission
Washington, D.C. 20207

Cohn: Earlier, Ron Hart and Bill Farland talked about the various steps in risk assessment. I am going to focus on the dose-response assessment part of this process so that I can later talk about the potential use of pharmacokinetic data in the risk assessment process, and especially its effect on dose-response assessment.

The traditional methodology that federal agencies have used is to obtain, usually from bioassays, animal high-dose data which is input into dose-response models. The data are in the form of applied dose and the response observed. The mathematical risk extrapolation models usually used are those that have been described earlier, such as the ones that Kenny Crump has developed involving a multistage model with low-dose linearity. Some people use safety factors, but the point is that, based on applied dose, we are trying to assess response at lower doses.

The other part, and to me one of the most controversial and uncertain ones, is species-to-species extrapolation. Once you have, for example, an estimated risk to an animal at a low dose, various assumptions are used to estimate what the human response could be. One method used is based on mg/kg/day. Another method applies the "surface" area correction to that.

Then, there are other considerations in the dose-response assessment, such as a proportion of lifetime correction. On the basis of a two-year bioassay with six hours' inhalation, five days a week, such a correction would be used to assess risk for example from one week's inhalation of one hour a day. Other factors include analysis of data from multiple sexes and species. Are they averaged, or is the most sensitive utilized? Once you have considered these and other factors, the results feed into the rest of the risk assessment process.

Well, it looks pretty easy. However, the problem with such a procedure is that every component of the process relies upon an assumption. A major goal is to reduce the uncertainty of the assumptions whenever possible.

In the case of pharmacokinetic data, we have something that may help us reduce the uncertainty of the dose-response assessment process. The bottom line in the use of pharmacokinetic data is to obtain an actual measurement or an indication of the concentration-over-time profile of a relevant compound or a metabolite at an "important" site, as opposed to using the traditional assumption based on applied dose.

These are three very important terms. The measurements giving the concentration-over-time profile provide what is known as an area-under-the-curve analysis. Ascertaining the relevant compound or metabolite requires knowing or deducing the important compound that is causing an effect such as carcinogenic response. The important site is another problem: if there is a response in liver in animals, what does that mean for humans?

However, there are a lot of clues that one can get from the data that allow some of these parameters that I have just described to be estimated or ascertained and used in the risk assessment process. Thus, risk assessment in humans could be based on delivered dose, the amount of dose that is actually at a target site, as opposed to the applied dose to the whole animal in a bioassay situation. Such a procedure could also be applied to human epidemiological studies as well.

The depth of information available for various compounds varies dramatically. I'll talk about two of them as examples. In the case of perchloroethylene, the only data that are available right now is the measurement of total body metabolism; a given dose is administered and the total urinary metabolites are measured. It has been assumed by some that total urinary metabolite is a measure of delivered dose, and the risks are adjusted accordingly. However, the important compound or metabolite is unknown, so there is no active site modeling. The mechanism of action is also unknown. Thus, rather large assumptions have to be made.

In the case of methylene chloride, much more work has been done. There have been some very sophisticated, physiologically based pharmacokinetic models that have been developed, mainly by Reitz at Dow Chemical and Andersen at the Air Force. Angelo at General Foods has been looking at these types of models as well.

These models utilize information obtained for methylene chloride, such as partition coefficients between blood and various tissues and between air and blood; blood flow rates, respiratory rates; and various metabolic constants that are actually derived from animals and humans. We try to put this all together into a living model, so to speak, to try to predict, upon either ingestion, inhalation, or even injection, what the time versus concentration profiles might be for a target tissue (e.g., the liver), of not only the parent compound, but metabolites by one or more pathways.

There has been a lot of information developed to try to verify such models for methylene chloride: for example, comparing how levels decrease in experimental animal chambers with that predicted by the model, and also, examining how the model predicts animal blood levels and metabolism after appropriate dosing.

There are several ways in which pharmacokinetic information might be used in the risk assessment process. First is for route-to-route extrapolation. One of the best examples I can think of is paradichlorobenzene. This compound was assayed by gavage in an NTP bioassay, but we are interested in human exposure by the inhalation route. If we have a pharmacokinetic model that estimates concentration in the blood and in a specific target site (e.g., the liver) in animals, via ingestion and then by inhalation, one should be able to derive estimates of risk for the route of inhalation, even though the bioassay is by gavage not by inhalation.

A second use of pharmacokinetic information is in time pattern extrapolation. If treatment is for six hours by inhalation, how long does the compound remain in the bloodstream? Does it remain long enough that if there was another six-hour inhalation the next day there would be an additive effect and so on, until an equilibrium was reached? One can manipulate these computer models to try to understand what is happening. They might be useful in looking at the effects of prolonged exposure and how much metabolite might be at a target site, versus intermittent exposure and how much might be at the same target site.

The third use is high-dose to low-dose extrapolation. I think that this is one area where pharmacokinetic information is going to be of great use, because there are a lot of systems where pathways saturate, where there are competing pathways, and where there is metabolic activation/deactivation; all may have an effect on the shape of the dose-response curve when extrapolating from high-dose to low-dose.

The example that Dr. Guengerich gave for methylene chloride would serve as a good example. In this case, he showed methylene chloride is metabolized by two pathways, the GST and the MFO pathway. The MFO pathway is thought not to be involved in the carcinogenic process; the GST pathway is thought to be involved in the carcinogenic response. The important fact is that the MFO pathway tends to saturate at levels below which the bioassay was conducted and the GST pathway does not. At high levels, as you increase the amount of methylene chloride to the animal or to the human, the risk, which is related to GST pathway output, would be projected to be proportional to the increase in applied dose, since the MFO pathway is saturated. At lower levels, when the MFO pathway is not saturated, as you increase the amount of methylene chloride, the MFO pathway is going to eliminate some methylene chloride so that it is not available to the GST pathway, so you expect a nonlinearity in the high-to-low dose-response curve. As a matter of fact, recent methylene chloride risk assessments done by various federal agencies have tried to take this into account. It actually reduces the risk, I think, by a factor of some twofold at low doses because nonlinearity is imposed on the dose-response curve by these competing pathways. So, that's a third use for pharmacokinetic information.

The fourth one, and the one that I want to spend the most time on is, again, the most controversial: species-to-species extrapolation. The problem here is that species-to-species extrapolation involves a number of components. I am not even going to begin to try to identify them all, but I can try to guess at some examples: obviously, pharmacokinetic differences between species, differences in DNA repair, and differences in the number of cells exposed to a given concentration. A mouse has much fewer cells in the liver compared to the human, yet in some cases, total risks to an organ are assumed to be similar. This can be offset by the fact that mice might have a higher cell turnover rate which can fix mutations faster or cause a tumor to progress faster. So, you have a number of components in what I term a "black box" when you try to extrapolate from a mouse or a rat or any other rodent to the human situation.

The point, however, is that now we are identifying species differences using pharmacokinetic data. Such information might, for example, estimate that for specific exposure for a specific compound, a mouse might metabolize that compound ten times faster than a human does.

What do we do with these data? Let's try to make this simplistic and say that one always uses a factor F to extrapolate between rodents and humans. As I said before, this factor might be 1 on a mg/kg/day basis. The factor might be 12.7, if you use the surface area correction for the differences between a mouse and a human. And then, F is a function, as I said, of a number of components. This equation could be very simple or it could be very difficult. I hope that Curtis Travis will embellish this a little bit later on as a discussant, but certainly, one of the terms is pharmacokinetic information and many other terms that fill up that box.

So, now that we know a pharmacokinetic term, how is it used? There are several choices: One is you can make an assumption for the value of all components, other than the pharmacokinetic term, and determine F accordingly. This is an approach at which some are seriously looking.

My feeling is that making an assumption for all other terms is no more certain than making an assumption for F itself. So, I don't know how to use pharmacokinetic data for species extrapolations. I feel more research is necessary before this type of approach is taken.

The bottom line is that I think the use of pharmacokinetic information is extremely valuable. It can be used, as I said before, in four different aspects of the dose-response assessment process. I think that the species-to-species component of it is one of the most exciting, but I think that a lot of research must be done in that area.

Estabrook: I'd like to know, are the data treated the same in other countries, Japan, Europe, for example, as we treat them in this country, in terms of doing the risk assessment?

Cohn: I really can't answer that. I have seen some risk assessments from other countries that are making an attempt to utilize pharmacokinetic data. Using pharmacokinetic information is relatively new. It has only been done, I think, in three cases at EPA, and it has only been done in two cases at my agency. FDA is just starting to look into it. We had an interagency group that met for about two years, trying to decide how to utilize this type of information in the risk assessment process. We came to a number of agreements and to a number of disagreements. We are just starting to try to fathom this out, so, I would doubt that other countries are to this point yet.

Wilson: Perhaps you should ask Dr. Clayson. He might have some first-hand experience.

Clayson: No.

Hart: I thought Murray on very short notice did an excellent job of summarizing how we are attempting to use pharmacokinetic and pharmacodynamic data in the regulatory process. The difficulties that we are really facing is that this is a very new area and that there is a diversity of the types of information that we are seeing. Species effects, age effects, sex effects, diet effects, which Wendell (Weber) and others brought out in their presentations earlier, really are confounding factors.

Part of the reason is the fact that there is a paucity of data on comparative toxicology. We have a large amount of data on compounds and analogs that are noncarcinogenic, carcinogenic, and so on, but we have really very few comparative studies on the toxicology done within the same labs under the same conditions. Without that comparative information, it is very hard to do the interspecies extrapolation about which Murray is talking.

The best you can do is go to the literature to try to pull out this data. Usually, it's mouse and rat, and sometimes, if you're lucky, hamster. Yet, at the same time, our ultimate goal is to make human extrapolations. I hope that the audience realizes that it is extremely difficult to be a regulatory scientist these days, while factoring in the mechanistic aspects of science.

Estabrook: I'll accept what you say, but it is difficult for me to understand the 50-plus years of pharmaceutical research that must have built up a huge backlog of data that would be directly applicable to this type of a problem.

Hart: It's almost impossible to get at. We have tried going to different pharmaceutical companies to get the information and have been unable to do so in many cases.

Enslein: There are really two aspects to this. One is that you are trying to deal with what in feedback theory one calls an "open loop" system, as contrasted to a "closed loop" system. That is, you are trying to project to an uncertain target from relatively uncertain data, and you have nothing to tell you when you are in error.

Cohn: The closest thing we have is studies like Dr. Crump is doing.

Enslein: I wonder whether one can learn something about making necessary adjustments from some of the approaches that have been used on noncarcinogenic data, modeling from mouse or rat or even from Daphne, and that have been developed from partition coefficients and structural parameters.

Cohn: It's certainly a possibility. The problem I have is that in some of the data presented earlier today, the responses in various species to the same compound are so diverse, so different, that it's tough to compare.

Enslein: Yes, however I'm not talking of measuring in human models. I think that would be going too far too soon.

Cohn: Comparing one animal to another?

Enslein: However, we have built models where the same end point was available in Daphne and in rat and where we were able to predict very effectively in either Daphne or rat. The Dapne work is only relatively recent.

Cohn: Which end point were you predicting?

Enslein: Acute toxicity, dose required for death, LD_{50}, as well as subchronic toxicity, 90-day toxicity.

Clayson: I recently accepted a paper for *Cancer Letters* from Dr. Hayden and Dr. Huff of the National Toxicology Program, in which they have analyzed the NCI/NTP database for the rat predicting for the mouse and the mouse predicting for the rat, and in each case it worked out about 75%. That's not terribly good.

Lijinsky: That's better than what I would have thought.

Enslein: What they didn't do was they didn't adjust for differences in structure. That's what we are trying to do.

Deasy: You mentioned that you were part of a work group on the use of pharmacokinetics in quantitative risk assessment. I wonder if you could comment about the composition and the purpose of that group and its outcome.

Cohn: The purpose of the group was to look at six specific chlorocarbons. The reason for establishing the pharmacokinetic work group was that, as I said, industry and Dr. Andersen at the Air Force have been starting to develop these pharmacokinetic models that have a strong effect on the way we perform risk assessment. That is new, and it required a lot of analysis. These compounds were of interest to all four agencies that were involved, my agency (CPSC), EPA, FDA, and OSHA. So, it was decided to form an interagency group to study these models in detail and to do it together so that we could try to come to a common understanding.

The outcome is that we wrote a rather large report, which is available from the EPA, discussing in much greater detail some of the concepts that I briefly described just now. The other outcome is that both EPA and CPSC have modified their applied dose risk assessments to include pharmacokinetic information: in both cases, incorporating high-to-low-dose differences, and in EPA's case, incorporating species-to-species differences.

Perera: Murray, you mentioned that EPA had incorporated pharmacokinetic data in risk assessments in three cases and CPSC in two. Are you saying that these were cases where you have done risk assessments for regulatory decision making? If so, what are these cases? I'm not aware that you have actually formally gone ahead and modified human risk assessments on the basis of pharmacokinetics.

Cohn: In the case of CPSC, one of them was for regulatory purposes, methylene chloride. The other one we did was perchloroethyelene, which we are currently studying. Bill can speak for EPA.

Farland: The process, of course, that we use is to develop health assessment documents for the various regulatory programs, like the air program and the water program. We now have three health assessment documents that incorporated the pharmacokinetic concept. They are in various stages of review. They have been turned over to the programs. They will be the basis for the health assessment component of the regulatory decision once they have gone through the full review.

The Science Advisory Board met in August to look at the assessment on methylene chloride. The assessment document on perchloroethylene was reviewed in May of 1986. We are expecting a response from them very shortly, but we got a very positive response at the meeting on the application of the pharmacokinetics in those two cases.

Perera: I'm aware that OSHA very recently rejected that concept as too speculative in doing a risk assessment on formaldehyde. I know we don't have time to go into this now, but maybe there will be some time later.

Singer: The human has so many different things being metabolized, so many different types of exposures, besides different genetics. What experiment would help to go, not from mouse to rat, but from any animal to human? What data would be needed?

Cohn: That's a difficult question. First of all, you're right about emphasizing human variation. I'll give you an example that relates to methylene chloride. You talked about glutathione S-transferase and that's the important pathway. That varies in humans for methylene chloride. I think Ron Pero's lab indicated that the Mu isozyme of GSH is in about 50% of humans, and he told me that he thinks that might be the one that will apply to methylene chloride. It's interesting, when data on human livers came in, the GSH pathway acting on methylene chloride was absent in almost 50% of the cases and present in the others. So, it does vary in humans quite a bit, as you suggest. That indicates that research is needed on target populations to which a risk assessment would apply.

My biggest problem, as you say, is to try to understand the relationship of the various factors in interspecies extrapolation. If we only have pharmacokinetic information right now, the relationship of it to all the other factors in coming up with a value for F is important. Some of the biological models that people are proposing might be one way to answer this, to try to actually get a handle on each of these other parameters and factor it into a model.

Another way that is harder is we actually have some 30 known human carcinogens, where we may have an idea of what F is already. If we can do pharmacokinetic studies on those compounds in the appropriate rodents and in humans, we might get an idea of the relationship of those other factors.

Singer: That's the only experiment that would mean anything, having a group of humans, then?

Cohn: That would be one thing I would like to see done. Of course, the human studies would have to be done in vitro. However, I think biological modeling might be helpful as well.

Guengerich: We simply did the study where we took samples from a group of different humans and actually measured that reaction directly, the conjugation with methylene chloride, and compared that with numbers that were used for the same strains of rats and mice that had been used in the bioassays for the assessment of cancer risk.

Panel Discussion

CURTIS C. TRAVIS
Oak Ridge National Laboratory, Tennessee
DAVID B. CLAYSON
Health and Welfare of Canada, Ontario, Canada
PETER FU
National Center for Toxicological Research, Arizona
MIRIAM C. POIRIER
National Cancer Institute, Maryland

Travis: The cancer process can be separated into a pharmacokinetic phase and a pharmacodynamic phase. The former relates applied dose to effective dose at target tissue, whereas the latter relates effective dose with biological effect. A recent development in the cancer risk assessment area is the advent of biologically based pharmacokinetic and pharmacodynamic models. Relying on actual physiological parameters such as body weight, cardiac output, breathing rates, tissue volumes, etc., to describe the metabolic process, pharmacokinetic models can predict chemical transport and metabolism across routes of administration, across species, and through temporal variations in exposure. Biologically based pharmacodynamic models relate fundamental cellular processes to the epidemiology of cancer in animal and human populations.

The focus of the previous talk was pharmacokinetics. The question that arises is: Can we incorporate pharmacokinetic data (and models) into the risk assessment process, and what kind of data do we need to accomplish this? I believe the answer depends on the type of risk assessment question one is attempting to answer. For example, in the classical health assessment methodology, inhaled dose (mg/kg/day) is calculated as the air concentration an animal is exposed to (mg/l) times a breathing rate (1/day) divided by the body weight (kg) of the animal. However, it is known that in realistic situations this calculation overestimates dose. When an animal is exposed to a volatile organic, the blood saturates fairly quickly and soon the animal is breathing out as much chemical as it is breathing in. Over a period of time the chemical moves from the blood to other parts of the body, but eventually the entire body will saturate. After that, the quantity of chemical entering the body per day depends entirely on the rate at which the chemical is metabolized and excreted from the body. Can we presently use pharmacokinetic

Banbury Report 31: Carcinogen Risk Assessment: New Directions in the Qualitative and Quantitative Aspects © Cold Spring Harbor Laboratory. 0-87969-231-6/88. $1.00 + .00

models to compute the actual daily amount of the chemical that stays in the body? I believe the answer is yes.

The question is what kind of data would you use to accomplish this? Well, for chemicals like methylene chloride, tetrachloroethylene, and trichloroethylene, we have pharmacokinetic data in mice, rats, *and* humans. In controlled exposure situations, we know blood concentrations over time, we know exhaled air concentrations over time, and sometimes we know total metabolite production over time. From data such as these, metabolic parameters can be estimated in mice, rats, and humans. They are not perfect data, but generally good enough to get started on the more realistic risk assessment.

What other type of data would make the use of pharmacokinetic models in risk assessment more acceptable? An important contribution would be the relative enzymatic activities for specific chemical substrates across animal species. Data like these were recently gathered for methylene chloride, and they proved to be very useful in increasing the acceptability of incorporating pharmacokinetics into the risk assessment process for methylene chloride.

Pharmacokinetic models can also be used to help answer questions like what is the proper measure of applied dose. It is frequently assumed that experimental results can be extrapolated between species when applied dosage is standardized as either mg/kg/day (body weight scaling) or as mg/surface area/day (surface area scaling). Pharmacokinetic models can be used to gain insight into this problem. Assume for the present that the proper measure of dose to target tissue is the area under the tissue-concentration curve of the toxic moiety (which could be either the parent compound or a metabolite). If one accepts this definition of dose to target tissue, then one can ask, "How can I measure applied dose so that I can get the same area under the curve of the toxic moiety in all species?"

I have used pharmacokinetic models to answer this question. The answer turns out to depend on whether the parent compound or a metabolite is the carcinogenic moiety. If the parent compound is the carcinogenic agent, then $mg/kg^{0.75}/day$ should be used as the proper measure of applied dose. If this measure of applied dose is used, the area under the curve of the parent compound will be the same in all species.

The above discussion points out that there are two ways that pharmacokinetic models can be used to improve the risk assessment process. The first is through the general investigation of the scientific bases for assumptions used in risk assessment (like interspecies extrapolation or the effect of doses that are variable in time). This application can proceed immediately. The other area where pharmacokinetic models can be used is to actually modify quantitative estimates of risk for specific chemicals like methylene chloride or tetrachloroethylene. This application of pharmacokinetic models is more speculative but certainly within reach if the proper metabolic data are obtained.

It should be pointed out that even if our knowledge of pharmacokinetics was perfect, it would not solve all problems with quantitative risk assessment. Suppose we knew how to extrapolate pharmacokinetic data across species, that is we knew how to go from applied dose to effective dose to target tissue. We still have the problem of pharmacodynamics, and we are almost back to square one. The question then becomes, "What is the proper measure of dose to target tissue so that pharmacodynamic effect is the same across species?" In other words, for a given measure of dose, is the liver tissue in a mouse just as sensitive as liver tissue in a human? Since we do not know the answer to this question, pharmacokinetics can only get us half-way to the answer of how to do interspecies extrapolations.

Before we are going to make significant improvements in the risk assessment process, we must recognize that there are two pieces to the interspecies extrapolation problem: pharmacokinetics and pharmacodynamics. We need more fundamental research in both areas! Hopefully, such efforts will help us answer the question of how we should go from applied dose to effective dose to target tissue and finally to effect.

Estabrook: Thank you. We have a couple of questions.

Beland: I think that if you are going to measure metabolites or parent compound, or genetic variations, you are sort of evading the central issue. I think people could concentrate on going in and measuring DNA damage. Let's assume for right now that if you go in and measure DNA damage, you are filtering out all the problems of detoxification, and genetic variation, and inactivation, and so forth, and you are getting to an end point that can be useful. There are a number of us who have developed nice postlabeling techniques that are now capable of measuring damage in humans. Mimi (Poirier), I think, is going to talk about measuring with antibodies. I would think if you people who were going to do pharmacokinetics would go one step further and start looking at DNA damage, you would have an easier time.

Travis: We don't know the relationship between exposure and DNA damage in humans. We can measure pharmacokinetics in mice, in rats, and you can obtain in vitro measurements of metabolic parameters in mice, rats, and humans. From that we want to predict what the metabolism in humans would be. The question is can we do it?

* Now, we could measure adduct levels in mice and rats and maybe be able to predict adduct levels in humans. I don't know. To me, that's part of the pharmacodynamic process. At least, it's at the interface.

Singer: Measurements of DNA damage in humans is being done, actually. It has been done with aflatoxin, for one thing.

Hart: However, there you excrete the adduct, so that's a little different.

Singer: However, it is being done.

Beland: They're measuring diethylnitrosamine-induced damage in Chinese populations.

Hart: There are a number of compounds where they have actually done that.

Cohn: I have one question. Even if we followed your suggestions, and we found that person A has 20 adducts per amount of tissue assayed, person B has 10, person C has 1, and person D has 50, what do you do with that information in terms of trying to predict human risk?

Beland: I don't have the faintest idea.

Estabrook: With that, we'll go to David Clayson.

*　　　*　　　*

Clayson: First of all, I would like to thank the organizers of this conference for an invitation. I want to change the pace and the direction of the discussion slightly. We have heard a lot of very good science today. The point I want to make is that in carcinogenesis, we may be chasing not one route to an end point but a multitude of routes to the end point of cancer. We may need different parts of this science for different parts of the process.

The first difficulty is the operational definition of a carcinogen at the moment: merely as an agent or process that increases the rate of formation of tumors. Now, we have already stated that carcinogenesis is a multistage process. It is my experience, in reading the literature, that anything that does enhance one of these stages may well result in an increase in the incidence of cancer. In other words, we have carcinogens that do the whole job, and we now also have carcinogens that may only do part of the job. If we are going to assess the risk from these, we really need to know with what we are going to be dealing.

Let's take an example. Cancer consists of initiation and promotion. Or, since the term "promotion" has become so debased, I prefer to call it initiation and tumor development. There are examples where we would expect to find preinitiated cells within a tissue and which are just sitting there waiting for something to come along and develop them. We would expect to find this where there is a background incidence of tumors, as, for example, in the B6C3F1 mouse liver. In that case, if you look at Soderman's data base of carcinogens, now six years out of date but nevertheless a very useful compilation, you will find there are nearly 30 examples of chemicals that have increased the incidence of liver tumors in male mice without producing any other tumor. One must begin to wonder whether these agents are the sort of "real" carcinogens people have been talking about and working on more than anything, or are they mainly things that push over tumor appearance using high levels of the agent. I don't know how we are going to be sure.

I am optimistic enough to believe that we may be able to sort out this mess by the use of the short-term genotoxicity tests, once we can get rid of the present confusion that I think has surrounded them. We assume that a single line of approach to cancer is sufficient, and we haven't begun to consider the innate sensitivity of things like the Ames test. What we call a carcinogen at the moment may be a number of different entities.

We have another problem. We use the maximum tolerated dose (MTD) for our cancer bioassays. We do a cancer bioassay, let the product onto the market because it failed to give us an increase in tumors, and then, to our embarrassment, someone repeats that bioassay with a slightly higher dose and finds the thing is a carcinogen. It's embarrassing to everybody. We define our MTD on three principles: (1) the animal still survives in good clinical condition; (2) the animal doesn't lose more than 10% in body weight as the result of this agent; and (3) the animal doesn't show morphological evidence of lesions that might interfere in the cancer process.

High-dose toxicity can be an important factor in the induction of tumors. We have done a little work in Canada on an agent called butylated hydroxyanisole (BHA), which is an important antioxidant used to prevent rancidization in food during transport and shelf storage. It was shown by Dr. Ito in Japan that if you introduce 2% of this compound in the diet of rats for two years, the forestomach will be full of carcinomas and papillomas mainly arising along the lesser curvature of the forestomach.

We were asked to see if we could do anything about contradicting this evidence to suggest that the compound was safe, since it is one of only three compounds which we use for that purpose in Canada. We fed some 2% BHA to the rats for 9 days and 27 days. We injected tritiated thymidine at the end of the study. We found not only florid proliferative lesions in the forestomach along the lesser curvature after this time, but we also found a marked increase in the tritiated thymidine labeling index. We had a look at the dose response of this effect, and we found the no-effect level very appreciably above what humans are exposed to. We went on and did a 91-day experiment, and we found the same no-effect level. We found, after that, that the tritiated thymidine labeling index fell to normal values very, very rapidly but the lesions regressed more slowly.

We have just completed a reversibility study in which we have found that if you treat for 3 months or 6 months and take the substance away, you don't get tumors as a result. After 12 months, the situation is getting far more complicated. We hope we will have the data in press very shortly.

Now, all of this makes it appear that what BHA is doing is increasing cellular proliferation at high doses and this, in some way, is leading to the tumors. We don't know what the initiating factor is: the result of the compound, the result of nitrosamine reflux, or the result of some nasty things in the animals' food that we don't know about.

What has been done is that we and people in other countries, including the U.S. and Japan, have looked in species without a forestomach, and we have given the highest tolerated dose of BHA for 3–18 months. We have found absolutely no biologically significant events using BHA at all. It looks as though there is something rather toxic specifically in the forestomach. Whether this is true or not, we will need to find out as the result of further work.

What I forgot to say is that Dr. Ito, when he did his carcinogenicity studies, omitted to report that he had been working above the MTD. We found this out as a result of the 91-day study and confirmed it in the reversibility study.

Tennant: Actually, among over 200 of the rodent assays that have been done in two species, there are a total, I think, of 21 that were mouse liver only. Of those studies, half of those were carcinogenic and half were not. Not only were there liver tumors induced by those 21 chemicals, but it is only one of those, as I recollect, in which the tumors occurred only in male mouse liver. Mouse liver is the primary site for tumorigenesis both in the rat and the mouse. Most often, the tumors occurred not only in the liver but at other sites. So, it's true, that 21 of those chemicals out of 112 or so carcinogens were mouse liver only.

However, the liver is such a high-frequency site of tumorigenesis for chemicals that it appears that it is logically a product of both the routes of administration and that these animals are dosed for a significant portion of their lifespan.

Now, it is therefore possible to indict the mouse as being supersensitive, but between the male and the female mouse there is possibly a 30-fold differential and at least a 10-fold differential. Male B6C3F1 mice have a 30% background liver tumor incidence, and the female has about a 3%. However, in none of the studies is there any proportionality between the effect of the chemical and the two sex species. Very often liver tumors are induced in rats that show a background liver tumor incidence that is more like the female B6C3F1 mouse, and again there is no proportionality involved in the response to the chemical. Although the genetics favors one or more genes in the C3H parent that may influence that tumorigenesis, it doesn't appear to account for the level of sensitivity accorded to the mouse in identifying carcinogens.

The second point that you raised has to do with the MTD. The MTD as a principle of exposure for identifying carcinogens has been universally embraced by the OECD, the OSTP, and other groups. I think we have to decide whether there is a scientific consensus about the use of the MTD. If we're not to use the MTD, then what?

Clayson: I agree with your comments. What I said was that I worked with Soderman's data base and I found somewhere between 25 and 30 compounds that left me wondering about the male mouse liver. We've got to look at that mouse liver tumor extraordinarily carefully. If the compound was genotoxic and gave an increasing amount of liver tumors, I would have no worry at all. If it doesn't show genotoxicity, then I am going to suggest that maybe it is helping tumor development rather than a whole, complete, genotoxic carcinogen.

Now, on the question of the MTD, I hope I never said one shouldn't use it. All I am saying is that one has got to define it perhaps even more tightly than the NTP has done already, and we then ought to find a way of staying with it. If I may remind you, in the NCI part of the bioassay program, you will find that there are many compounds that were started at one dose level that proved too high for the continued survival of the animal. The dose level was then reduced, sometimes once, sometimes twice, and very occasionally more than twice. The question that arises there and is very much on my mind is: Did that initial toxic dose have an adverse effect on the animal and shouldn't we be considering that part of the bioassay program as potentially flawed?

Tennant: I think you judge that on an individual study basis.

Michejda: There is another thing with the MTD, which I think arises from Druckey's original experiments. He did them one way, and then everyone else did them that way.

Clayson: And we want to do them, I don't deny that. We've got to define the term toxic dose more specifically.

Michejda: Yes, but it leads to some really kind of silly inconsistencies, as Willy Lijinsky found with nitrosodiethanolamine. It is perhaps the most toxic nitroso compound to which humans are exposed, and yet Druckey fed it to rats at gal/kg, because the substance was simply nontoxic.

Lijinsky: The total dose altered the weight of the animals.

Michejda: That's right. The animals died of liver cancer, but Druckey concluded that it is a weak carcinogen.

Lijinsky: It isn't.

Michejda: It now turns out that it's a very strong carcinogen. It's slightly less carcinogenic than diethylnitrosamine but in that order of carcinogenicity. It's simply nontoxic, and it's tolerated extremely well. Insects live on it. Everything lives on it.

Lijinsky: It isn't genotoxic.

Weisburger: I have a question about BHA. If it affects forestomach, why doesn't it affect the naturally rapidly proliferating tissues in the animal, like the intestinal tract?

Lijinsky: Esophagus.

Clayson: It doesn't. You do remember that the forestomach is not a rapidly proliferating tissue. In the younger animal, it's quite low, and it gets a bit more rapid in old age. The only other affected tissue, out of the ones we've studied, is the bladder, where at 2% BHA we found about a sixfold increase in proliferation without any obvious pathological changes. What we think is the cause of this is very simply that the forestomach and the bladder are to some extent storage organs, and the substance remains there long enough to exert its damaging effects.

Weisburger: It just goes through the intestinal tract.

Clayson: Yes. I believe Dr. Grice of Can Tox gave a paper on this subject to the Toxicology Forum last summer, which more or less suggested that BHA goes through the esophagus like an express train.

Lijinsky: If you give nitrosamines by mouth, and they just bathe the esophagus very casually, you get esophageal tumors. If you give the same compound by gavage, you don't get the esophageal tumors. So, there is obviously a local effect, even though it's very transient.

Stevenson: Rat forestomach seems to be heavily populated in bacteria and appears to be the source of bacteria further back in the gut. It is also extremely anaerobic. I think Goldman at Harvard has studied this.

Clayson: This is the first time I've heard of the forestomach being anaerobic. I thought that was a good deal further down the GI tract.

Perera: I was part of the ad hoc panel reviewing the extensive data available at that time, seven years ago, and we did come up with a definition, as you described, of MTD. I am not aware of data or reports of a consensus of experts since then that would invalidate that definition. Our panel also pointed to the problem of the lack of sensitivity in the bioassay using MTD. So, I think you are between a rock and a hard place. You want to have the most sensitive possible model. If anyone is aware of a better definition of MTD or a better method, I think we should discuss that.

Clayson: I agree with you completely, but we have a way further to go if we can. The phrase, "morphological lesion," raises a big question mark in my mind. I am not quite sure whether it means anything or everything. With BHA, as an example, would the morphological lesions you are seeing early in the forestomach invalidate the use of that dose as the MTD?

Lijinsky: I think it probably would if the proper studies were done.

Estabrook: Now to Dr. Fu.

*   *   *

Fu: As a panelist, I would like to congratulate Dr. Guengerich and Dr. Weber for their excellent presentations and their leading research in metabolism. Both human cytochrome P-450 polymorphisms and human acetylation polymorphisms are crucial determinants in the detoxification of xenobiotics, and conceivably, in the metabolic detoxification as well as activation of chemical carcinogens. It is apparent that both of these studies have great potential for human carcinogen risk assessment.

I would like to comment on their presentations in relation to our work with nitroaromatics. It is estimated that nitroaromatics account for a significant portion of the world's industrial chemical products. Nitro-aromatics have been prepared as dye intermediates, human and veteri-nary medicines, and food additives. Recently, nitroaromatics have been found as environmental pollutants and contaminants in the food chains. Unfortunately, many of these compounds are mutagenic in bacteria and mammalian cells and tumorigenic in experimental animals. Examples include 5-nitrofurans, nitroimidazoles, and nitro-polycyclic aromatic hydrocarbons (nitro-PAHs).

Recently, we have studied the rat liver microsomal metabolism of a series of nitro-PAHs and several 5-nitrofurans. In collaboration with R.H. Heflich at NCTR, we have also determined the mutagenicity of these compounds and their metabolites in *Salmonella typhimurium* tester strains TA98 and TA100. Several interesting observations have been obtained and are summarized as follows:

1. Nitro substitution can drastically affect the regio- and stereo-selectivity of the microsomal cytochrome P-450 isozymes toward metabolism of nitro-PAHs.
2. On determination of the mutagenicity of these compounds and their metabolites, we have found that there exist at least five activation pathways. They are nitroreduction, nitroreduction followed by esterification, ring-oxidation, ring-oxidation followed by nitroreduction, and ring-oxidation followed by nitroreduction and esterification. Similar results have also been obtained by Dr. Beland and other groups.
3. The orientation of the nitro substituent has been found to be an important structural feature that affects the reductive metabolism of nitro-PAHs and the direct-acting mutagenicity of nitro-PAHs in *S. typhimurium* tester strains TA98 and TA100. Nitro-PAHs with their nitro substituents perpendicular or nearly perpendicular to the aromatic rings are not reduced by the rat liver microsomal enzymes and are either weak or non-direct-acting mutagens. However, nitro-PAHs with their nitro substituents parallel or nearly parallel to the aromatic rings are, in general, readily reduced to the corresponding amino-PAHs under anaerobic conditions and are metabolized to form ring-oxidized metabolites under aerobic conditions. For example, 1-, 3-, and 6-nitrobenzo[a]pyrene are a set of isomeric nitro-PAHs derived from the potent PAH, benzo[a]pyrene. 1- and 3-nitrobenzo[a]pyrene, both of which have their nitro groups parallel to the benzo[a]pyrenyl ring, are facily reduced to 1- and 3-aminobenzo[a]pyrene, respectively, and are potent direct-acting mutagens. On the other hand, the 6-nitrobenzo[a]pyrene isomer, with a perpendicular nitro group, cannot be reduced by the rat liver microsomal cytochrome P-450 enzymes and is a non-direct-acting mutagen.
4. The ease of nitroreduction of the nitro-PAHs varies among compounds and in different enzymatic systems. Based on our findings, we have hypothesized that the ease of nitroreduction of nitro-PAHs by the reduc-

tive enzymes, including microsomal P-450 enzymes, in an enzymatic system is a potential biomarker for correlation with the mutagenicity and/or carcinogenicity of this class of nitroaromatics.

Based on the results summarized above, it is reasonable that rat liver microsomal cytochrome P-450 isozymes exhibit markedly different substrate specificities on the oxidative and reductive metabolism of nitro-PAHs. Thus, nitro-PAHs can serve as a set of model compounds for exploring the polymorphisms of human cytochrome P-450 isozymes and acyltransferases. In addition, at the present time, little is known concerning the reduction capability of any of the cytochrome P-450 enzymes, either those of humans or rodents. Since nitroaromatics account for a significant portion of the world's industrial chemical products and since many of them are genotoxic, it is timely and important to study metabolic activation of these compounds. Hopefully, these studies will eventually enhance our understanding of the human cytochrome P-450 and actylation polymorphisms.

Estabrook: A year ago I was invited to consult with a drug company who had great concern because one of the compounds, in which they had invested a large amount of money in developing, turned out to be a good inducer of what we call P-448, the aryl hydrocarbon hydroxylase form of cytochrome P-450. This company was going to terminate their further development of this drug on the basis that this drug may have potentially carcinogenic activity. I think those of us in the field are aware that you cannot simply classify P-450s as good P-450s and bad P-450s, and you simply can't categorize a compound on the basis of the type of P-450 that is induced. Unfortunately, I think that type of generalization is being accepted.

Weisburger: Dr. Fu, what are the actual levels of these nitro-PAHs that are found in the food supply? You can find them with HPLC, I'm sure, but what are the actual levels? How many mg/lb of food?

Fu: They are very low.

Weisburger: What is "very low?"

Fu: Well, I know they are too low, but the problem is that a significant portion of the industrial products in the world are nitrogen-containing compounds. Nitro-PAH is only one example.

Weisburger: However, you still didn't answer my question. How much is there per pound of food that I eat?

Fu: It depends on how the foods are cooked. A paper published in Japan indicated that toasted chicken contains nitrated pyrene.

Weisburger: I don't eat toasted chicken.

Beland: The quantities are very low in the μg/kg range. Nitro-PAHs are not particularly good inducers of cytochrome P-450. However, some of these compounds are quite potent carcinogens. For example, 6-nitro-chrysene and the dinitropyrenes induce tumors at very low levels.

Weisburger: If I am going to ingest it, has it been fed to animals and produced tumors?

Beland: Charles King has administered the dinitropyrenes intraperitoneally and subcutaneously and obtained mammary gland tumors.

Weisburger: However, people don't take it IP or subcutaneously; they would take it by ingestion. If we're going to look at risk assessment, let's look at a realistic model. It should be by ingestion.

Beland: Or by inhalation.

Fu: Last month I attended a meeting in D.C. where Dr. Ohnishi had a finding that was very interesting. It is that when rats were fed with pyrene and inhaled nitrogen dioxide, 1-nitropyrene was formed in the body.

Weisburger: That nitrated the pyrene, yes. These are all very interesting experiments, but you still have not answered my question. I'm sorry.

Lijinsky: Is there as much of these nitro compounds in food as there is methyl nitrosamine in beer?

Fu: They are present in similar quantities.

Estabrook: Dr. Poirier will speak now.

*   *   *

Poirier: I would like to make a couple of generalizations based on animal studies that people have done and then discuss DNA adduct dosimetry in the human population.

   As far as the animal models go, there are generally two different kinds of dosing. There is the situation where you give increasing amounts of compound in a single dose to different animals over a large dose range, and you generally get a curve that is a linear increase in adducts with increasing single-exposure doses.

   This kind of study has been done, for example, with benzo[a]pyrene, aflatoxin, NNK, and many compounds in a variety of different organs. Some studies have come out of Marshall Anderson's lab and Bruce

Dunn has done others. Many people have looked at benzo[a]pyrene-DNA adducts in mouse skin. The increase in adducts is linear over many doses. Basically, this kind of dosing simply reflects adduct formation; it doesn't reflect adduct removal.

On the other hand, if you want to model what is going on in human exposure, you really have to look at chronic dosing. The assumption is that you are continuously feeding or you're giving something in drinking water, so you get continuous carcinogen administration. What you get, then, in many different model systems is a situation where adduct concentrations reach a steady state. Adducts accumulate to a certain point until the adduct formation rates equal the adduct removal rates, and you get plateaus at a particular adduct levels. We have done these kinds of studies with chronic feeding of AAF, but they have also been done with feeding of aflatoxin and NNK.

More recently, Jim Swenberg published a very elegant study, in which he chronically fed a number of different doses. His study shows that a plateau will occur at a certain level of adducts based on the dose that the animal is being given chronically.

One of the things that one would like to do is extrapolate back to the dose that the animal has received. In the case of human exposure, you would take an adduct measurement and extrapolate back to what the person has received. You would also like to then predict tumors. I'm not going to deal with tumors as an end point today. Fred (Beland) will present tumor data in a study that we have done with mice.

What I am addressing right now are the following questions: Can you say from an adduct measurement that a person or an animal has been exposed? Yes, you can say they have been exposed. Can you say what the extent of the exposure has been? It depends. If you have a chronic exposure and you're not on the linear portion of the dose-response curve, there really isn't very much that you can do. Also, there are a lot of confounding factors when you are dealing with human samples. Since you don't have an inbred population, you can get differences in metabolism repair and other complications.

In the animal models, we are in a position to do DNA adduct measurements, we can do chronic dosing, we can do single dosing, we can look at the adducts, we can then later on look at tumors as an end point, and we can say something about what DNA adducts mean in this whole process of carcinogenesis.

The animal model system is obviously much better defined than the human system. So, over the past few years we have developed some immunoassays that are specific for carcinogen DNA adducts, and we have attempted to look in the human population. First of all, we wanted to know if we could measure adducts, because this was an uncertainty in the beginning, and, secondly, we wanted to explore the biological significance of adduct formation.

When we first started looking at adducts in human tissues, we were investigating benzo[a]pyrene. This study was in collaboration with Frederica Perera. We thought it would be interesting to look at the lungs of lung cancer patients and to see if we could measure benzo[a]pyrene DNA adducts. We did manage to find a few positive people, but we realized very early that we weren't able to validate the assay system because we had no dose-response. We didn't really know for sure to what doses these individuals had been exposed, and it was very difficult to obtain a nonexposed control.

So, we turned to a chemotherapeutic agent, cisplatin, which is known to damage DNA. It does so through the displacement of the chlorides, or, in the case of the analog carboplatin, you get binding to DNA through a hydrolysis of the ester linkages. Most of the adducts on DNA are the G-G or analogous A-G, bidentate intrastrand adducts. We have made antibodies to DNA that has the G-G and the A-G adducts, we have established immunoassays and used them to assay tissues of cancer patients.

The major advantage of this kind of system is the known dosages. These individuals are being treated at the NCI in the clinical center and are primarily patients with ovarian and testicular cancers. The people are followed for their lifetime, and it is easy to obtain unexposed controls. As controls, we have used tissues from individuals on other chemotherapy, individuals who have never been exposed to any chemotherapy, and tissues from some of the patients before they receive therapy. The controls are always negative.

In following these individuals for a long term we have been able to correlate a biological effect, a disease response, with adducts. I am really not going to go into detail on that. One of our goals is to produce some information for the clinician that would help in the management of the neoplastic disease.

The only data that I am going to present is dose-response. The way treatment is done at NCI for the platinum drugs, the individual receives five days of drug infusion, and then for three or four weeks they remain untreated. Subsequently, they go back and receive second, third, and fourth monthly cycles. This is kind of quasi-chronic exposure, if you will.

We took 97 blood samples from 77 individuals. We took approximately 50 ml of blood, centrifuged the blood, and separated out the buffy coat (nucleated blood cells) between the serum and the hemoglobin. We have extracted DNA and have measured this DNA by our immuno-assay.

We measured the increasing cumulative cisplatin dose occurring over a period of months in the one-month cycles that these people were undergoing. The adducts were measured from blood samples from testicular and ovarian cancer patients who had not received any prior therapy. It complicates the picture if the individuals have received prior therapy.

What we find is that only about half of the samples are positive. Half of the samples have adducts that are high enough for us to measure in this assay. If you do a linear regression, the correlation coefficient is about 0.85. On the other hand, for about half of the blood samples, we still are not able to find evidence of adduct formation, even when the doses are really quite high.

This has intrigued us as a possible heterogeneity in the human population. Cisplatin is a compound that is not supposed to undergo any sort of extensive metabolic activation. On the other hand, it is known that things like glutathione and sulfhydryl compounds can affect the drug efficacy. You can imagine that metallothionine also would perhaps play a part. Another possibility is that there may be a heterogeneity in the human population with respect to cisplatin repair. Some individuals may remove the adducts very rapidly, and others may remove them slowly.

To take the whole thing a step further than this, we find that there is a correlation between the individuals who do not form adducts and a lack of ability to respond to therapy. Conversely, the individuals who do respond, generally, have the highest adduct levels.

Mostly I wanted to explain to you the dose response for adduct formation in cancer patients, where the doses are known. Also, I wanted to mention the heterogeneity, where some individuals do not form adducts.

Singer: Are the samples five days after treatment?

Poirier: The treatment is for five days. We take the blood samples on the morning of day six. Based on some studies that the Dutch group has done, there is probably an early phase of repair that is actually finished by that time.

Enslein: If I understand you correctly, some of these measurements were taken on the same individuals at several points in time.

Poirier: No. We never really had more than two blood samples on the same individual. If the person was positive, both samples were generally positive.

Enslein: That's the problem, because that means there is serial correlation really, and your 0.85 is probably substantially lower. Your correlation is probably not as well as you think it is because you have multiple observations on the same individuals.

Cohn: I think data of this nature are very useful for risk assessment purposes. We are looking at high-to-low-dose extrapolation within humans themselves. You could take the steady-state levels that you have, correlate them with dose, and look for linearity or nonlinearities.

Poirier: Except that you have this heterogeneity.

Cohn: That's what makes it even more valuable, because now you can see the effect of heterogeneity on the dose response. I think you have utilized statistics to try to get a handle on that part of it, but if you get enough patients in there, I think you are going to be able to see a pattern that might be useful in high-to-low-dose extrapolation.

Barsotti: This may be very obvious, but did you in your population of testicular and ovarian cancer patients, separate the males and the females to see if there was any difference?

Poirier: Yes. For the disease response data, we have disease response on 55 ovarian patients and 17 testicular patients. The correlation with disease response holds very well for both. However, there are only 17 testicular patients, so, although there is a correlation, you can't calculate an impressive correlation coefficient.

Lijinsky: May I ask the mathematicians among us a question? This is related to Mimi's linear relation of adduct formation. Many years ago, I did an experiment in which I applied different doses of dibenzanthracene to mouse skin, and I got a linear tumor response with no plateau.

Recently, I did a dose-response study with nitrosomorpholine done over a very large range of dose, and, again, no plateau and a linear response. Now, how do you interpret this response in relation to a linear formation of adducts as the dose increases? I don't know enough mathematics to interpret this, but it is amazing that I got the same response for a single dose of a polycyclic hydrocarbon put on mouse skin and for chronic dosing of nitrosomorpholine.

Crump: Was there a background tumor response?

Lijinsky: The background tumor response was zero for—well, it was 1% in the case of nitrosomorpholine—liver tumors in Fischer rats. That goes up to 100%. The skin tumor incidence was zero.

Singer: I found a linear response with tumors but with a nonmetabolized carcinogen. That may be the difference.

Lijinsky: So you think it's the metabolism? The fact that this compound has to be metabolized doesn't affect the linearity. I'm trying to get a feel for why you have linearity in adduct formation, but nonlinearity in tumor response.

Singer: The difference is that ours are also tumors. Mimi's is DNA adducts.

Poirier: I'm only dealing with adducts.

Lijinsky: Yours are adducts. The tumors that you see, what I'm doing is laying the two alongside each other.

Poirier: I know. Fred will have some comments on this later. I think the bottom line is that adducts are a component, as has been said many times. They are necessary, but not sufficient. I think tissue-specific differences come into play, and species-specific differences are also important. Often you have adducts in tissues that never form a tumor. It's complex.

Lijinsky: It's the response measurements that intrigued me.

Travis: Willy, do you know that you're not getting increased cellular proliferation at that point? Are you turning on a toxic dose?

Lijinsky: No. The doses here ranged from 10–200 μm.

Hart: However, that's still not the point. The point is are you starting to get toxicity at the same point that you started to get increases in tumors?

Lijinsky: I don't know. We didn't look. This dibenzanthracene study was done 25 years ago.

Hart: Curtis has a very valid point, and I think Jim was trying to say the same thing. If you induce proliferation or cellular replacement, then you may be getting fixation of the damage that may change the effects. That's the question. Did you or did you not measure that end point?

Lijinsky: No, we did not measure the end point.

Pfitzer: Willy, I think the answer to your question, from a mathematician's standpoint, is that you are measuring two different things. You are measuring percent response, so you are seeing population distribution. Here we are measuring individual responses, which are linear. It simply is that you are taking individuals and expressing them as a percentage.

It's a standard either normal or log-normal distribution, which produces a nonlinear response.

Hart: We have a paucity of comparative data, and I don't know how we can make risk assessment analysis without it. We have had some elegant science presented, but we still haven't completely tackled the really difficult questions. Can we use pharmacokinetics and pharmacodynamics in making risk assessments? If so, what aspects of pharmacokinetics and pharmacodynamics can we use, and how can we do it better? We still are not addressing that question.

Estabrook: We have only asked part of the question. How do you use the data from animals to humans?

Cohn: We have used it for high-to-low-dose extrapolation but not for interspecies.

Hart: Exactly correct.

Molecular Biological Data

Human Carcinogens and DNA Modification: The First Step in Risk Assessment

B. SINGER
Donner Laboratory
Lawrence Berkeley Laboratory
University of California
Berkeley, California 94720

OVERVIEW

Carcinogens can be classified according to their site(s) of reaction with nucleosides or DNA and the biological consequences of reaction. Among those for which there is good evidence about in vivo products formed, repair enzymes, and effect of adducts on DNA structure, are the N-nitrosamines and N-nitrosoureas. The human carcinogen, vinyl chloride, is only now being studied at this level. In other instances, a compound which is found to be a carcinogen in animals, e.g., formaldehyde or acetaldehyde, has been long studied chemically, but no direct evidence has been obtained regarding reactions with DNA in vivo. Finally, there are carcinogens that apparently do not form covalent bonds to DNA but without doubt contribute to human cancer. These include asbestos and ethanol. The lack of any uniformity in the mode of action of the carcinogens to be discussed in this paper supports the concept that no single DNA adduct can be used as an indicator of exposure or risk.

INTRODUCTION

The first chemical evidence for an in vivo product resulting from a carcinogen was obtained by Magee and Farber in 1962. Radioactive-labeled dimethylnitrosamine, a liver carcinogen in rodents, formed radioactive 7-methylguanine in the target organ. In the 25 succeeding years, theory after theory was examined in an effort to equate mutagenesis and carcinogenesis with formation of specific derivatives.

One of the difficulties in attempting correlations was that initially the only alkylation products generally quantitated were 7-alkyl G and 3-alkyl A, since these could be depurinated at neutral pH. When Loveless (1969) suggested that O^6-alkyl G could be a mutagenic product, the analyses began to also include this derivative, since it could be depurinated in weak acid. This is not to say that it was not known that other alkylation sites included the N-1 and

Banbury Report 31: Carcinogen Risk Assessment: New Directions in the Qualitative and Quantitative Aspects © Cold Spring Harbor Laboratory. 0-87969-231-6/88. $1.00 + .00
   123

N-7 of A, the N-3 of G, and the N-3 of C. Nevertheless, they were considered "minor" products and were seldom analyzed for.

The finding that O^6-alkyl G was formed in DNA, and the apparent correlation of its presence with mutation in bacteria (Cairns 1980) was a turning point. Lindahl's laboratory isolated a new type of enzyme from bacteria that transferred the methyl group (and less efficiently the ethyl group) to the cysteine of an acceptor protein, termed O^6-methylguanine DNA methyltransferase (MT) (for review, see Lindahl 1982). Pegg et al. (1983) found the same type of enzyme in rat liver. These proteins were inactivated by the alkyl group. The MT was therefore termed a "suicide" enzyme and thus quantitation of the MT in various cells could predict the maximal amount of error-free repair of O^6-alkyl G in DNA (Pegg and Singer 1984; Yarosh 1985). Unrepaired O^6-alkyl G, when incorporated into synthetic polynucleotides, was found to act as G or A in in vitro transcription or replication (Mehta and Ludlum 1978; Snow et al. 1984). The ability to direct this changed incorporation represented a mutagenic event, and much work ensued in an effort to correlate the presence of O^6-alkyl G in a target organ with carcinogenesis.

When the pyrimidine oxygens were also found to react in vivo with the same simple alkylating agents, they were able to act as either pyrimidine, which also would be mutagenic, causing transitions as did O^6-alkyl G (Singer et al. 1978, 1979, 1981, 1983; Preston et al. 1986, 1987). However, few investigators were interested enough to use the more laborious procedures necessary to quantitate these acid- and alkali-labile products, notwithstanding the fact that they were not repaired efficiently in mammalian cells (Singer et al. 1981) and, thus, had a high potential to cause mutations. More recently, O^4-alkyl T has been found to be highly persistent in rat liver hepatocytes that, although capable of repairing O^6-alkyl G, become transformed (Swenberg et al. 1984; Dyroff et al. 1986).

Vinyl chloride differs completely from the N-nitroso compounds in its reaction and spectrum of products (Singer and Grunberger 1983). A new derivative, N^2,3-etheno G, not formed in vitro from guanosine by vinyl chloride metabolites, has now been found in vivo (Laib 1986) and is highly mutagenic, also causing transitions (Singer et al. 1987). The present interest in N^2,3-etheno G stems from the fact that this product can be formed also by other carcinogens, such as acrylonitrile and vinyl carbamate, and may represent a common mechanism of carcinogenesis for this group.

In the most recent work in this laboratory, we are employing the same approaches to study how ethanol and acetaldehyde cause their biological effects. We usually start by first looking at in vitro reactions with nucleosides using large amounts of material. When products are detected by UV or fluorescence, these are purified using various separation procedures and identified by mass spectrometry and nuclear magnetic resonance (NMR). If the products are sufficiently stable, deoxynucleoside triphosphates are synthesized and polymers prepared that are used as templates for replication with polymerases. Both changed base incorporation and structure can be determined. When feasible, site-directed mutation experiments are used that can confirm that a specific mutation occurs solely as a result of the single, incorporated modified base. It is, of course, essential to administer these chemical compounds to animals and search for carcinogen-derived products in the DNA. Finally, repair studies can be done both in vitro and in vivo and persistence in vivo can be determined. Such studies may indicate how a carcinogen initiates malignant transformation.

When metabolites are not completely known or when DNA structure plays a significant role, e.g., intercalation or cross-links, then preliminary experiments can utilize mammalian cells in culture, identifying possible products by sensitive methods, such as radioimmune assay, postlabeling techniques, isotope dilution, or fluorescence, when applicable.

RESULTS

Simple Alkylating Agents

The earliest and most studied class of mutagens and carcinogens are the monofunctional dialkyl sulfates, alkyl alkane sulfonates, dialkylnitrosamines, N-alkyl-N-nitrosoureas, and N-alkyl-N'-nitro-N-nitrosoguanidines (Fig. 1).

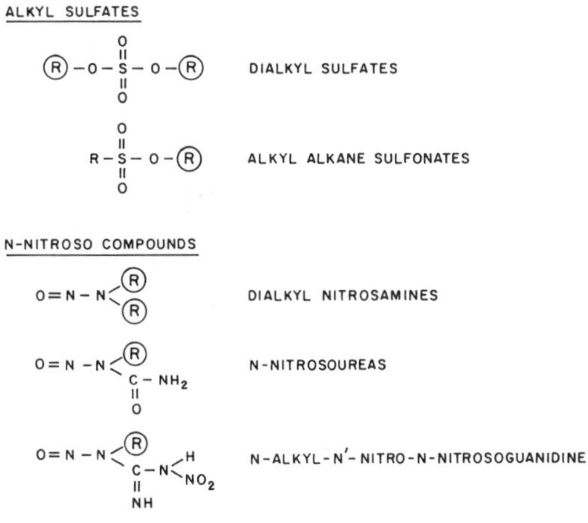

Figure 1

Structural formulas of representative simple aliphatic alkyl sulfates and N-nitroso compounds. R indicates the alkyl group.

Only the dialklynitrosamines require metabolic activation. The bifunctional sulfur and nitrogen mustards (Fig. 2) resemble dialkyl sulfates in their reactions, except that they can also form inter- and intrastrand cross-links through the N-7 of G.

The products of these compounds with nucleic acids have been studied in vitro and, for the N-nitroso compounds, in vivo as well. Although all oxygens and nitrogens are capable of reacting, the extent of reactions at each site is a function of the type of carcinogen and of the alkyl group. The dialkyl sulfates, alkylalkane sulfonates, and mustards react with double-stranded nucleic acids almost exclusively at the N-7 of G and the N-3 of A. Complete analyses are summarized in Singer and Grunberger (1983).

In contrast, the N-nitroso compounds react to a high extent with oxygens, but the proportion is a function of the alkyl group. Figure 3 shows both the sites of reaction and the initial proportion of total alkylation for several methylating and ethylating carcinogens in vivo. It should be noted that methylation of nucleic acids occurs primarily on nitrogens (80%), whereas ethylation occurs primarily on oxygens (80%).

The mutagenic effect of each derivative has been assayed by using various techniques. The N-3 alkyl purines are chemically very labile and become depurinated rapidly. In vivo there are glycosylases that also act to increase the formation of apurinic sites (Lindahl 1982), and are found to be occasional miscoding lesions (Loeb and Preston 1986). N-7 alkylguanine, the major product of methylation (70%) is per se not mutagenic (Ludlum 1970; Singer and Kuśmierek 1982), but the instability conferred by the quaternary structure leads to ring-opening of the imidazole ring as well as depurination. There are enzymes in bacteria or animal cells which either depurinate 7-alkyldeoxyguanosine (Laval et al. 1981; Margison and Pegg 1981; Singer and Brent 1981) or can excise the ring-opened product (Margison and Pegg 1981; Boiteux et al. 1984). The derivatives that are found most mutagenic and are, by implication, potential initiators of cancer are those which have an O-alkyl group: O^6-alkylguanine, O^4-alkylthymine, O^2-alkylcytosine, and O^2-alkylthymine. The first two have been extensively studied, and it appears that O^6-methylguanine (O^6-MeG) can be a causatory factor in carcinogenesis by methylating agents, whereas O^4-ethylthymine (O^4-EtT) may be the more important chemical event in carcinogenesis by ethylating agents (Pegg and

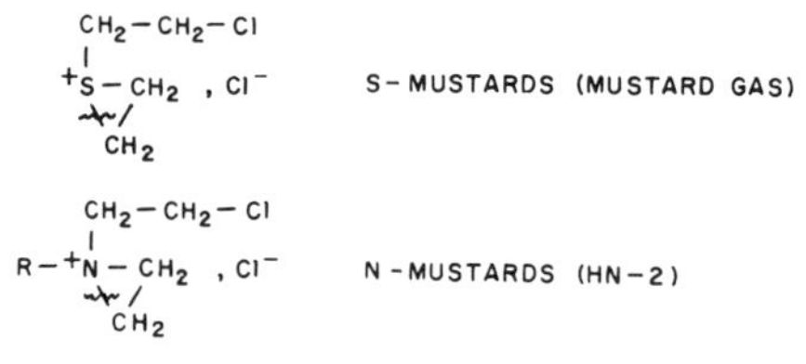

$$CH_2-CH_2-Cl$$
$$|$$
$$^+S-CH_2 \ , \ Cl^-$$
$$\overset{\curlywedge/}{CH_2}$$
S-MUSTARDS (MUSTARD GAS)

$$CH_2-CH_2-Cl$$
$$|$$
$$R-^+N-CH_2 \ , \ Cl^-$$
$$\overset{\curlywedge/}{CH_2}$$
N-MUSTARDS (HN-2)

Figure 2

Structural formulas of sulfur and nitrogen mustards. Note that they are cyclic compounds that are only activated when the unstable ring is opened, as shown by the wavy line.

INITIAL *IN VIVO* ALKYLATION

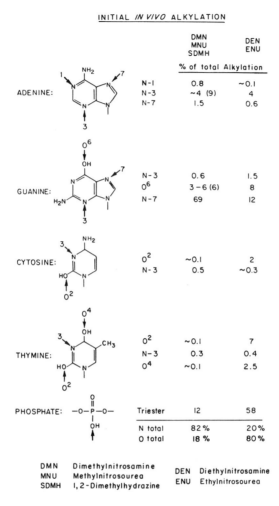

		DMN MNU SDMH	DEN ENU
		% of total Alkylation	
ADENINE:	N-1	0.8	~0.1
	N-3	~4 (9)	4
	N-7	1.5	0.6
GUANINE:	N-3	0.6	1.5
	O^6	3-6 (6)	8
	N-7	69	12
CYTOSINE:	O^2	~0.1	2
	N-3	0.5	~0.3
THYMINE:	O^2	~0.1	7
	N-3	0.3	0.4
	O^4	~0.1	2.5
PHOSPHATE:	Triester	12	58
	N total	82%	20%
	O total	18%	80%

DMN	Dimethylnitrosamine	DEN	Diethylnitrosamine
MNU	Methylnitrosourea	ENU	Ethylnitrosourea
SDMH	1,2-Dimethylhydrazine		

Figure 3
The arrows on the structural formulas indicate sites of modification of nucleic acids. The proportion of alkylation in vivo at each site is shown for both methylating and ethylating agents. The numbers in parentheses are expected alkylation, if no repair occurs. The initial time point (up to 5 hr) varies with the carcinogen.

Singer 1984). More information is needed on the other O-alkyl compounds, although their potential mutagenicity has been established (Singer 1986).

The relative importance of O^6G or O^4T alkylation in carcinogenesis is complicated by the fact that O^6-alkylguanine is, as stated above, repaired by an enzyme (MT) that transfers the alkyl group to a cysteine and inactivates the enzyme. In bacteria, this same enzyme can also dealkylate O^4-alkyl thymine (Ahmed and Laval 1984; McCarthy et al. 1984). However, the analogous mammalian enzyme does not act on O^4-alkylthymine (Dolan et al. 1984), nor has any enzyme been found in eukaryotes capable of removing/ repairing this derivative (Brent et al. 1988). Furthermore, the amount of the O^6-alkylguanine-DNA methyltransferase in specific species and in different cells vary by orders of magnitude (Domoradzki et al. 1984; Pegg 1984), so that in some cells O^6-MeG is repaired almost instantly and in others not detectably. Thus, the relative proportions of O^6-alkylguanine and O^4-alkyl- thymine (Fig. 3), over a time period, can be found to change more than 50-fold, in favor of O^4-alkyl T, when the former is repaired and the latter accumulates (Swenberg et al. 1984).

O^6-MeG, O^4-methylthymine (O^4-MeT), O^4-EtT, and O^4-isopropylthy- mine have been site-specifically incorporated into phage DNA and evidence for specific changed base pairing obtained by sequencing of progeny DNA from mutants (Loechler 1984; Preston et al. 1986, 1987). Although each can act as the unmodified base, in each case, mutations resulted from transitions.

Physical studies on the structures of $m^6G \cdot C$, $m^6G \cdot T$, $m^4T \cdot A$, and $m^4T \cdot G$, using oligonucleotides, indicate that there is helix distortion and weakened hydrogen bonding for all these pairings (Gaffney et al. 1984; Kalnik et al. 1988a,b). Nevertheless, in DNA replicated in vivo such bonds can occur, perhaps stabilized by stacking or flanking sequences. Hot spots, or sequences found to be highly mutable, have been reported for both m^6G and m^4T mutations (Richardson et al. 1987). This latter fact may reflect structural impediments in enzymatic repair.

Vinyl Halides

In the case of vinyl chloride, the most studied of this class, in vitro products from reaction of the stable metabolite, chloroacetaldehyde, with nucleosides or bases were identified and studied in detail long before there was interest in the biological consequences (for review, see Leonard 1984). The metabolic pathway is shown in Figure 4 and the products identified in liver RNA or DNA after vinyl chloride administration to rodents are shown in Figure 5.

The first metabolite, chloroethylene oxide, is rapidly rearranged ($t_{1/2} \approx 8.5$ seconds) to chloroacetaldehyde. Nevertheless, it was shown in vitro and in vivo that this metabolite alkylated the N-7 of G (Laib et al. 1981; Scherer et al. 1981). A simple epoxide should also alkylate the same sites as any alkylating agent (see Fig. 3), but only 7-(2-oxoethyl)G has been identified.

The stable metabolite, chloroacetaldehyde, forms cyclic etheno products between the amino group and an adjacent endo nitrogen. There is also good evidence that this bifunctional aldehyde forms cross-links in DNA (Singer et al. 1986). Vinyl chloride is a gas at room temperature, so that almost all in

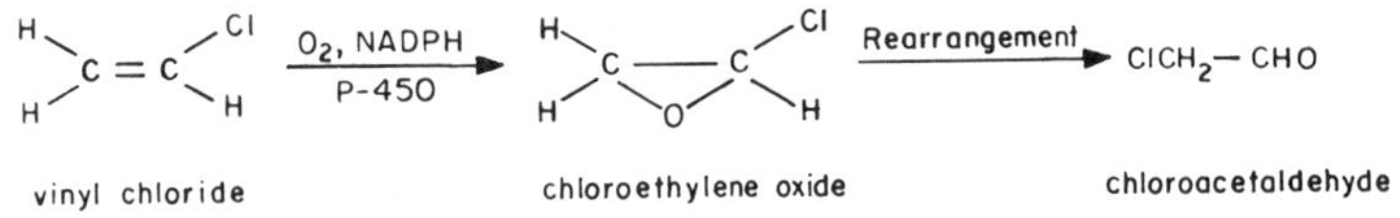

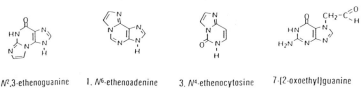

(structures: vinyl chloride → chloroethylene oxide → chloroacetaldehyde, with O$_2$, NADPH, P-450 and Rearrangement arrows)

Figure 4
Postulated mechanisms for the metabolism of vinyl chloride (adapted from Zajdela et al. 1980). The same mechanism occurs for vinyl bromide metabolism. Acrylonitrile is activated by epoxidation to 2-cyanoethylene oxide by the same pathway (Guengerich et al. 1986). (Reprinted, with permission, from Singer and Grunberger 1983.)

vivo studies have used inhalation as the mode of administration to rats or mice. Under conditions leading to angiosarcomas, the primary type of tumor in humans exposed to vinyl chloride (Creech and Johnson 1974), the expected etheno products were not observed in DNA by the detection methods used. This is not unexpected since 1,N^6-etheno A, 3,N^4-etheno C, and 1, N^2-etheno G cannot be formed in a double-stranded nucleic acid where one of the positions necessary for cyclization is blocked (Kuśmierek and Singer 1982). However, presumably due to small single-stranded regions (or thermal denaturation), etheno compounds were detected in DNA reacted in vitro with chloroacetaldehyde (Bedell et al. 1986). Most recently, N^2,3-etheno G was also found in vivo (Laib 1986). This latter compound does not form from guanosine or guanine unless the O^6 is substituted to direct ring closure to the N-3, rather than the N-1. Kuśmierek et al. (1987) have now synthesized the nucleoside and its triphosphate which has enabled us to synthesize polynucleotides for mutagenesis studies.

N^2,3-etheno G was thus found to pair with either C or T (Singer et al. 1987). The formation of N^2,3-etheno G·T pairs represents the only mutagenic event found to date to result from chloroacetaldehyde reaction. The ratio of C/T incorporation in the complementary chain is 4/1, which is similar to the extent of changed incorporation directed by O^6-methyl G. N^2,3-etheno G is likely to be involved in initiation of vinyl halide carcinogenesis, since it has been shown to form in a double-stranded structure.

N^2,3-ethenoguanine   1. N^6-ethenoadenine   3. N^4-ethenocytosine   7-[2-oxoethyl]guanine

Figure 5
Vinyl chloride products found in vivo in RNA or DNA (to date). All structures are shown as bases. Not shown is the in vitro product of guanosine with chloroacetaldehyde, 1,N^2-ethenoguanine, which has not been reported as a product in vivo.

In contrast to many other modifications, N^2,3-etheno G can form two hydrogen bonds with either C or T, which closely resemble the wobble base pair (Fig. 6). This feature makes it likely that enzymatic repair will not occur. So far, there have not been long term studies following this adduct.

Acetaldehyde and Ethanol

These two carcinogens, although not classified as strong carcinogens (Peto 1985; Ames et al. 1987 and references therein), become of importance in human risk because of the widespread use of ethanol which is metabolized to acetaldehyde by alcohol dehydrogenase (with the cofactor nicotinamide adenine dinucleotide). In addition, acetaldehyde results from many metabolic and other oxidative processes, including baking of bread.

We have recently found that stable adducts on the amino groups of nucleosides result only when both compounds are present. Acetaldehyde, like formaldehyde (Fraenkel-Conrat 1954), is known to add reversibly to amino groups in aqueous solution at ambient temperature. The resulting alkylol groups (-NH-CHR-OH) are known to be highly reactive (Fraenkel-Conrat and Olcott 1948) and become stabilized by secondary condensation reactions. We now find that this type of compound, formed at the exocyclic group of nucleosides and acetaldehyde (R= $-$ CH$_3$), reacts readily with alcohols, also

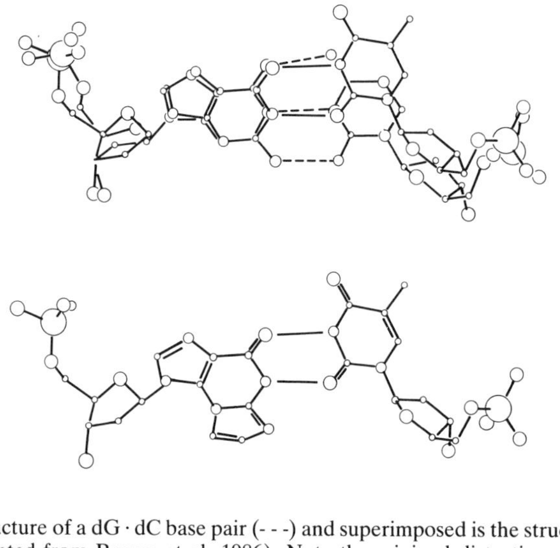

Figure 6

(*Top*) Crystal structure of a dG · dC base pair (- - -) and superimposed is the structure of a dG · dT wobble pair (adapted from Brown et al. 1986). Note the minimal distortion of a wobble pair. (*Bottom*) Drawing of possible structure of N^2,3-etheno dG with dT. This pair is identical to the dG · dT pair above.

at ambient temperature. Mass spectra and NMR indicate the resulting product with ethanol to be:

base-NH-CH(CH$_3$)-O-C$_2$H$_5$

The reaction is understandably favored by high concentrations of alcohol and high yields of products are obtained.

In neutral aqueous solution containing low amounts of acetaldehyde and ethanol, deoxycytidine is modified almost instantly, forming N^4-ethoxyethyldeoxycytidine (Fraenkel-Conrat and Singer 1988). The level of reaction, although limited, rapidly reaches a steady state due to competitive hydrolysis with water. Studies on mutagenicity and formation in DNA are in progress.

DISCUSSION

The three types of carcinogen interaction with models and DNA that are discussed illustrate why it is difficult or impossible to predict the mechanism by which chemicals initiate carcinogenesis. Whereas simple alkylating agents react with DNA predictably, repair processes are unique to cell type and adduct. Although there is a considerable literature on enzymatic repair in bacteria, parallel enzymes or mechanisms do not always exist, qualitatively or quantitatively, in animal cells. What can be termed a "minor" adduct, e.g., O^4-methyl T, is not repaired rapidly or efficiently in rat liver hepatocytes after dimethylnitrosamine or 1,2-dimethylhydrazine administration, whereas these cells are highly competent to repair O^6-methyl G. Both derivatives are miscoding lesions, yet in this specific case, the increased level of O^4-methyl T makes it a probable initiator of hepatocellular carcinogenesis. "Probable" is used because other promutagenic derivatives have not been quantitated in the same way. Similarly, in ethylnitrosourea-induced brain tumors in susceptible rats, the brain cells lack the ability to repair O^4-ethyl T and also repair other O-ethylpyrimidines poorly.

Numerous examples can be given indicating that metabolism, species, mode of carcinogen administration, cell type, and replication influence the organ specificity of each carcinogen. The situation with vinyl chloride carcinogenesis is somewhat different. The compound has been known as a human carcinogen for many years but only in 1985 was a potential initiator found in vivo. The amount of N^2,3-etheno G, under a carcinogenic regimen in rats, is reported to be 0.25 moles/10^6 moles G. Is this minor? Or can a single modified base/10^7 nucleotides be the biologically significant event? If so, methodologies must be far more sensitive to identify other, yet unknown products, particularly when they are not found in the usual model experiments.

Finally, no mechanism exists for alcohol carcinogenesis. We suggest that this is an unusual case in which the ingested chemical, ethanol, must react together with its metabolite, acetaldehyde, to form a nucleic acid derivative.

Virtually all nucleic acid modifications perturbate DNA structure and may inhibit replication or cause errors that are termed mutations. So far the implications of helix distortion, handedness, or changes in stacking interactions have not generally been considered in carcinogenesis. Advances in biology, chemistry, and biophysics should be correlated in order to obtain a more balanced picture of carcinogen action.

Risk is, at a minimum, a composite of genetic susceptibility, exposure, metabolism, chemical reaction, target organ or cell type, repair, and expression. Given that only a few cells ever become foci of transformation, the presence of a metabolite or reaction product in urine or blood is not likely to measure target-specific risk but only exposure. This returns to the question of whether formation and excretion of any single derivative can be useful in risk assessment for carcinogens, inasmuch as this type of analysis does not give information whether the critical derivative exists in an essential transcribed or regulatory gene.

ACKNOWLEDGMENTS

This work was supported by grants CA-12316 and CA-42736 from the National Institutes of Health, Bethesda, Maryland. The author gratefully acknowledges the helpful discussions and critical reading of the manuscript by S.J. Spengler and H. Fraenkel-Conrat.

REFERENCES

Ahmed, Z. and J. Laval. 1984. Enzymatic repair of O-alkylated thymidine residues in DNA: Involvement of a O^4-methyl-thymine-DNA methyltransferase and a O^2-methylthymine-DNA glycosylase. *Biochem. Biophys. Res. Commun.* **120**: 1.

Ames, B.N., R. Magaw, and L.S. Gold. 1987. Ranking possible carcinogenic hazards. *Science* **236**: 271.

Bedell, M.A., M.C. Dyroff, G. Doerjer, and J.A. Swenberg. 1986. Quantitatiton of etheno adducts by fluorescence detection. *IARC Sci. Publ.* **70**: 425.

Boiteux, S., J. Belleney, B.P. Rogues, and J. Laval. 1984. Two rotameric forms of open ring 7-methylguanine are present in alkylated polynucleotides. *Nucleic Acids Res.* **12**: 5430.

Brent, T.P., M.E. Dolan, H. Fraenkel-Conrat, J. Hall, P. Karran, F. Laval, G.P. Margison, R. Montesano, A.E. Pegg, P.M. Potter, B. Singer, J.A. Swenberg, and

D.B. Yarosh. 1988. Repair of O-alkylpyrimidines in mammalian cells: A present consensus. *Proc. Natl. Acad. Sci.* **85:** 1759.

Brown, T., W.N. Hunter, G. Kneale, and O. Kennard. 1986. Molecular structure of the G · A basepair in DNA and implications for the mechanism of transversion mutations. *Proc. Natl. Acad. Sci.* **83:** 2402.

Cairns, J. 1980. Efficiency of the adaptive response of Escherichia coli to alkylating agents. *Nature* **286:** 176.

Creech, J.L. and M.N. Johnson. 1974. Angiosarcoma of the liver in the manufacture of polyvinyl chloride. *J. Occup. Med.* **16:** 150.

Dolan, M.E., D. Scicchitano, B. Singer, and A.E. Pegg. 1984. Comparison of repair of methylated pyrimidines in poly(dT) by extract from rat liver and *Escherichia coli.* *Biochem. Biophys. Res. Commun.* **123:** 324.

Domoradzki, J., A.E. Pegg, M.E. Dolan, V.M. Maher, and J.J. McCormick. 1984. Correlations between O^6-methylguanine-DNA methyltransferase activity and resistance of human cells to the cytotoxic and mutagenic effect of N-methyl-N'-nitro-N-nitrosoguanidine. *Carcinogenesis* **5:** 1641.

Dyroff, M.C., F.C. Richardson, J.A. Popp, M.A. Bedell, and J.A. Swenberg. 1986. Correlation of O^4-ethyldeoxythymidine accumulation, hepatic initiation and hepatocellular carcinoma in rats continuously administered diethylnitrosamine. *Carcinogenesis* **7:** 241.

Fraenkel-Conrat, H. 1954. Reaction of nucleic acid with formaldehyde. *Biochim. Biophys. Acta* **15:** 307.

Fraenkel-Conrat, H. and H.S. Olcott. 1948. The reaction of formaldehyde with proteins. V. Crosslinking between amino and primary amide or guanidyl groups. *J. Am. Chem. Soc.* **70:** 2673.

Fraenkel-Conrat, H. and B. Singer. 1988. Nucleoside adducts are formed by cooperative reaction of acetaldehyde and alcohols: A possible mechanism for ethanol's role in carcinogenesis. *Proc. Natl. Acad. Sci.* (in press).

Gaffney, B.L., L.A. Marky, and R.A. Jones. 1984. Synthesis and characterization of a set of four dodecadeoxyribonucleoside undecaphosphates containing O^6-methylguanine opposite adenine, cystosine, guanine, and thymine. *Biochemistry* **23:** 5686.

Guengerich, F.P., L.L. Hogy, P.B. Inskeep, and D.C. Liebler. 1986. Metabolism and covalent binding of *vic*-dihaloalkanes, vinyl halides and acrylonitrile. *IARC Sci. Publ.* **70:** 255.

Kalnik, M.W., M. Kouchakdjian, B.F. Li, P.F. Swann, and D.J. Patel. 1988a. Base pair mismatches and carcinogen-modified bases in DNA: An nmr study of G · T and G · O⁴meT pairing in dodecanucleotide duplexes. *Biochemistry* **27:** 108.

———. 1988b. Base pair mismatches and carcinogen-modified bases in DNA: An nmr study of A · C and A · O⁴meT pairing in dodecanucleotide duplexes. *Biochemistry* **27:** 100.

Kuśmierek, J.T. and B. Singer. 1982. Chloroacetaldehyde-treated ribo- and deoxyribopolynucleotides. 1. Reaction products. *Biochemistry* **21:** 5717.

Kuśmierek, J.T., D.E. Jensen, S.J. Spengler, R. Stolarski, and B. Singer. 1987. Synthesis and properties of N^2,3-ethenoguanosine and N^2,3-ethenoguanosine 5'-diphosphate. *J. Org. Chem.* **52:** 2374.

Laib, R.J. 1986. The role of cyclic base adducts in vinyl chloride-induced carcinogenesis: Studies on nucleic acid alkylation *in vivo*. *IARC Sci. Publ.* **70:** 101.

Laib, R.J., L.M. Gwinner, and H.M. Bolt. 1981. DNA alkylation by vinyl chloride metabolites: Etheno derivatives or 7-alkylation of guanine? *Chem.-Biol. Interact.* **37:** 219.

Laval, J., J. Pierre, and F. Laval. 1981. Release of 7-methylguanine residues from alkylated DNA by extracts of *Micrococcus luteus* and *Escherichia coli*. *Proc. Natl. Acad. Sci.* **78:** 852.

Leonard, N.J. 1984. Etheno-substituted nucleotides and coenzymes: Fluorescence and biological activity. *CRC Crit. Rev. Biochem.* **15:** 125.

Lindahl, T. 1982. DNA repair enzymes. *Annu. Rev. Biochem.* **51:** 61.

Loeb, L.A. and B.D. Preston. 1986. Mutagenesis by apurinic/apyrimidinic sites. *Annu. Rev. Genet.* **20:** 201.

Loechler, E.L., C.L. Green, and J.M. Essigmann. 1984. *In vivo* mutagenesis by O^6-methylguanine built into a unique site in a viral genome. *Proc. Natl. Acad. Sci.* **81:** 6271.

Loveless, A. 1969. Possible relevance of O-6 alkylation of deoxyguanosine to the mutagenicity and carcinogenicity of nitrosamines and nitrosamides. *Nature* **223:** 206.

Ludlum, D.B. 1970. The properties of 7-methylguanine-containing templates for ribonucleic acid polymerase. *J. Biol. Chem.* **245:** 477.

Magee, P.N. and E. Farber. 1962. Toxic liver injury and carcinogenesis. Methylation of rat-liver nucleic acids by dimethylnitrosamine *in vivo*. *Biochem. J.* **83:** 114.

Margison, G.P. and A.E. Pegg. 1981. Enzymatic release of 7-methylguanine from methylated DNA by rodent liver extracts. *Proc. Natl. Acad. Sci.* **78:** 861.

McCarthy, T., P. Karran, and T. Lindahl. 1984. Inducible repair of O-alkylated DNA pyrimidines in *Escherichia coli*. *EMBO J.* **3:** 545.

Mehta, J.R. and D.B. Ludlum. 1978. Synthesis and properties of O^6-methyldeoxyguanylic acid and its copolymers with deoxycytidylic acid. *Biochim. Biophys. Acta* **521:** 770.

Pegg, A.E. 1984. Properties of the O^6-alkylguanine-DNA repair system of mammalian cells. *IARC Sci. Publ.* **57:** 575.

Pegg, A.E. and B. Singer. 1984. Is O^6-alkylguanine necessary for initiation of carcinogenesis by alkylating agents? *Cancer Invest.* **2(3):** 221.

Pegg, A.E., L. Wiest, R.S. Foote, S. Mitra, and W. Perry. 1983. Purification and properties of O^6-methylguanine-DNA transmethylase from rat liver. *J. Biol. Chem.* **258:** 2327.

Peto, R. 1985. Epidemiological reservations about risk assessment. In *Assessment of risk from low level exposure to radiation and chemicals* (ed. A.D. Woodhead et al.), p. 3. Plenum Press, New York.

Preston, B.D., B. Singer, and L.A. Loeb. 1986. Mutagenic potential of O^4-methylthymine *in vivo* determined by an enzymatic approach to site-specific mutagenesis. *Proc. Natl. Acad. Sci.* **84:** 8501.

———. 1987. Comparison of the relative mutagenicities of O-alkylthymines site-specifically incorporated into ϕX174 DNA. *J. Biol. Chem.* **262:** 13821.

Richardson, K.K., F.C. Richardson, R.M. Crosby, J.A. Swenberg, and T.R. Skopek.

1987. DNA base changes and alkylation following *in vivo* exposure of *Escherichia coli* to N-methyl-N-nitrosourea or N-ethyl-N-nitrosourea. *Proc. Natl. Acad. Sci.* **84:** 344.

Scherer, E., C.J. Van der Laken, L.M. Gwinner, R.J. Laib, and P. Emmelot. 1981. Modification of deoxyguanosine by chloroethylene oxide. *Carcinogenesis* **2:** 671.

Singer, B. 1986. O-Alkyl pyrimidines in mutagenesis and carcinogenesis: Occurrence and significance. *Cancer Res.* **46:** 4879.

Singer, B. and T.P. Brent. 1981. Human lymphoblasts contain DNA glycosylase activity excising N-3 and N-7 methyl and ethyl purines but not O^6-alkylguanines or 1-alkyladenines. *Proc. Natl. Acad. Sci.* **78:** 856.

Singer, B. and D. Grunberger. 1983. *Molecular biology of mutagens and carcinogens.* Plenum Press, New York.

Singer, B. and J.T. Kuśmierek. 1982. Chemical mutagenesis. *Annu. Rev. Biochem.* **52:** 655.

Singer, B., R.G. Pergolizzi, and D. Grunberger. 1979. Synthesis and coding properties of dinucleoside diphosphates containing alkyl pyrimidines which are formed by the action of carcinogens on nucleic acids. *Nucleic Acids Res.* **6:** 1709.

Singer, B., J. Sagi, and J.T. Kuśmierek. 1983. *Escherichia coli* polymerase I can use O^2-methyldeoxythymidine or O^4-methyldeoxythymidine in place of deoxythymidine in primed poly(dA-dT)·poly (dA-dT) synthesis. *Proc. Natl. Acad. Sci.* **80:** 4884.

Singer, B., S. Spengler, and W.J. Bodell. 1981. Tissue-dependent enzyme-mediated repair or removal of O-ethylpyrimidines and ethyl purines in carcinogen-treated rats. *Carcinogenesis* **2:** 1069.

Singer, B., S.R. Holbrook, H. Fraenkel-Conrat, and J.T. Kuśmierek. 1986. Neutral reactions of haloacetaldehydes with polynucleotides: Mechanisms, monomer and polymer products. *IARC Sci. Publ.* **70:** 45.

Singer, B., S.J. Spengler, F. Chavez, and J.T. Kuśmierek. 1987. The vinyl chloride-derived nucleoside, N^2,3-ethenoguanosine, is a highly efficient mutagen in transcription. *Carcinogenesis* **8:** 745.

Singer, B., W.J. Bodell, J.E. Cleaver, G.H. Thomas, M.F. Rajewsky, and W. Thon. 1978. Oxygens in DNA are main targets for ethylnitrosourea in normal and Xeroderma pigmentosum fibroblasts and fetal rat brain cells. *Nature* **276:** 85.

Snow, E.T., R.S. Foote, and S. Mitra. 1984. Kinetics of incorporation of O^6-methyldeoxyguanine and monophosphate during *in vitro* DNA synthesis. *Biochemistry* **23:** 4289.

Swenberg, J.A., M.C. Dyroff, M.A. Bedell, J.A. Popp, N. Huh, U. Kirstein, and M.F. Rajewsky. 1984. O^4-Ethyldeoxythymidine, but not O^6-ethyldeoxyguanosine, accumulates in hepatocyte DNA of rats exposed continuously to diethylnitrosamine. *Proc. Natl. Acad. Sci.* **81:** 1692.

Yarosh, D.B. 1985. The role of O^6-methylguanine-DNA methyltransferase in cell survival, mutagenesis and carcinogenesis. *Mutat. Res.* **145:** 1.

Zajdela, F., A. Croisy, A. Barbin, C. Malaveille, L. Tomatis, and H. Bartsch. 1980. Carcinogenicity of chloroethylene oxide, an ultimate reactive metabolite of vinyl chloride, and bis(chloromethyl)ether after subcutaneous administration and in initiation-promotion experiments in mice. *Cancer Res.* **40:** 352.

COMMENTS

Beland: Why doesn't O^6 methyl-G transferase work with O^4-methyl-thymine?

Singer: In *Escherichia coli*, the enzyme that repairs O^6-alkyl G does work on the O-alkyl pyrimidines, but that is not the case for enzymes isolated from mammalian cells. In a paper to be published in *PNAS* called "Repair of O-alkyl Pyrimidines in Mammalian Cells - A Present Concensus," this subject is discussed. These facts have now been so well documented that the paper has 14 authors from 10 institutions.

Setlow: That wasn't really an answer to the question. He asked why.

Singer: The O-alkyl pyrimidines are repaired in vivo, but presumbly by different enzymatic mechanisms.

Beland: You said Jim Swenberg is getting increasing levels of O^4-methyl-thymine.

Singer: Those experiments use continuous dosage and measure steady state. However, the half-lives have been determined in single dose experiments. For m^4T Swenberg finds a $t_{1/2}$ of 20 hours, and for e^4T, 11 weeks. This cannot be a result of dilution or synthesis of DNA. It is repair. Generally, ethylated products are repaired more slowly than methylated. Regarding orientation of the alkyl group, I could talk about antibody recognition also. Only half of the O^4T's are recognized by specific antibodies in a polymer, so that can be interpreted to mean that half of them have the alkyl group in the groove and half of them have the alkyl group in the opposite direction. It's hard to say what groove the alkyl group is in when half of them are orientated in one direction and half of them in the other.

Michejda: I think this whole discussion of repair has been focusing on only part of the repair process, particularly on the alkyl transferase. Chances are there are many other repair systems waiting to be discovered. Most recently, the excision repair of O^6-alkyl groups is larger than methyl has been suggested.

Singer: In mammalian cells?

Michejda: Yes, in mammalian cells.

Singer: They are just different pathways, and we have not yet elucidated the pathways. Is that simple? If you keep looking at the same enzyme, you are not going to find anything different than anybody else. People have to start with a fresh approach.

Hoerger: Bea, would you comment on the significance of the metabolites of vinyl chloride cross-linking, perhaps from the standpoint of dose response?

SINGER: I can't comment on dose response since we work in vitro and thus have not done dose response. However, we know the conditions it takes to form one cross-link per 50 bp. Generally, cross-links in vivo are found at very, very low levels. In all the cross-links that I know about, the alkylation-induced cross-links, with nitrogen mustards and similar agents that are used chemotherapeutically, all occur at extremely low levels: 1 in 10^4 bases, 1 in 10^5, something like that. We cannot look at 1 in 10^4 or 10^5 in our in vitro polymeric systems. We need to produce higher levels. However, there is definitely a dose response.

Hart: Could we go back to the alcohol work your laboratory has done?

Singer: The day or night alcohol?

Hart: Could we go back to the form of damage induced and any additional information you have on that?

Singer: On the basis of other work that we have done, work that doesn't give us the same derivative but very similar derivatives, this new type of base modification indicates that the new class of compounds turn out to be mutagenic.

Hart: How have you tested that?

Singer: We haven't yet, since this work is still in early stages. The first paper, now in preparation, is on characterization of these derivatives.

Hart: What would you expect the repair capability to be, based upon what you would project to be the frequency of reduction of this type of damage at the doses that you discussed? Would you expect a fairly high repair capability for derivatives modified on exocyclic amino groups?

Singer: No. These kinds of derivatives apparently are not repaired according to Celina Janion who has looked for repair of N^4-hydroxy C in *E. coli*. I find it very interesting that an ingested normal chemical has to react with its metabolite to modify nucleic acids. Neither of the chemicals (CH_3CHO and C_2H_5-OH) has unequivocaly been shown to be a carcinogen. There is evidence for sister chromatid exchange resulting from alcohol. Acetaldehyde, over a long period of inhalation, can produce nasal tumors in rats. We show that this cooperative reaction occurs at low levels of reagents not yet studied in vivo, you understand, but we still find the products, and they appear stable. We have followed reaction now for 24 hours, and that's a long time for something that you would expect to reverse in water.

Hart: Alcohol has, indeed, been called a carcinogen.

Singer: It has been called a carcinogen, but nobody has found covalent binding, have they?

Hart: No, not to my knowledge.

Singer: You see, that's the point.

Weisburger: There was an article in *Cancer Research* in 1979 where Tuyns ascribed as much as 8% of human cancers to alcohol.

Singer: I'll bet that such data have about as much effect on drinking habits as saying that smoking is bad. With that, I will leave.

Setlow: Can I summarize by saying you should dilute your alcohol when you drink it, that bourbon and water is better?

Singer: I'm sure it's better.

Nongenotoxic Mechanisms in Carcinogenesis: Role of Inhibited Intercellular Communication

JAMES EDWARD TROSKO AND CHIA-CHENG CHANG
Department of Pediatrics/Human Development
Center for Environmental Toxicology
Michigan State University
College of Human Medicine
East Lansing, Michigan 48824

OVERVIEW

Carcinogenesis is a multistep process, involving several distinct mechanisms, involving the conversion of a normal stem-like cell to a cell resistant to terminal differentiation (i.e., initiation), followed by the clonal expansion of this initiated cell (i.e., promotion), during which time additional changes occur allowing the cell to become malignant (i.e., progression). Each of these distinct operational stages of carcinogenesis probably involves several mechanisms (i.e., many mechanisms for initiation and promotion).

The assessment of risk from exposure to radiation and chemicals is hindered by the basic lack of scientific knowledge concerning the complex nature of the multiple levels of interactions between the chemicals and biological organism. Since gene and chromosomal mutations, cell death, and modulation of gene expression are the biological consequences of chemical exposure, many genetic, biological, and environmental factors can modulate how a given chemical can induce these changes. In addition, complicating the risk assessment process are the inadequacies of the bioassay systems and the limitations of in vitro short-term tests to assess the "carcinogenicity" of various chemicals. The general paradigm of "carcinogenesis as mutagens" is considered totally inadequate to design the test protocol for animal bioassays and to interpret the data from these tests.

The role of inhibited intercellular communication has been postulated to play a role in the tumor promotion and progression phases. Examination of experimental results of known tumor promoters as inhibitors of intercellular communication is presented. Implications of these results suggest a new paradigm is needed to approach the problem of a "biological risk assessment" model. "Science progresses more by the introduction of new world views or 'pictures' than by the steady accumulation of information." (Eldredge and Gould 1972)

Banbury Report 31: Carcinogen Risk Assessment: New Directions in the Qualitative and Quantitative Aspects © Cold Spring Harbor Laboratory. 0-87969-231-6/88. $1.00 + .00

INTRODUCTION

Mutagenesis Is Carcinogenesis: A Failed Paradigm

Raw observations in science must be interpreted to be understood. In all scientific disciplines, the prevailing paradigm helps the scientific community to interpret the results of experiments. In cancer research, the paradigms, "carcinogens are mutagens" (Ames et al. 1973) and "genotoxicity" (Ehrenberg et al. 1973) have shaped most of the present thinking in the area of understanding the mechanism(s) of carcinogenesis and the practical issue of risk assessment to human beings to cancer after exposure to radiation and chemical agents. Although we wish to make it clear we feel mutagenesis does play a significant role in carcinogenesis, as is evident from genetic predispositions to human cancer (Trosko et al. 1985) and from all the evidence that mutagens and mutations found in experimental studies on mammalian and human cells (somatic mutation theory of cancer; see [Trosko and Chang 1978]), we must emphasize that carcinogenesis is more than mutagenesis. These are two independent and nonequivalent biological processes, one taking place in an organism (the former), whereas the other takes place within a single cell.

The multistep nature of the cancer process has been noted, both in experimental animals and in the normal clinical course of tumor development in human beings (Foulds 1975; Nowell 1976; Cairns 1981). Conceptually, the initiation, promotion, and progression stages have been developed to explain the multistep nature of carcinogenesis (Boutwell 1974; Pitot et al. 1981). Clearly, these operational concepts on the whole animal level do not imply any specific mechanism, nor is it yet known what the mechanism(s) is (are) that underlie each of these steps. However, one thing appears perfectly clear, initiation and promotion are two distinct processes, and, therefore, the underlying cellular and molecular mechanisms must be different (Trosko et al. 1983a). Several working hypotheses have been advanced, suggesting that initiation, an irreversible process, involves a mutagenic event, promotion involves a mitogenic event (Trosko and Chang 1983), whereas progression might involve another event, possibly requiring either another mutagenic hit (Trosko and Chang 1980; Potter 1981; Trosko and Chang 1986) and/or another epigenetic process (Frost and Kerbel 1983). Therefore, the objective of this report is to suggest that biological data, related to the multistep carcinogenic process, must be incorporated into any risk assessment process and that the current paradigm shaping the design of the bioassay and of short-term assays for carcinogen testing must be challenged to include the nongenotoxic properties of chemicals that could influence the ultimate appearance of cancers in humans (Trosko and Chang 1985).

RESULTS

Limitations of Current Bioassay and Short-term Assays to Detect Carcinogens

In several recent evaluations of the predictability of chemical carcinogenicity in rodents from in vitro genetic toxicity assays, it has been noted that the results have been extremely disappointing (Tennant et al. 1987). However, in light of the benefit of hindsight, it should now be evident that the results are, indeed, not surprising, based on the assumptions that mutagens are carcinogens; that carcinogenesis is a one step process; that a single chemical can induce all the steps and mechanisms needed to complete the carcinogenic process; that all in vitro assays, designed to detect point and chromosomal mutations, only detect mutations; that all mutations are the result of DNA-damaging chemicals; that the biology of the test animal is sufficiently similar to the human situation so as not to influence the carcinogenic potential of the chemical in humans; and that there is no threshold for carcinogens. The lack of concordance between the results of short-term genotoxicity assays and the bioassays for carcinogen testing is, most likely, the result of the short-term tests being inadequate and the bioassay protocol not being designed to accomodate the multistage nature of carcinogenesis (Trosko 1984).

In the former case, there are all kinds of problems with short-term genotoxicity assays. They are (1) inadequate to detect the nongenotoxic components of carcinogenesis (e.g., cytotoxic and epigenetic mechanisms); (2) frequently misinterpreted due to the many potential artifacts associated with each test; (3) unable to recreate, in vitro, the higher order biological functions found in vivo (e.g., endocrine and immune mechanisms) that could modify carcinogenesis; and (4) used in ways that do not represent the true in vivo situation (e.g., interaction of mixtures of chemicals used at unrealistic concentrations (Clayson 1987).

Since carcinogenesis is clearly not a one-hit process, whereby a single normal cell, by being exposed to a single molecule of a carcinogen, is converted directly to a full-blown, metastasizing cancer cell, a bioassay system that is fundamentally based on that assumption is doomed to fail. By assuming a nonthreshold basis for carcinogenesis, by using animals hypersensitive to cancer induction, by ignoring the multiple genotoxic and nongenotoxic mechanisms involved in the multistage nature of carcinogenesis, and by using extremely high levels of chemicals in order to reduce the number of animals to be used, the current animal bioassay strategy introduces multiple artifacts. For example, tissue necrosis due to cytotoxic levels of chemical exposure can lead to compensatory hyperplasia, which, itself, might be a promoting condition for spontaneously initiated cells (Frei

1976; Jones et al. 1983; Trosko et al. 1983a; Argyris 1985). In other words, a chemical might not have any genotoxic (i.e., initiating) or noncytotoxic, epigenetic (i.e., promoting) activity. However, at a level where it can kill cells, the stimulation of regenerative hyperplasia could promote a single cell, initiated by some other spontaneous event. The tumors in such animals would be assumed to have been caused by the tested chemical and thereby labeled as a carcinogen (Trosko et al. 1983b). When tested in a short-term assay, it might be shown to be nongenotoxic (see next section for example). In addition, high levels of chemical exposure might lead to immune suppression, altered drug metabolism and/or hormone imbalances, which, in turn, could influence the appearance of tumors that, under normal conditions, would never have appeared.

Carcinogenesis Is More Than Mutagenesis: Mutagenesis and Mitogenesis

Because of the clonal nature of the multistep carcinogenic process (Fialkow 1974; Nowell 1976), it is assumed that a single stem or progenitor cell, once exposed to an initiator, is unable to terminally differentiate (Yuspa and Morgan 1981; Kawamura et al. 1985; Scott and Maercklein 1985; Miller et al. 1987). However, if left unstimulated to proliferate, it can be held in check by the surrounding normal cells. After stimulated to divide, (i.e., by growth factors, chemical tumor promoters, solid objects, wounding, cell necrosis, etc. [Trosko et al. 1983a]), the initiated stem cell, as well as other noninitiated stem cells, will proliferate. That appears to be a necessary facet of the tumor promotion phase, namely the clonal expansion and selective accumulation of the initiated cell. The normal progenitor cell, upon removal of the mitogenic stimuli, has the potential to terminally differentiate, whereas the initiated cell seems to be unable to terminally differentiate. As a result, in time, a clone of proliferable, but undifferentiatable, cells selectively accumulates. The enzyme-altered foci of rat liver, the papilloma of mouse skin, and the polyps of colon might all represent the tissue manifestation of this phase of carcinogenesis. After continued growth to a critical mass, other genetic (Trosko and Chang 1980; Potter 1981) or epigenetic alterations (Frost and Kerbel 1983) could confer the appropriate phenotype needed for a cell's ability to invade and metastasize. In other words, the promotion phase of carcinogenesis (which has been considered an important rate-limiting step in carcinogenesis [Trosko and Chang 1983]) is a mitogenic, not a mutagenic, process. If additional changes occur in the genome as a result of the initiated cells mitotic activity, then a conversion or progression step to the malignant state can occur (Trosko et al. 1988) (Fig. 1).

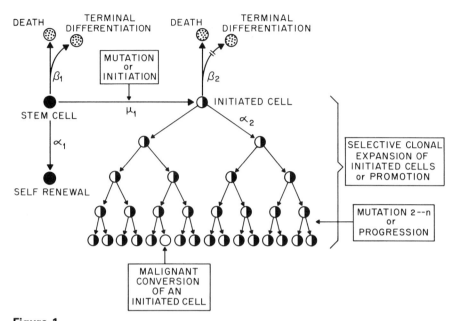

Figure 1

The initiation/promotion/progression model of carcinogenesis. β_1 is the rate of terminal differentiation and death of stem cell; β_2 is the rate of death, but not of ($-\|\rightarrow$) terminal differentiation of the initiated cell; α_1 is the rate of cell division of stem cells; α_2 is the rate of cell division of initiated cells; μ_1 is the rate of the molecular event leading to initiation (i.e, possibly mutation); μ_2=rate at which second event occurs within an initiated cell. (Reprinted, with permission, from Trosko et al. 1988.)

Inhibited Gap Junctional Communication: A Nongenotoxic Mechanism in Carcinogenesis

When an organism is exposed to chemicals, three potential biological responses are possible: (1) gene or chromosomal mutations, (2) cell death, and/or (3) an epigenetic event (Trosko et al. 1983b). Whereas these are not necessarily mutually exclusive end points (i.e., a chemical might induce a lethal mutation, leading to the death of the cell, thereby causing a surviving, neighboring cell to divide in the wound-healing process by activating genes for mitogenesis), it is possible to alter gene expression without killing cells or inducing mutations (i.e., such as tumor promoter and growth factor induction of genes).

Most stem and precursor cells in an organism are in a quiescent, "G_0" state, held there by various intercellular communications processes, involving either the transfer of negative growth factors from one cell to another over a cellular space or the transfer of ions and small molecular weight molecules via the membrane-protein channel, the gap junctions. Gap junctional intercellular communication (GJIC) appears to be a fundamental process needed for the regulation of tissue hemostasis, cell growth and differentiation, as well as synchronization of tissue reactions and tissue regeneration (Loewenstein 1979; MacDonald 1985; Schultz 1985; Neyton and Trautmann 1986; Pitts and Finbow 1986). Their role in the control of normal differentiation has been demonstrated by experiments in which antibodies directed against the gap junction protein are introduced into cells of developing systems, showing that development is altered (Warner et al. 1984; Fraser et al. 1987).

The possible role of gap junctions in the carcinogenic process comes from a wide range of observations. Cancer, which has been characterized as a stem cell disease (Cairns 1975; Nowell 1976; Fialkow 1977), a disease of differentiation (Markert 1968; Pierce 1974; Potter 1978), or a disease of dysfunctional growth control (Potter 1980), appears, in many cases, to be associated with dysfunctional GJIC (Loewenstein 1979; Kanno 1985).

In addition, since gap junction function is known to be modulated by many endogenous and exogenous factors (Larsen 1983; Trosko and Chang 1984; Spray and Bennett 1985), the demonstration that chemicals that are known tumor promoters can reversibly inhibit GJIC helped to support the hypothesis that inhibited intercellular communication would release suppressed initiated cells from surrounding normal cells allowing them to clonally amplify (Yotti et al. 1979). More recently, several oncogenes (*src, mos, ras*) and the middle T antigen of the polyoma virus have been shown to inhibit intercellular communication (Azarnia and Loewenstein 1984, 1987; Chang et al. 1985; Atkinson et al. 1986; El-Fouly et al. 1986). In addition, when transformed noncommunicating cells are induced to communicate, they lose their transformed phenotype (Mehta et al. 1986).

Cytotoxicity, another cellular end point, can involve the modulation of gap junctions by an indirect process. Gap junction regulation has been speculated to play a significant role in preventing death in a gap junctionally coupled tissue (Saez et al. 1987). When a cell is killed by any mechanism, to prevent ions such as calcium to pass from the nonfunctioning dying or dead cell to the coupled living cells, the gap junctions can be closed down. In addition, release of many cellular products for lyzed cells could inhibit more gap junctional communication in the immediate surrounding tissue to induce regenerative hyperplasia or wound healing.

Finally, the placement of solid inert materials into tissues could be conceived as not providing "contact inhibition" to the cells neighboring the object, leading to hyperplasia in that region. "Solid state" carcinogenesis might simply be a promoting stimulus involving the lack of cell-cell communication between the object and neighboring tissue (Trosko et al. 1983b).

Polybrominated Biphenyls: A Case in Point to Challenge the Current Risk Assessment Paradigm

In their recent assessment of the results of the National Toxicology Program's effort to evaluate 300 chemicals in a standard in vitro/in vivo protocol, Tennant et al. (1987) noted that ". . . . the three most potent carcinogens produced no genetic toxicity in any of the four short term tests studied." Working within the genotoxicity paradigm, one might conclude that the assays used were not the right ones to detect these three chemicals (2,3,7,8-tetrachlorodibenzo-p-dioxin [TCDD], polybrominated biphenyls, and reserpine) and others like it. We feel the time has come to say, "the Emperor wears no clothes" (Trosko 1985) and to try to force chemicals such as these to be mutagens, where the weight of existing evidence points to their acting by nongenotoxic mechanisms, is like trying to fit square pegs into round holes.

To illustrate how mechanisms, such as inhibition of intercellular communication, by either cytotoxic or noncytotoxic pathways, can contribute to the understanding of the basic mechanism of carcinogenesis and to point out the failure of current bioassay and in-vitro short-term assay batteries, we have examined the results of studies on polybrominated biphenyls (PBBs) and a few other similar carcinogens.

In several studies, PBB has been shown to induce liver cancers in rats (Kimbrough et al. 1981). Based on these results and the idea that anything that causes cancers in animals is a carcinogen, it was assumed that it had to be a genotoxic mixture. However, exhaustive studies to test the gene and chromosomal mutation potential have failed to demonstrate any genotoxicity in a wide variety of short-term tests (Kavanagh et al. 1987). On the other hand, when PBB (and purified congeners) were tested in initiation/promotion protocols in rats, these were shown to be powerful liver tumor promoters (Jensen et al. 1982). In fact, they were predicted to be in vivo tumor promoters on the bases of short-term assays designed to test if PBBs could inhibit gap junctional intercellular communication in a manner similar to the powerful skin tumor promoter, 12-O-tetradecanoylphorbol-13-acetate (TPA) (Trosko et al. 1981). These studies were designed to test the hypothesis that inhibition of gap junction function would allow for the clonal expansion of initiated cells by releasing them from a suppressive effect of surrounding normal cells.

These in vitro studies on PBBs ability to inhibit gap junctional communication also demonstrated several other important features associated with the in vivo tumor promotion process. First, there was a structure/function relationship (Tsushimoto et al. 1982). Second, with the use of two purified congeners of PBB, one could see that there are at least two basic mechanisms by which inhibition of intercellular communication could take place, namely via noncytotoxic and cytotoxic mechanisms. The congener, 2,2,',4,4',5,5'-hexa-bromobiphenyl (HBB) was noncytotoxic in vitro when it inhibited gap junctional communication, and it also produced no liver necrosis in vivo when shown to be a tumor promoter (Jensen and Sleight 1986). On the other hand, the 3,3',4,4',5,5'-HBB, was relatively cytotoxic (yet not mutagenic [Kavanagh et al. 1987]) in vitro and did not inhibit gap junction function in vitro at noncytotoxic levels (Tsushimoto et al. 1982). In vivo, when tested at non-cytotoxic levels it was not a carcinogen or tumor promoter (Jensen and Sleight 1986). However, at cytotoxic levels in vivo, it was shown to be a tumor promoter (Jensen and Sleight 1986). The plausible explanation is that cell killing in vivo, in a manner similar to wounding or partial hepatectomy, could itself act as a promoting stimulus by forcing surviving initiated cells to go into regenerative hyperplasia (Frei 1976; Trosko et al. 1983a; Argyris 1985).

PBBs ability to block gap junction function has also been shown to be reversible and dose-dependent (Evans et al. 1988), showing a "no-effect" or threshold level in vitro (Tsushimoto et al. 1982). These are all characteristics of tumor promoters in vivo. Although for PBBs the no-effect level and dose-dependence of PBB have not been demonstrated in vivo, they have been for polychlorinated biphenyls (PCB), a chemical that acts similarly to PBBs (Tsushimoto et al. 1983; Deml and Oesterle 1987).

Many other chemicals, shown to be carcinogens in various bioassays, have been shown on detailed examination, to be tumor promoters, nongenotoxi-cants and inhibitors of intercellular communication. TCDD and reserpine, as carcinogens, have not been shown to be genotoxic, yet TCDD is definitely a tumor promoter (Pitot et al. 1980; Poland et al. 1982). It has not yet been shown to inhibit intercellular communication, probably because the correct target cells have not been used to study its effects. Reserpine has been shown to inhibit intercellular communication (Bohrman et al. 1987).

Chemicals, such as phenobarbital, unsaturated fatty acids, cholesterol epoxides, valium, DDT, dieldrin, saccharin, butylated hydroxytoluene, di-(2-ethylhexyl)phthalate, trisodium nitrilotriacetate monohydrate (NTA), among many others (see Table 1 at end of this chapter) have been shown to be inhibitors of intercellular communication and tumor promoters. These chemicals, in spite of interpretation of results from some short-term genotoxic assays that they might be weak mutagens, are not likely to be genotoxic. The fact that all short-term genotoxicity assays are indirect indicators of DNA damage or mutation induction prevents one from discriminating between mutagenic from epigenetic changes or from artifacts due to the nature of measuring the effects (Trosko 1984, 1985).

Unfortunately, most chemicals tested in the bioassays have not been tested specifically as either tumor initiators or tumor promoters. Also, many chemicals tested in a cell-cell communication system have not been tested, in vivo, as tumor promoters. It is becoming clear that no one in vitro cell system or one technique to measure gap junction function can be used as a universal screen for potential tumor promoters for all species.

Mechanisms of Chemical Inhibition of Gap Junction Function: Implications to Biological Risk Assessment

Assuming inhibition of intercellular communication plays some role in carcinogenesis, as is inferred from the facts that most tumor promoting conditions inhibit gap junctions (Trosko et al. 1983a, 1988), that many tumor cells lack GJIC (Loewenstein 1979; Kanno 1985), that several oncogenes, when expressed, seemed to inhibit gap junction function (Azarnia and Loewenstein 1984; Chang et al. 1985; Atkinson et al. 1986; El-Fouly et al. 1986), and that there seems to be a correlation between the decrease in gap junction function and tumor metastasis (Nicolson et al. 1988), one would be forced to examine how gap junction function can be modulated. It is a fact that there are genetic/developmental and environmental modulators of gap junction structure and function (Larsen 1983; Lo 1985; Schultz 1985). Changes in intracellular Ca^{++} ions, pH, C-AMP, activation of protein kinase C, and oxygen free radical production (Spray and Bennett 1985; Saez et al. 1987) can modulate gap junction function. Clearly, the TPA model of tumor promotion, with its focus on the activation of protein kinase C and generation of oxygen radicals, cannot be the universal model for all tumor promoters, since there is little evidence that all non-TPA type of tumor promoters activate protein kinase C and some evidence that these chemicals work by different mechanisms (Saez et al. 1987).

Consequently, the exact mechanisms by which chemicals can block gap junctions in various cell types from various species will have to be elucidated for risk assessment purposes. In addition, with preliminary data showing various kinds of interactions between chemicals, it is going to prove extremely difficult to make mono-risk assessments for the real life situation, based on single chemical data, since some interactions will synergize, others will be additive, and still others will be antagonistic.

There is, of course, the major problem of the existence of possible thresholds for initiators and promoters (Scherer and Emmelot 1975; Fry 1981; Burns et al. 1983; Ehling et al. 1983; Maekawa et al. 1984; Tazima et al. 1984). Although the answer to either is unresolved, there does seem to be indirect evidence indicating threshold levels for tumor promoters (Verma and Boutwell 1980; Goldsworthy et al. 1984; Oesterle and Deml 1984; Shirai et al. 1985; Ito et al. 1986; Pereira et al. 1986), if one assumes that inhibition of gap junctions plays a role in tumor promotion. All tested inhibitors of intercellular communication seem to have a "no-effect" level. In addition, tumor promotion seems to be a rate-limiting process in carcinogenesis (Trosko and Chang 1983).

There are, of course, many complicating factors, such as species, tissue and cell-type specificity, receptor/nonreceptor dependent promoters, and interaction with other chemicals. Lastly the "good news/bad news" phenomenon has been observed with many chemicals tested as carcinogens or anticarcinogens (i.e., TCDD, DDT, PCB, butylated hydroxytoluene, phenobarbital) (Cohen et al. 1979; Tsuda et al. 1984; Bailey et al. 1987; Birt et al. 1987; Manson et al. 1987; Shirai et al. 1987; see also Williams 1984). Under one set of biological conditions the chemical can block induction of cancers, and under another set they can enhance the production of tumors in experimental animals. Therefore, the goal of being able to develop a quantitative risk assessment model, without understanding the mechanisms of actions or without integrating biological factors into a risk assessment model, would seem to be impossible to attain.

ACKNOWLEDGMENTS

Authors wish to thank Drs. B.V. Madhukar, S.Y. Oh, D. Bombick, and M. El-Fouly for their helpful discussions during the preparation of the manuscript and to acknowledge the contributions of Mrs. Beth Lockwood and Mrs. Darla Conley for helping to prepare the manuscript. Research was supported by grants from the National Cancer Institute (CA-21104), the Air Force Office of Scientific Research (AFOSR-86-0084), and the R.J. Reynolds/Nabisco Company.

REFERENCES

Ames, B.N., W.E. Durston, E. Yamaski, and F.D. Lee. 1973. Carcinogens are mutagens: A simple test system combining liver homogenates for activation and bacteria for detection. *Proc. Natl. Acad. Sci.* **70:** 2281.

Argyris, T.S. 1985. Regeneration and the mechanism of epidermal tumor promotion. *CRC Crit. Rev. Toxicol.* **14:** 211.

Atkinson, M.M., S.K. Anderson, and J.D. Sheridan. 1986. Modification of gap junctions in cells transformed by a temperature-sensitive mutant of Rous sarcoma virus. *J. Membr. Biol.* **9:** 53.

Azarnia, R. and W.R. Loewenstein. 1984. Intercellular communication and the control of growth: Alteration of junctional permeability by the *src* gene: A study with temperature-sensitive mutant Rous sarcoma virus. *J. Membr. Biol.* **82:** 191.

———. 1987. Polyoma virus middle T antigen down regulates junctional cell to cell communication. *Mol. Cell. Biol.* **7:** 946.

Bailey, G.S., J.D. Hendricks, D.W. Shelton, J.E. Nixon, and N.E. Pawlowski. 1987.

Enhancement of carcinogenesis by the natural anticarcinogen indole-3-carbinol. *J. Natl. Cancer Inst.* **78:** 931.

Birt, D.F., J.C. Pelling, P.M. Pour, M.G. Tibbels, L. Schweickert, and E. Bresnick. 1987. Enhanced pancreatic and skin tumorigenesis in cabbage-fed hamsters and mice. *Carcinogenensis* **8:** 913.

Bohrman, J.S., J. Burg, E. Elmore, D. McGregor, R. Langenbach, and M. Toraason. 1987. Effect of carcinogens and non-carcinogens on metabolic cooperation in V79 cells. *In Vitro Cell. Dev. Biol.* **23:** 13A.

Boutwell, R.K. 1974. The function and mechanism of promoters of carcinogenesis. *CRC Crit. Rev. Toxicol.* **2:** 419.

Burns, F., R. Albert, B. Altshular, and E. Morris. 1983. Approach to risk assessment for genotoxic carcinogens based on data from the mouse skin initiation-promotion model. *Environ. Health Perspect.* **50:** 309.

Cairns, J. 1975. Mutation selection and the natural history of cancer. *Nature* **255:** 197.

———. 1981. The origin of human cancers. *Nature* **289:** 353.

Chang, C.C., J.E. Trosko, H.J. Kung, D. Bombick, and F. Matsumura. 1985. Potential role of the *src* gene product in inhibition of gap junctional communication in NIH 3T3 cells. *Proc. Natl. Acad. Sci.* **82:** 5360.

Clayson, D.B. 1987. The need for biological risk assesment in reaching decision about carcinogens. *Mutat. Res.* **185:** 243.

Cohen, G.M., W.H. Bracken, R.P. Iyer, D.L. Berry, J.K. Selkirk, and T.J. Slaga. 1979. Anticarcinogenic effects of 2,3,7,8-tetrachlorodibenzo-p-dioxin on benzo(a)pyrene and 7,12-dimethyl-benz(a) anthracene tumor initiation and its relationship to DNA binding. *Cancer Res.* **39:** 4027.

Deml, E. and D. Oesterle. 1987. Dose response of promotion by polychlorinated biphenyls and chloroform in rat liver foci bioassay. *Arch. Toxicol.* **60:** 209.

Ehling, U.H., D. Averbeck, P.A. Cerutti, J. Friedman, H. Greim, A.C. Kolbye, and M.L. Mendelson. 1983. Review of the evidence for the presence or absence of thresholds in the induction of genetic effects by genotoxic chemicals. *Mutat. Res.* **123:** 281.

Ehrenberg, L., P. Brookes, H. Druckrey, B. Lagerlof, J. Litwin, and G. Williams. 1973. The relation of cancer induction and genetic damages. *Ambio. Spec. Rep.* **3:** 15.

Eldredge, N. and S.J. Gould. 1972. Punctuated equilibria: An alternative to phyletic gradualism. In *Models in paleobiology* (ed. T.J.M. Schoph). Freeman and Cooper, San Francisco.

El-Fouly, M.H., S.T. Warren, J.E. Trosko, and C.C. Chang. 1986. Inhibition of gap junction-mediated intercellular communication in cells transfected with the human H-*ras* oncogene. *Am. J. Hum. Genet.* **39:** A30.

Evans, M.G., M.H. El-Fouly, J.E. Trosko, and S.D. Sleight. 1988. Anchored cell analysis/sorting coupled with the scrape-loading/dye transfer technique to quantify inhibition of gap junctional intercellular communication in WB-F344 cells by 2,2′,4,4′,5,5′-hexabromobiphenyl. *J. Toxicol. Environ. Health* (in press).

Fialkow, P.J. 1974. The origin and development of human tumors studied with cell markers. *N. Engl. J. Med.* **291:** 26.

————. 1977. Clonal origin and stem cell evolution of human tumors. In *Genetics of human cancer* (ed. J.J. Mulvihill et al.), p. 439. Raven Press, New York.

Foulds, L. 1975. *Neoplastic development.* Academic Press, New York.

Fraser, S.E., C.R. Green, H.R. Bode, and N.B. Gilula. 1987. Selective disruption of gap junctional communication interferes with a patterning process in Hydra. *Science* **237**: 49.

Frei, J.V. 1976. Some mechanisms operative in carcinogenesis, a review. *Chem.-Biol. Interact.* **13**: 1.

Frost, P. and R.S. Kerbel. 1983. On the possible epigenetic mechanism(s) of tumor cell heterogeneity: The role of DNA-methylation. *Cancer Metast. Rev.* **2**: 375.

Fry, R.J.M. 1981. Experimental radiation carcinogenesis: What have we learned? *Radiat. Res.* **87**: 224.

Goldsworthy, T., H.A. Campbell, and H.C. Pitot. 1984. The natural history of enzyme-altered foci in rat liver following phenobarbital and diethylnitrosamine administration. *Carcinogenesis* **5**: 67.

Ito, N., S. Fukushima, S. Tamano, M. Hirose, and A. Hagiwara. 1986. Dose response in butylated hydroxyanisole induction of forestomach carcinogenesis in F344 rats. *J. Natl. Cancer Inst.* **77**: 1261.

Jensen, R.K. and S.D. Sleight. 1986. Sequential study on the effects of 2,2',4,4',5,5'-hexabromobiphenyl and 3,3',4,4',5,5'-hexabromobiphenyl on hepatic tumor promotion. *Carcinogenesis* **7**: 1771.

Jensen, R.K., S.D. Sleight, J.I. Goodman, S.D. Aust, and J.E. Trosko. 1982. Polybrominated biphenyls as promoters in experimental hepatocarcinogenesis in rats. *Carcinogenesis* **3**: 1183.

Jones, T.D., G.D. Griffin, and P.J. Walsh. 1983. A unifying concept for carcinogenic risk assessments. *J. Theor. Biol.* **105**: 35.

Kanno, Y. 1985. Modulation of cell communication and carcinogenesis. *Jpn. J. Physiol.* **35**: 693.

Kavanagh, T.J., C.C. Chang, and J.E. Trosko. 1987. Effect of various polybrominated biphenyls on cell-cell communication in cultured human teratocarcinoma cells. *Fundam. Appl. Toxicol.* **8**: 127.

Kawamura, H., J.E. Strickland, and S.H. Yuspa. 1985. Association of resistance to terminal differentiation with initiation of carcinogenesis in adult mouse epidermal cells. *Cancer Res.* **45**: 2748.

Kimbrough, R.D., D.F. Groce, M.P. Lorver, and V.W. Burse. 1981. Induction of liver tumors in female Sherman strain rats by polybrominated biphenyls. *J. Natl. Cancer Inst.* **66**: 535.

Larsen, W.J. 1983. Biological implications of gap junction structure, distribution and composition: A review. *Tissue Cell* **15**: 645.

Lo, C.W. 1985. Communication compartmentation and pattern formation in development. In *Gap junctions* (ed. M.V.L. Bennett and D.C. Spray), p. 251. Cold Spring Harbor Laboratory, Cold Spring Harbor, New York.

Loewenstein, W.R. 1979. Junctional intercellular communication and the control of growth. *Biochim. Biophys. Acta* **605**: 33.

MacDonald, C. 1985. Gap junctions and cell-cell communication. *Essays Biochem.* **21**: 86.

Maekawa, A., T. Ogiu, C. Matsuoka, H. Onodera, K. Furuta, Y. Kurokawa, M. Takahashi, T. Kokubo, T. Tanigawa, Y. Hayashi, M. Nakadate, and A. Tanimura. 1984. Carcinogenicity of low doses of N-ethyl-N-nitrosourea in F344 rats: A dose response study. *Gann* **75**: 117.

Manson, M.M., J.A. Green, and H.E. Driver. 1987. Ethoxyquin alone induces preneoplastic changes in rat kidney whilst preventing induction of such lesions in liver by aflatoxin β_1. *Carcinogenesis* **8**: 723.

Markert, C. 1968. Neoplasia: A disease of cell differentiation. *Cancer Res.* **28**: 1908.

Mehta, P.P., J.S. Bertram, and W.R. Loewenstein. 1986. Growth inhibition of transformed cells correlates with their junctional communication with normal cells. *Cell* **44**: 187.

Miller, D.R., A. Viaje, C.M. Aldaz, C.J. Conti, and T.J. Slaga. 1987. Terminal differentiation-resistant epidermal cells in mice undergoing two-stage carcinogenesis. *Cancer Res.* **47**: 1935.

Neyton, J. and A. Trautmann. 1986. Physiological modulation of gap junction permeability. *J. Exp. Biol.* **124**: 93.

Nicholson, G.L., K.M. Dulski, and J.E. Trosko. 1988. Highly metastatic mammary adenocarcinoma cells show loss of intercellular junctional communication. *Proc. Natl. Acad. Sci.* (in press).

Nowell, P.C. 1976. The clonal evolution of tumor cell populations. *Science* **194**: 23.

Oesterle, D. and E. Deml. 1984. Dose-dependent promoting effect of polychlorinated biphenyls on enzyme-altered islands in livers of adult and weanling rats. *Carcinogenesis* **5**: 351.

Pereira, M.A., S.L. Herren-Freund, and R.E. Long. 1986. Dose-response relationship of phenobarbital promotion of diethylnitrosamine initiated tumors in rat liver. *Cancer Lett.* **32**: 305.

Pierce, G.B. 1974. Neoplasms, differentiation and mutations. *Am. J. Pathol.* **77**: 103.

Pitot, H.C., T. Goldsworthy, and S. Moran. 1981. The natural history of carcinogenesis: Implications of experimental carcinogenesis in the genesis of human cancer. *J. Supramol. Struct. Cell. Biochem.* **17**: 133.

Pitot, H.C., T. Goldsworthy, H.A. Campbell, and A. Poland. 1980. Quantitative evaluation of the promotion by 2,3,7,8-tetrachlorodibenzo-p-dioxin of hepatocarcinogenesis from diethylnitrosamine. *Cancer Res.* **40**: 3616.

Pitts, J.D. and M.E. Finbow. 1986. The gap junction. *J. Cell Sci.* (suppl.) **4**: 239.

Poland, A., D. Palen, and E. Glover. 1982. Tumor promotion by TCDD in skin of HRS/J hairless. *Nature* **300**: 271.

Potter, V.R. 1978. Phenotypic diversity in experimental hepatomas: The concept of partially blocked ontogeny. *Br. J. Cancer* **38**: 1.

———. 1980. Initiation and promotion in cancer formation: The importance of studies on intercellular communication. *Yale J. Biol. Med.* **53**: 367.

———. 1981. Commentary: A new protocol and its rationale for the study of initiation and promotion of carcinogenesis in rat liver. *Carcinogenesis* **2**: 1375.

Saez, J.C., M.V.L. Bennett, and D.C. Spray. 1987. Carbon tetrachloride at hepatotoxic levels blocks reversibly gap junctions between rat hepatocytes. *Science* **236**: 967.

Scherer, E. and P. Emmelot. 1975. Kinetics of induction and growth of precancerous liver-cell foci, and liver tumour formation by diethylnitrosamine in the rat. *Eur. J. Cancer* **11:** 689.

Schultz, R.M. 1985. Roles of cell to cell communication in development. *Biol. Reprod.* **32:** 27.

Scott, R.E. and P.B. Maercklein. 1985. An initiation of carcinogenesis selectively and stably inhibits stem cell differentiation: A concept that initiation of carcinogenesis involves multiple phases. *Proc. Natl. Acad. Sci.* **82:** 2995.

Shirai, T., K. Hosoda, K. Hirose, M. Hirose, and N. Ito. 1985. Promoting effects of phenobarbital and 3'-methyl-4-dimethylaminoazobenzene on the appearance of γ-glutamyltranspeptidase positive foci in rat liver pretreated with varying doses of diethylnitrosamine. *Cancer Lett.* **28:** 127.

Shirai, T., H. Tsuda, T. Ogiso, M. Hirose, and N. Ito. 1987. Organ specific modifying potential of ethinyl estradiol on carcinogenesis initiated with different carcinogens. *Carcinogenesis* **8:** 115.

Spray, D.C. and M.V.L. Bennett. 1985. Physiology and pharmacology of gap junctions. *Annu. Rev. Physiol.* **47:** 281.

Tazima, Y., S. Kondo, and Y. Kuroda. 1984. *Problems of threshold in chemical mutagenensis.* Kokusai-bunken, Tokyo.

Tennant, R.W., B.H. Margolin, M.D. Shelby, E. Zeiger, J.K. Haseman, J Spalding, W. Caspary, M. Resnick, S. Stasiewicz, B. Anderson, and R. Minor. 1987. Prediction of chemical carcinogenicity in rodents from in vitro genetic toxicity assays. *Science* **236:** 933.

Trosko, J.E. 1984. A new paradigm is needed in toxicology evaluation. *Environ. Mutagen.* **6:** 767.

———. 1985. Adaptive and non-adaptive consequences of chemical inhibition of cellular communication by toxic substances. In *Proceedings of the 15th Annual Conference on Environmental Toxicology*, AFAMRL-TR-84-002 (ed. J.D. MacEwen and E.H. Vernot), p. 169. Air Force Aerospace Medical Research Lab., W-PAFB, Ohio.

Trosko, J.E. and C.C. Chang. 1978. Environmental carcinogenesis: An integrative model. *Q. Rev. Biol.* **53:** 115.

———. 1980. An integrative hypothesis linking cancer, diabetes and atherosclerosis: The role of mutations and epigenetic changes. *Med. Hypotheses* **6:** 455.

———. 1983. Potential role of intercellular communication in the rate-limiting step in carcinogenesis. In *Cancer and the environment: Possible mechanisms of thresholds for carcinogens and other toxic substances* (ed. J.A. Cimino), p. 5. Mary Ann Liebert, New York.

———. 1984. Adaptive and non-adaptive consequences of chemical inhibition of intercellular communication. *Pharmacol. Rev.* **36:** 137.

———. 1985. Role of tumor promotion in affecting the multi-hit nature of carcinogenesis. In *Assessment of risk from low level exposure to radiation and chemicals* (ed. A.D. Woodhead et al.), p. 261. Plenum Press, New York.

———. 1986. Role of intercellular communication in modifying the consequences of mutations in somatic cells. In *Antimutagenesis and anticarcinogenesis mechanisms* (ed. D.M. Shankel et al.), p. 439. Plenum Press, New York.

Trosko, J.E., C.C. Chang, and A. Medcalf. 1983a. Mechanisms of tumor promotion: Potential role of intercellular communication. *Cancer Invest.* **1:** 511.

Trosko, J.E., B. Dawson, and C.C. Chang. 1981. PBB inhibits metabolic cooperation in Chinese hamster cells in vitro: Its potential as a tumor promoter. *Environ. Health Perspect.* **37:** 179.

Trosko, J.E., C. Jone, and C.C. Chang. 1983b. The role of tumor promoters on phenotypic alterations affecting intercellular communication and tumorigenesis. *Ann. N.Y. Acad. Sci.* **407:** 316.

Trosko, J.E., V.M. Riccardi, C.C. Chang, S. Warren, and M. Wade. 1985. Genetic predispositions to initiation or promotion phases in human carcinogenesis. In *Biomarkers, genetics, and cancer* (ed. H. Anton-Guirgis and H.T. Lynch), p. 13. Van Nostrand Reinhold, New York.

Trosko, J.E., C.C. Chang, B.V. Madhukar, S.Y. Oh, D. Bombick, and M.H. El-Fouly. 1988. Modulation of gap junction intercellular communication by tumor promoting chemicals, oncogenes and growth factors during carcinogenesis. In *Gap junctions* (see E.L. Hertzberg and R. Johnson). A.R. Liss, New York. (In press.)

Tsuda, H., T. Sakata, T. Masui, K. Imaida, and N. Ito. 1984. Modifying effects of butylated hydroxyanisole, ethoxyquin and acetaminophen on induction of neoplastic lesions in rat liver and kidney initiated by N-ethyl-N-hydroxyethylnitrosamine. *Carcinogenesis* **5:** 525.

Tsushimoto, G., S. Asano, J.E. Trosko, and C.C. Chang. 1983. Inhibition of intercellular communication by various congeners of polybrominated biphenyl and polychlorinated biphenyl. In *PCB's human and environmental hazards* (ed. F.M. D'Itri and M.A. Kamrin), p. 241. Butterworth, Boston.

Tsushimoto, G., J.E. Trosko, C.C. Chang, and S.D. Aust. 1982. Inhibition of metabolic cooperation in Chinese hamster V79 cells in culture by various polybrominated biphenyl (PBB) congeners. *Carcinogenesis* **3:** 181.

Verma, A.K. and R.K. Boutwell. 1980. Effects of dose and duration of treatment with the tumor-promoting agent, TPA on mouse skin carcinogenesis. *Carcinogenesis* **1:** 271.

Warner, A.E., S.C. Guthrie, and N.B. Gilula. 1984. Antibodies to gap junctional protein selectively disrupt junctional communication in the early amphibian embryo. *Nature* **311:** 127.

Williams, G.M. 1984. Modulation of chemial carcinogenesis by xenobiotics. *Fundam. Appl. Toxicol.* **4:** 325.

Yotti, L.P., C.C. Chang, and J.E. Trosko. 1979. Elimination of metabolic cooperation in Chinese hamster cells by a tumor promoter. *Science* **206:** 1089.

Yuspa, S.H. and D.L. Morgan. 1981. Mouse skin cells resistant to terminal differentiation associated with initiation of carcinogenesis. *Nature* **293:** 72.

COMMENTS

Munro: There *is* a great deal of concern, particularly in the regulatory agencies, about mechanisms and means for regulatory control of carcinogens such as dioxin, PPBs, reserpine, and for chemicals that are not what one might call classical genotoxic carcinogens. Your assay, as you have demonstrated, seems to detect at least the activity with respect to those substances regarding cell-to-cell communication. I take it the implication is that this assay can be used to identify certain classes of nongenotoxic carcinogens?

Trosko: Epigenetic carcinogens. I have no problem using the word.

Munro: The question I raise relates primarily to the use of this model in a regulatory setting, and its validation for that purpose. You listed among the substances that are active in the system a number of nutrients and other materials. How does one deal with the question of use of this assay in a regulatory setting, particularly dealing with the question of the specificity to detect these particular groups of substances that are of concern?

Trosko: That is an important question. I'm not going to skirt it, because it is the real issue. The question relates to what Bruce Ames and others have said, that is, let's put into perspective the risk of things to which we are normally exposed. There is no doubt, with all the concern of diet and cancer, that there is a link between the two. In fact, the animal carcinogenesis story is very clear. The tumor-promoting effects of dietary fat have been well documented using many experimental mammary tumor systems. Is the exposure to unsaturated fatty acids any less a risk than exposure to PBBs? In fact, there is probably a greater risk to high fat diets than to PBBs. Right now, on the basis of 9 million people being exposed to PBBs in Michigan, I am more concerned about the huge amounts of unsaturated fatty acids that I find in my doughnut than I am about the few pg of PBB that are in my tissues.

Molecules are molecules. The cell doesn't know that it's made by me, i.e., some essential fatty acid, as opposed to a chemical that an organic chemist, like Willy (Lijinsky), has synthesized and has found its way into my body. The cell can't make that distinction.

The point is, both those cells work by this important mechanism. I can't underscore that point enough: intercellular communication is a fundamental biological process that makes you a multicellular organism. The adaptive and nonadaptive consequences of the modulation of intercellular communication can be illustrated by drinking coffee in the morning, taking in the caffeine, that blocks the breakdown of cyclic-AMP, which then opens the gap junctions, so that we can sit here wide awake and listen to me talk, as opposed to drinking alcohol, which closes the gap junctions, and we drowse.

All I'm saying is that all kinds of chemicals have the potential of blocking gap junctions. That includes those that we call pollutants, industrial, and drug, or the natural ones that we make or the ones animals and plants make that we eat. It is a question now of putting these things in perspective.

Lijinsky: Jim, do the genotoxic carcinogens also block gap junctions? If they do, how do they compare in potency or effectiveness in doing this with the nongenotoxic ones?

Trosko: That is now being analyzed by a few people, like Gary Williams, Hiroshi Yamasaki, and James Klaunig. The few that have been tested, the so-called real genotoxic carcinogens, do not seem to be very potent at noncytotoxic concentrations. However, and I underscore this point, most of these genotoxic carcinogens, by damaging DNA, kill cells, and in that manner, they block communication in a very indirect way. If you use these chemicals at doses that kill cells, it's inhibiting intercellular communication in an indirect way.

There is one report (*Carcinogenesis* [1986] **7**: 885), however, in which dimethylbenzanthracene does seem to block cell-cell communication in vivo at doses where the pathologists do not see much cytotoxicity. However, I can't answer the question adequately because this area is so new.

Weber: You said the gene that is responsible for these gap junctions has been cloned. Are there any mutations in that gene?

Trosko: That's one of the most interesting lines of work right now. A paper came out in *Science* 1987 (**236**: 1920), where the investigators injected the mRNA from the cloned gap junction gene into cells that did not have gap junctions, and cell-cell channels were induced. Right now, the race is on to put it in a cancer cell. It will have no relevance to the cure of cancer, but it is going to be of academic interest to see whether a cancer cell that does not communicate by having functional gap junctions will become normal. That also leads to the question whether during the cancer process, mutations occur in genes that alter the structure of gap junctions or in the regulation of gap junctions.

Clayson: I think, if I have understood your method correctly, you have told us that one of the consequences of the inhibition of the gap junctions is what you called hyperplasia and I think I call cellular proliferation. Phenobarbital is one of the gap junction inhibitors, and yet, Peraino in 1980 pointed out that in the living animal there was a very time-limited period of cellular proliferation, following the start of phenobarbital feeding, which then quieted down. I have seen the same pattern again with a peroxisome inhibitor, I think it was diethyhexylphthalate, that gave a time-limited wave of cellular proliferation. Would you tell us a little bit about what you think the biological significance is of that wave of cellular proliferation and why it quiets down?

Trosko: It turns out the first naive picture we had was that, by blocking contact inhibition, by blocking gap junctions, cells should divide. That is basically what happens when you add TPA to the skin. Both the initiated cell and the normal cell divide. In the case of the skin, the normal cell goes on to terminally differentiate, whereas the initiated cell, which proliferates also, cannot terminally differentiate. Therefore, it selectively accumulates.

In the liver treated with phenobarbital, sustained massive cell division of the hepatocytes does not occur. However, by definition, sustained division of the initiated cell must occur. So, here is a case where the promoter, by blocking communication, seems to give selective mitogenic stimuli to the initiated cell, by definition, because how can you go from one initiated cell in the liver to that enzyme-altered focus that has millions of cells?

Then, that leads to the second question: Are there cell-type specific responses to chemical modulators of gap junctions? Recently, we have taken a number of cells from liver, lung, skin, kidney, etc. We then took one chemical of those five classes of mechanisms by which gap junctions are modulated: calcium changes, pH changes, activated PKC, free radicals, cAMP. A beautiful pattern seems to have emerged. For example, the cigarette tar condensate, which we know blocks gap junctions and is a tumor promoter, does nothing to liver cells. You could add the condensate to such a high level that you could see the membranes bleb and the cells died, but the gap junctions were still functional. However, when you added it to lung cells, it blocked gap junctions at noncytotoxic doses. What I'm saying is, there seems to be a cell-type, if not a species-type reaction to chemical modulators of gap junctions.

Now, we get to another question: Do all promoters act alike on the same cell? Our data clearly show that not all promoters act like TPA, the classic tumor promoting chemical. TPA does seem to activate PKC, which implies that it phosphorylates things. However, dieldrin, which also blocks gap junctions, doesn't activate PKC. So we can now find synergisms. If we add, for example, TPA at a low level, which just barely blocks communication, and then add dieldrin, we find they synergise. If we add TPA to a cell and then posttreat it with quercetin, an inhibitor of PKC, we ameliorate the effect of TPA. If we add dieldrin and DDT, which seems to work by the same mechanism, we get additivity.

So, what we are finding now on the phenomenology of gap junctions is that chemicals, working by different mechanisms, are giving us what we observe in animals given mixtures of chemicals: additivity, synergism, and antagonisms.

Clayson: Could I just follow that up very briefly? I have been puzzled about this for some time. What I wonder is, Kinzel and Slaga have reported two stages of promotion in the mouse skin. Are we looking at the same thing here?

Trosko: I have problems with their view of promotion but not their observation. The observation is real. Many times when you have reports in the literature that seem to be different, it's because people do different experiments. When you do the initiation/promotion model in the liver, Henry Pitot claims you don't find the two stages of promotion, although you do find it in the skin. One interpretation is that the skin's architecture is different, because it's an open-ended cell proliferation system, as opposed to the liver, which is a closed system. Maybe that phenomenology of two stages of promotion is simply related to the architecture of the skin as opposed to the liver. I don't see it here in this system.

Michejda: Your whole concept doesn't really conflict with the "mutagen is a carcinogen" idea. I mean, you still need an initiated cell.

Trosko: It doesn't conflict. There are some people who feel that mutagens are the whole answer. All I'm saying is, let's modify the paradigm.

Michejda: Your whole concept doesn't really conflict with the "mutagen as a carcinogen" idea. I mean, you still need an initiated cell.

Trosko: I wish you were right.

Michejda: The other question is what happens in cells such as 3T3 cells and 10T1/2 cells in terms of gap junctions? They are frequently thought of as being almost 90% transformed. Are their gap junctions disturbed when they're in confluent cultures?

Trosko: In those kinds of cells, the answer is yes. Yamasaki has clearly shown that. However, they do communicate under certain conditions. There is another observation that is coming out of this field. As you learn more, you fine-tune. One of the things they are fine-tuning is the fact that normal stem cells don't communicate. Cells that start down the differentiation pathway as normal cells do start to communicate. If you block the cells from differentiating, they still communicate, but it seems that they selectively communicate. In other words, the initiated cells within enzyme-altered foci in the liver or in the transformed foci communicate with themselves but not with normal neighbors. Yamasaki has demonstrated this beautifully. However, when the cell is metastasizing, it doesn't communicate with itself or anything else.

In fact, Garth Nicholson has a paper that is coming out in *Proc. Natl. Acad. Sci.* (in press), in which he has measured gap junctional communication in nonmetastatic mammary carcinomas, intermediate metastatic carcinomas, and highly metastatic carcinomas. He found that the nonmetastatic carcinomas communicate with themselves beautifully but not with normal neighbors. The intermediate cells had intermediate communication ability. The highly metastatic cells did not communicate with any cells. When he took the nonmetastatic cells and transfected them with the *ras* gene, which blocked communication, they became metastatic.

Neal: Could I expand on that? That is Craig Boreiko's work at CIIT, who was using TPA and examining gap junction or cell-cell communication with the 10T1/2 cells. He noted that in the first 24 hours that TPA is present in the media, there is a decrease in cell communication.

Trosko: Transient blockage.

Neal: Transient blockage with the 3T3 cells. However, with TPA still in the media, after 24 hours, they start communicating normally, but you require TPA in the media for six weeks for the transformation to take place. So, the TPA has to be there (for 6 weeks), but it only blocks communication for approximately the first 24 hours and then they start communicating normally. However, the TPA has to be there in order to do the transformation.

Michejda: Was Nicholson's experiment with mammary carcinoma or melanoma? Isn't he using Fidler's melanoma lines?

Trosko: I don't remember which one it is, but it's his line, whichever it is.

Barsotti: Could you comment on the theory of dedifferentiation, and how this fits into your work?

Trosko: I understand there is the retrodifferentiation/dedifferentiation model that exists somewhere, but let me just say I'm wedded to the Barry Pierce, the Markert, the Van Potter model, where you start with a stem cell that has a block in its way to differentiation. I do not believe there is convincing evidence that N-stage differentiated cells can dedifferentiate.

Guengerich: There's one thing you touched on, Jim, on which I want to follow up. How heterogeneous do you think the gap junction proteins are? Are we going to be dealing with 25 of these that respond to different chemicals that are tissue-specific, or what?

Trosko: The analysis done by the Cal Tech group seems to indicate, by and large, with the exception of the lense gap junction protein, that the gap junction found in the primitive multicellular organisms is the same as what is found in most of your tissues. The difference, however, might be—and this refers to Dr. Neal's point—in fact, the regulation of gap junctions. In a soon-to-be-published paper, we show that you can add TPA to hepatocytes, and it blocks gap junctions. However, within hours they recommunicate even in the presence of TPA. They up-regulate. The PKC is activated, inactivated, and becomes insensitive to mobilization to the membrane. However, you add TPA to human keratinocytes, and their gap junctions down for almost 24 hours. So, the regulation from cell type to cell type is very, very different.

Wilson: I'll be interested to hear your results on TCDD, especially observing the differences you did between 2,2,' and 3,3' hexabromobiphenyls. The 3,3' hexabromobiphenyls are thought to operate by a similar mechanism. TCDD is known to stimulate terminal differentiation of skin cells, so that it could be operating by a different mechanism. It also has the opposite effect on protein kinase C that TPA does, so it will be interesting to see what it does to the gap junction.

The critical question is what does it mean with regard to risk assessment. What you have provided us with, I think, is a very intriguing mechanism that explains a lot of the eight different classes that Williams and Weisburger proposed for nongenotoxic chemicals.

I think the risk assessment that we have to deal with here is when this information is applicable to the human use situation.

Trosko: Right. To answer your question very briefly, I have some privileged information which I have been given permission to use. The James Klaunig group in Toledo has done a matrix like this with liver cells and phenobarbital on a whole variety of mouse and rat strains, and they find a difference. Of all the chemicals to which we should apply risk assessment and that might be a promoter in the human population, it's phenobarbital. We can show that there is a threshold level in terms of cell-cell communication in many cell types.

Stevenson: How does the TCDD, which apparently is anticarcinogenic with hormonally related tumors, fit in with your work?

Trosko: So is phenobarbital, so is PBB, and so is BHA. Every one of these chemicals that can block cell-cell communication is a promoter under one set of conditions and prevents cancer formation under another set of conditions. That's the good news/bad news for you regulators. PBB clearly will block certain types of carcinogen action. On the other hand, it will promote it also. It depends on the biological condition.

Wilson: The good news is there is a very sharp dose response.

Table 1
Chemicals That Inhibit GJIC in Several In Vitro Assays and That Are Either Carcinogens, Tumor Promoters, Neurotoxins, or Reproductive Toxicants

Biological toxins	Modulator of intercellular communication[a]	Toxic end point[a]
Phorbol	− (1)	− mouse skin tumor promoter (2)
12-O-Tetradecanoylphorbol-13-acetate (TPA)	+ + + + (1–7)	+ strong mouse skin tumor promoter (8)
Phorbol-12,13-didecanoate (PDD)	+ + + (1)	+ moderate mouse skin tumor promoter (9)
4-α PDD	− (1)	− mouse skin tumor promoter (9)
4-O-Methyl TPA	− (1–10)	− mouse skin promoter (11)
Phorbol-12,13-diacetate (PDA)	+ (1)	+ weak mouse skin promoter (12)
Phorbol-12,13-dibutyrate (PDBu)	+ + (1)	+ moderate mouse skin promoter (13)
Teleocidin	+ + + + (14)	+ skin tumor promoter (15)
Teleocidin B	+ + + + (14)	+ skin tumor promoter (15)
Hydrolyzed teleocidin	+ (14)	?
Palytoxin	− (16)	+ mouse skin promoter[b] (17)
Mezerein	+ + + + (18)	+ second stage tumor promoter (19)
Aplysiatoxin	+ + + + (17)	+ tumor promoter (20)
Anhydrodebromoaplysiatoxin	+ + (17)	?
Debromoaplysiatoxin	+ + (17)	+ tumor promoter (20)
T2 toxin	+ + (17)	+ rat carcinogen (21)
Vomitoxin	+ + + (17)	?

Food additives/nutrients	Modulator of intercellular communication	Toxic end point[a]
Linoleic acid	+ + + (44, 45)	+ rat mammary tumor promoter (46, 47)
Stearic acid	− (45)	− mouse skin tumor promoter (48)
cis-Palmitoleic acid	+ + + (45)	+ rat mammary tumor promoter (46)

Drugs	Modulator of intercellular communication[a]	Toxic end point[a]
Palmitic acid	− (45)	− rat mammary tumor promoter (46)
Palmitelaidic acid	++ (45)	+ rat mammary tumor promoter (49)
Myristoleic acid	+++ (45)	+ rat mammary tumor promoter (46)
Myristic acid	− (45)	− rat mammary tumor promoter (46)
Oleic acid	+++ (45)	+ mouse skin tumor promoter (50)
Linolenic acid	+++ (45)	+ rat mammary tumor promoter (46, 47)
cis-Oleic acid	++++ (45)	+ rat mammary tumor promoter (46, 47)
Elaidic acid (Trans)	++ (45)	+ promotes mammary carcinogenesis and metastasis (51)
Undecanoic acid	++ (45)	?
Undecylenic acid	++ (45)	?
Butylated hydroxytoluene	+ (18, 22)	+ mouse lung tumor promoter (23); rat liver tumor promoter (24); + bladder tumor promoter (25)
Saccharin	+ (26, 27)	+ rat urinary bladder (28, 29)
Sodium cyclamate	+ (22, 30)	+ bladder tumor promoter (28)
Cholesterol	+ (31)	?
Cholesterol 5α, 6α epoxide	++ (32)	?
Cholesterol 5β, 5β epoxide	++ (32)	?
Cholestone 3β, 5α, 6β triol	++ (32)	?
Deoxycholic acid	++ (18)	+ rat liver tumor promoter (33); + rat colon promoter (34)
Lithocholic acid	++ (27, 18)	+ rat colon tumor promoter (35)
Taurodeoxycholic acid	− (18)	?
Retinoic acid	+ (36–39)	+ mouse skin tumor promoter (40)
1-Oleoyl-2-acetylglycerol	+ (41–43)	?
Phenobarbital	++ (52–55)	+ rat liver tumor promoter (24, 56)
Diphenylhydantoin	+ (52)	+ teratogen (57)

(*Continued on next page*)

Drugs	Modulator of intercellular communication[a]	Toxic end point[a]
Valium	++ (58)	+ mouse liver tumor promoter (59)
Methyl clofenapate	− (18)	?
Nafenopin	++ (18)	+ rat liver promoter (60)
[4-Chloro-(2,3-xylidino)2-pyrimidinylthio]acetic acid (Wy-14643)	++ (18)	+ hepatocellular carcinogen (61)
Gossypol	++ (62)	+ male reproductive toxicant (63) + rainbow trout liver tumor promoter (131)
Diethylstilbestrol	+ (132)	+ human vaginal adeno carcinoma (133); + promotion-like phenotypic effects on human endometrial stromal cells (134)
Reserpine	+ (135)	+ breast tumor promoter in pinealectomized rats (136)

Pollutants	Modulator of intercellular communication[a]	Toxic end point[a]
Polybromobiphenyls (mixture)	+++ (64)	+ rat liver tumor promoter (65–67)
2,4,5,2',4',5'-Hexabromobiphenyl	+++ (68)	+ rat liver tumor promoter (69)
2,4,5,3',4',5'-Hexabromobiphenyl	++ (68)	?
2,4,5,3',4'-Pentabromobiphenyl	+ (68)	?
3,4,5,3',5'-Pentabromobiphenyl	+ (68)	?
3,4,5,3',4',5'-Hexabromobiphenyl	− (68)	− rat liver tumor promoter at noncytotoxic levels; + rat liver tumor promoter at cytotoxic levels (70)
2,3,4,5,2',4',5'-Heptabromobiphenyl	+++ (68)	?
2,3,4,5,2',3',4',5'-Octobromobiphenyl	+++ (68)	?

Compound		
2,4,5,2',4',5'-Hexachlorobiphenyl	+++ (71)	+ rat liver tumor promoter (72)
3,4,5,3',4',5'-Hexachlorobiphenyl	– (71)	+ rat liver tumor promoter at cytotoxic levels (73)
Aroclor 1254 (polychlorinated biphenyl) (mixture)	+++ (55)	+ rat liver tumor promoter (74–77)
DDT	++ (54, 78–83)	liver tumor promoter (84–86), rat breast tumor promoter (87)
1,1-Dichloro-2,2-bis(p-chlorophenyl)ethane (TDE)	++ (80)	?
1,1,1-Trichloro-2-(O-chlorophenyl)-2-p-chlorophenyl)ethane (O-p'-DDT)	+ (80)	?
Methoxychlor	++ (80)	?
1,1-Dichloro-2,2-bis(p-chlorophenyl)ethane (DDE)	++ (80)	?
Dicofol	+ (79)	+ mouse liver carcinogen (88)
Phenol	– (22, 106, 107)	± non- or weak skin tumor promoter (108)[c]
Catechol	+ (22)	+ co-carcinogen in mouse skin (109)
Quinol	+ (22)	not a complete promoter in mouse skin (108)
Hydroxyquinol	+ (22)	?
Hydroquinone	+ (18)	?
Benzoyl peroxide	++ (110, 111)	+ mouse skin tumor promoter (110)
Ethylene glycol	+++ (112)	+ teratogen, reproductive toxicant (113–117)
Ethylene glycol monomethylether	+++ (112, 101)	+ teratogen, reproductive toxicant (113–117)
Ethylene glycol monoethylether	++ (112, 101)	+ teratogen, reproductive toxicant (113–117)
Ethylene glycol monobutylether	++ (112, 101)	+ teratogen, reproductive toxicant (113–117)
Ethylene glycol mono-n-propylether	++ (112, 101)	+ teratogen, reproductive toxicant (113–117)
Ethylene glycol mono-isopropylether	++ (101)	+ teratogen, reproductive toxicant (113–117)
Ethanol	+ (22, 106)	+ rat liver tumor promoter (118)
Anthralin	+ (119)	+ mouse skin tumor promoter (120)
Cigarette smoke condensate	+ (121)	+ mouse skin tumor promoter (122, 123)

(Continued on next page)

Pollutants	Modulator of intercellular communication[a]	Toxic end point[a]
α-Benzene hexachloride	+ (80)	+ rat liver tumor promoter (86)
γ-Benzene hexachloride	+ (80)	?
β-Benzene hexachloride	− (80)	?
Chlorobenzilate	+++ (79)	+ rat liver tumor promoter (86)
Bromopropylate	+++ (79)	?
Chloropylate	+++ (79)	?
Femarimol	+ (79)	?
Dieldrin	+++ (54, 80, 89)	+ rat liver tumor promoter (86, 90)
Aldrin	+++ (80, 89)	+ rat liver (86)
Endrin	+++ (80)	+ rat liver promoter (86)
Toxaphene	++ (89)	carcinogen (91)
Chlordane	++ (78, 82)	+ mouse liver tumor promoter (85)
Lindane	++ (78)	+ rat liver tumor promoter (86)
Heptachlor	++ (80, 82)	+ mouse liver tumor promoter (92)
Heptachlor epoxide	++ (18)	?
Trisodium nitrilotriacetate	++ (22)	+ kidney tumor promoter (93)
Kepone	++ (94)	+ rat and mouse liver carcinogen (95–97)
Mirex	++ (94)	+ rat and mouse liver carcinogen (96, 98)
2,4-Dinitrofluorobenzene	+++ (99)	+ skin tumor promoter (100)
Warfarin	++ (101)	+ human teratogen (102)
Di-(ethylhexyl)phthalate	+++ (103)	+ mouse liver tumor promoter (104, 105)
Carbon tetrachloride	+ (124)	+ rat liver tumor promoter (125)
n-Decane	+ (126)	mouse skin tumor promoter (127)
n-Tetradecane	+ (126)	mouse skin tumor promoter (127)

2,4,5-Trichlorophenoxyacetic acid	++ (128)	?
2,4-Dichlorophenoxyacetic acid	++ (128)	?
Lead acetate	++ (129)	+ rat renal tumor promoter (130)

The tabulation of chemicals has excluded several chemicals that have been tested in one of several cell-cell communications which have either tested negative or which have not been tested as carcinogens or tumor promoters. Because of the complexities of testing for inhibitors of intercellular communication in various types of assays (e.g., tissue, cell type and species specificities, metabolism of parent compounds, synergisms, antagonisms, receptor dependence, etc.), many negative results were not included. Moreover, several chemicals positive in the metabolic cooperation assay were not included because little in vivo toxicological studies have been made on these chemicals. In addition, no attempt was made to make an all-inclusive review of all the references related to the biological toxicities of each chemical.

[a]Numbers in parentheses indicate references.

[b]Intercellular communication can be inhibited by noncytotoxic or cytotoxic means. In the latter case, any chemical, by its cytotoxic action in the tissue, will cause surviving cells, because a decrease of intercellular communication, to go into regenerative hyperplasia.

[c]Some chemicals might need metabolism in order to inhibit intercellular communication.

References

1. Yotti, L.P., C.C. Chang, and J.E. Trosko. 1979. Elimination of metabolic cooperation in Chinese hamster cells by a tumor promoter. *Science* **206**: 1089.
2. Hecker, E. 1968. Cocarcinogenic principles from the seed oil of croton tiglium and from other Euphorbiaceae. *Cancer Res.* **28**: 2338.
3. Murray, A.W. and D.J. Fitzgerald. 1979. Tumor promoters inhibit metabolic cooperation in cocultures of epidermal and 3T3 cells. *Biochem. Biophys. Res. Commun.* **91**: 395.
4. Enomoto, T., Y. Sasaki, Y. Shiba, Y. Kanno, and H. Yamasaki. 1981. Tumor promoters cause a rapid and reversible inhibition of the formation and maintenance of electrical cell coupling in culture. *Proc. Natl. Acad. Sci.* **78**: 5628.
5. Newbold, R.F. and J. Amos. 1981. Inhibition of metabolic cooperation between mammalian cells in culture by tumor promoters. *Carcinogenesis* **2**: 243.
6. Mosser, D.O. and N.C. Bols. 1982. The effect of phorbols on metabolic cooperation between human fibroblasts. *Carcinogenesis* **3**: 1207.
7. Davidson, J.S., I.M. Baumgarten, and E.H. Harley. 1985. Effects of 12-O-tetradecanoylphorbol-13-acetate and retinoids on intercellular junctional communication measured with a citrulline incorporation assay. *Carcinogenesis* **6**: 645.
8. Hecker, E. and R. Schmidt. 1974. Phorbolesters: The irritants and cocarcinogens of croton Tiglium L. *Prog. Chem. Org. Nat. Prod.* **31**: 377.
9. Kreibich, G., R. Suss, and V. Kinzel. 1974. On the biochemical mechanism of tumorigenesis in mouse skin. V. Studies of the metabolism of tumor promoting and non-promoting phorbol derivatives in vivo and in vitro. *Z. Krebsforsch.* **81**: 135.
10. Rolin-Limbosch, S., W. Moens, and C. Szpirer. 1986. Effects of tumor promoters on metabolic cooperation between human hepatoma cells. *Carcinogenesis* **7**: 1235.
11. Hecker, E. 1978. Structure-activity relationships in diterpene esters irritant and cocarcinogenic to mouse skin. In *Carcinogenesis: Mechanisms of tumor promotion and cocarcinogenesis* (ed. T.J. Slaga et al.), vol. 2, p. 11. Raven Press, New York.
12. Schmidt, R. and E. Hecker. 1971. Untersuchungen uber die Bezidhungen zwischen struktur und wirkung von phorbolestern. In *Aktuelle Probleme aus dem Gebiet der Cancerologie* (ed. H. Lettre and G. Wagner). p. 98. Springer-Verlag, Berlin.
13. Thielmann, H.W. and E. Hecker. 1968. Beziehungen zwischen der struktur von phorbolderivaten und ihren entzundlichen und Tumorpromovierenden Eigenschaften, Fortschritte der Krebsforschung, p. 171. F.K. Schattauer, Verlag, Stuttgart.
14. Jone, C.M., J.E. Trosko, C.C. Chang, H. Fujiki, and T. Sugimura. 1982. Inhibition of intercellular communication in Chinese hamster V79 cells by teleocidin. *Gann* **73**: 874.
15. Fujiki, H., M. Suganuma, N. Matsukura, T. Sugimura, and S. Takayama. 1982. Teleocidin from streptomyces is a potent promoter of mouse skin carcinogenesis. *Carcinogenesis* **3**: 895.
16. Jone, C., L. Erickson, J.E. Trosko, and C.C. Chang. 1987. Effect of biological toxins on gap-junctional intercellular communication in Chinese hamster V79 cells. *Cell Biol. Toxicol.* **3**: 1.

(Continued on next page)

17. Fujiki, H., M. Suganuma, T. Tahira, A. Yoshioka, M. Nakayasu, Y. Endo, K. Shudo, S. Takayama, R.E. Moore, and T. Sugimura. 1984. New classes of tumor promoters: Teleocidin, aplysiatoxin and palytoxin. In *Cellular interactions by environmental tumor promoters* (ed. H. Fujiki et al.), p. 37. Japan Scientific Societies Press, Tokyo.

18. Trosko, J.E., L.P. Yotti, S.T. Warren, G. Tsushimoto, and C.C. Chang. 1982. Inhibition of cell-cell communication by tumor promoters. In *Carcinogenesis: Cocarcinogenesis and biological effects of tumor promoters* (ed. E. Hecker et al.), vol. 7, p. 565. Raven Press, New York.

19. Slaga, T.J., S.M. Fischer, K. Nelson, and G.L. Gleason. 1980. Studies on the mechanism of skin tumor promotion: Evidence for several stages in promotion. *Proc. Natl. Acad. Sci.* **72:** 3659.

20. Fujiki, H., M. Suganuma, M. Nakayasu, H. Hoshino, R.E. Moore, and T. Sugimura. 1982. The third class of new tumor promoters, polyacetates (debromoaplysiatoxin and aplysiatoxin), can differentiate biological actions relevant to tumor promoters. *Gann* **73:** 495.

21. Schoental, R., A.Z. Jaffe, and B. Yager. 1979. Cardiovascular lesions and various tumors found in rats given T-2 toxin, a trichotecane metabolite of Fusarium. *Cancer Res.* **39:** 2979.

22. Malcolm, A.R. and L.J. Mills. 1984. Effects of structurally diverse chemicals on metabolic cooperation in vitro. In *New approaches in toxicity testing and their application to human risk assessment* (ed. A.P. Li et al.), p. 79. Thomas, Springfield, Illinois.

23. Witschi, H.P. 1981. Enhancement of tumor formation in mouse lung by dietary butylated hydroxytoluene. *Toxicology* **21:** 95.

24. Peraino, C., R.J.M. Fry, E. Staffeldt, and J.P. Christopher. 1977. Enhancing effects of phenobarbitone and butylated hydroxytoluene on 2-acetyl-aminofluorene-induced hepatic tumorigenesis in the rat. *Food Cosmet. Toxicol.* **15:** 93.

25. Imaida, K., S. Fukushima, T. Shirai, T. Masui, T. Ogiso, and N. Ito. 1984. Promoting activities of butylated hydroxyanisole, butylated hydroxytoluene and sodium L-ascorbate on forestomach and urinary bladder carcinogenesis initiated with methylnitrosoureas in F344 male rats. *Gann* **75:** 769.

26. Umeda, M., K. Noda, and T. Ono. 1980. Inhibition of metabolic cooperation in Chinese hamster cells by various chemicals including tumor promoters. *Gann* **71:** 614.

27. Trosko, J.E., B. Dawson, L.P. Yotti, and C.C. Chang. 1980. Saccharin may act as a tumor promoter by inhibiting metabolic cooperation between cells. *Nature* **285:** 108.

28. Hicks, R.M., J.S. Wakefield, and J. Chowaniec. 1975. Evaluation of a new model to detect bladder carcinogens or co-carcinogens; results obtained with saccharin, cyclamate and cyclophosphamide. *Chem.-Biol. Interact.* **11:** 725.

29. Cohen, S.M., M. Arai, J.B. Jacobs, and G.H. Friedell. 1979. Promoting effect of saccharin and DL-tryptophan in urinary bladder carcinogenesis. *Cancer Res.* **39:** 1207.

30. Malcolm, A.R. and L.J. Mills. 1988. The potential role of bioactivation in tumor promotion: Indirect evidence from effects of phenol, sodium cyclamate and their metabolites on metabolic cooperation in vitro. In *Biochemical mechanisms and regulation of intercellular communication* (ed. H.A. Milman and E. Elmore). Princeton Scientific, Princeton, New Jersey. (In press.)

31. Meyer, R.A., B. Malewicz, W.J. Bauman, and R.G. Johnson. 1987. Changes in cell cholesterol alter gap junction function. In *Abstracts from the Symposium on gap junctions,* Asilomar, California.

32. Chang, C.C., C. Jone, J.E. Trosko, A.R. Peterson, and A. Sevanian. 1988. Effect of cholesterol epoxides on the inhibition of intercellular communication and on mutation induction in Chinese V79 cells. *Mutat. Res.* (in press).

33. Cameron, R., K. Imaida, and N. Ito. 1981. Promotive effects of deoxycholic acid on hepatocarcinogenesis initiated by diethylnitrosamine in male rats. *Gann* **72:** 635.

34. Reddy, B.S., T. Narasawa, J.H. Weisburger, and E.L. Wynder. 1976. Promoting effect of sodium deoxycholate on colon adenocarcinomas in germ free rats. *J. Natl. Cancer Inst.* **56:** 441.

35. Reddy, B.S. and K. Watanabe. 1979. Effect of cholesterol metabolites and promoting effect of lithocholic acid on colon carcinogenesis in germ-free and conventional F344 rats. *Cancer Res.* **39:** 1521.

36. Davidson, J.S., I.M. Baumgarten, and E.H. Harley. 1985. Effects of TPA and retinoids on intercellular junctional communication measured with a citrulline incorporation assay. *Carcinogenesis* **6:** 645.

37. Walder, L. and R. Lutzelschwab. 1984. Effects of TPA, retinoic acid and diazepam on intercellular communication in a monolayer of rat liver epithelial cells. *Exp. Cell Res.* **152:** 66.

38. Pitts, J.D., M.E. Finbow, T.E. Buultjens, A.E. Hamilton, and R.R. Burk. 1982. The gap junction channel. *Tokai J. Exp. Clin. Med.* **7:** 203.

39. Shuin, T., R. Nishimura, K. Noda, M. Umeda, and T. Ono. 1983. Concentration dependent differential effect of retinoic acid on intercellular metabolic cooperation. *Gann* **74**: 100.

40. Hennings, H., M.L. Wenk, and R. Donahoe. 1982. Retinoic acid promotion of papilloma formation in mouse skin. *Cancer Lett.* **16**: 1.

41. Davidson, J.S., I.M. Baumgarten, and E.H. Harley. 1985. Studies on the mechanism of phorbol ester-induced inhibition of intercellular junctional communication. *Carcinogenesis* **6**: 1353.

42. Gainer, H. St. C. and A.W. Murray. 1985. Diacylglycerol inhibits gap junctional communication in cultured epidermal cells: Evidence for a role of protein kinase C. *Biochem. Biophys. Res. Commun.* **126**: 1109.

43. Enomoto, T. and H. Yamasaki. 1985. Rapid inhibition of intercellular communication between BALB/c3T3 cells by diacylglycerol, a possible endogenous functional analogue of phorbol esters. *Cancer Res.* **45**: 3706.

44. Trosko, J., C. Jone, C. Aylsworth, and G. Tsushimoto. 1982. Elimination of metabolic cooperation is associated with the tumor promoters, oleic acid and anthralin. *Carcinogenesis* **3**: 1101.

45. Aylsworth, C.F., C.W. Welsch, J.J. Kabara, and J.E. Trosko. 1987. Effects of fatty acids on gap junctional communication: Possible role in tumor promotion by dietary fat. *Lipids* **22**: 445.

46. Carroll, K.K. and H.T. Khor. 1971. Effect of level and type of dietary fact on incidence of mammary tumors induced in female Sprague-Dawley rats by 7,12-dimethylbenz(a)anthracene. *Lipids* **6**: 415.

47. Ip, C., C.A. Carter, and M.M. Ip. 1985. Requirement of essential fatty acid for mammary tumorigenesis in the rat. *Cancer Res.* **45**: 1997.

48. VanDuuren, B.L. and B.M. Goldschmidt. 1976. Cocarcinogenic and tumor-promoting agents in tobacco carcinogenesis. *J. Natl. Cancer Inst.* **56**: 1237.

49. Reddy, B.S., T. Tanaka, and B. Simi. 1985. Effect of different levels of dietary trans fat or corn oil on azoxymethane-induced colon carcinogenesis in F344 rats. *J. Natl. Cancer Inst.* **75**: 791.

50. Holsti, P. 1959. Tumor promoting effects of some long-chain fatty acids in experimental skin carcinogenesis in the mouse. *Acta Pathol. Microbiol. Scand.* **46**: 51.

51. Erickson, K.L., D.S. Schlanger, D.A. Adams, D. Fregean, and J.S. Stern. 1984. Influence of dietary fatty acid concentration and geometric configuration on murine mammary tumorigenesis and experimental metastasis. *J. Nutr.* **114**: 1834.

52. Jone, C.M., L. Parker, J.E. Trosko, M. Netzloff, and C.C. Chang. 1986. Inhibition of metabolic cooperation by the anticonvulsants, diphenylhydantoin and phenobarbital. *Teratog. Carcinog. Mutagen.* **5**: 379.

53. Williams, G.M. 1980. Classification of genotoxic and epigenetic hepatocarcinogens using liver culture assays. *Ann. N.Y. Acad. Sci.* **349**: 273.

54. Ruch, R.J. and J.E. Klaunig. 1986. Effects of tumor promoter, genotoxic carcinogens and hepatocytotoxins on mouse hepatocyte intercellular communication. *Cell Biol. Toxicol.* **2**: 469.

55. Ruch, R.J., J.E. Klaunig, and M.A. Pereira. 1987. Inhibition of intercellular communication between mouse hepatocytes by tumor promoters. *Toxicol. Appl. Pharmacol.* **87**: 111.

56. Kitagawa, T. and H. Sugano. 1978. Enhancing effect of phenobarbital on the development of enzyme-altered islands and hepatocellular carcinomas initiated by 3'-methyl-4-(dimethylamino)azobenzene or diethylnitrosamine. *Gann* **69**: 679.

57. Hanson, J.W. and B.A. Buehler. 1982. Fetal hydantoin syndrome: Current status. *J. Pediatr.* **101**: 816.

58. Trosko, J.E. and D.F. Horrobin. 1980. The activity of diazepam in a Chinese hamster V79 lung cell assay for tumor promoters. *IRCS Med. Sci.* **8**: 887.

59. Diwan, B.A., J.M. Rice, and J.M. Ward. 1986. Tumor-promoting activity of benzodiazepine tranquilizers, diazepam and oxazepam in mouse liver. *Carcinogenesis* **7**: 789.

60. Preat, V., M. Lans, J. Gerlache, H. Taper, and M. Roberfroid. 1986. Comparison of the biological effects of phenobarbital and nafenopin on rat hepatocarcinogenesis. *Jpn. J. Cancer Res.* **77**: 629.

61. Rao, M.S., N.D. Lalwani, D.G. Scarpelli, and J.K. Reddy. 1982. The absence of γ-glutamyl transpeptidase activity in putative preneoplastic lesions and hepatocellular carcinomas induced in rats by the hypolipidemic peroxisone proliferator, Wy-14, 643. *Carcinogenesis* **3**: 1231.

62. Ye, Y.X., D. Bombick, K. Hirst, B.V. Madhukar, C.C. Chang, J.E. Trosko, and T. Akera. The effect of gossypol on cytotoxicity, mutagenicity and the modulation of gap junctional communication in various mammalian cell lines in vitro (in prep.)

63. Coutinho, E.M., J.F. Melo, I. Barbosa, and S.J. Segal. 1984. Antispermatogenic action of gossypol in men. *Fertil. Steril.* **42**: 424.

(*Continued on next page*)

64. Trosko, J.E., B. Dawson, and C.C. Chang. 1981. PBB inhibits metabolic cooperation in Chinese hamster cells in vitro: Its potential as a tumor promoter. *Environ. Health Perspect.* **37**: 179.

65. Jensen, R.K., S.D. Sleight, J.I. Goodman, S.D. Aust, and J.E. Trosko. 1982. Polybrominated biphenyls as promoters in experimental hepatocarcinogenesis in rats. *Carcinogenesis* **3**: 1183.

66. Jensen, R.K., S.D. Sleight, and S.D. Aust. 1984. Effect of varying the length of exposure to polybrominated biphenyls on the development of γ-glutamyl transpeptidase enzyme-altered foci. *Carcinogenesis* **5**: 63.

67. Rezabek, M.S., S.D. Sleight, R.K. Jensen, S.D. Aust, and D. Dixon. 1987. Short-term oral administration of polybrominated biphenyls enhances the development of hepatic-enzyme-altered foci in initiated rats. *J. Toxicol. Environ. Health* **20**: 347.

68. Tsushimoto, G., J.E. Trosko, C.C. Chang, and S.D. Aust. 1982. Inhibition of metabolic cooperation in chinese hamster V79 cells in culture by various polybrominated biphenyl (PBB) congeners. *Carcinogenesis* **3**: 181.

69. Jensen, R.K. and S.D. Sleight. 1986. Sequential study on the effects of 2,2′,4,4′,5,5′-hexabromomogiphenyl and 3,3′,4,4′,5,5′-hexabromogiphenyl on hepatic tumor promotion. *Carcinogenesis* **7**: 1771.

70. Jensen, R.K., S.D. Sleight, S.D. Aust, J.I. Goodman, and J.E. Trosko. 1983. Hepatic tumor-promoting ability of 3,3′,4,4′,5,5′-hexabromobiphenyl: The interrelationship between toxicity, induction of hepatic microsomal drug metabolizing enzymes, and tumor promoting ability. *Toxicol. Appl. Pharmacol.* **71**: 163.

71. Tsushimoto, G., S. Asano, J.E. Trosko, and C.C. Chang. 1983. Inhibition of intercellular communication by various congeners of polybrominated biphenyl and polychlorinated biphenyl. In *PCB's: Human and environmental hazards* (ed. F.M. D'Itri and M.A. Kamrin), p. 241. Butterworth, Boston.

72. Sleight, S.D., R.K. Jensen, and M.S. Rezabek. 1987. Enhancement of hepatocarcinogenesis in rats by simultaneous administration of 2,4,5,2′,4′,5′-hexachlorobiphenyl and 2,3,7,8-tetrachlorodibenzo-p-dioxin. *Toxicologist* **7**: 103.

73. Evans, M.G. and S.D. Sleight. 1984. Potential for 2,2′,4,4′,5,5′-hexachlorobiphenyl and 3,3′,4,4′,5,5′-hexachlorobiphenyl to induce hepatic enzyme-altered foci in rats. *Fed. Proc.* **43**(3): (Abstr. 1789).

74. Hirose, M., T. Shirai, H. Tsuda, S. Fukushima, T. Ogiso, and N. Ito. 1981. Effect of phenobarbital, polychlorinated biphenyl and sodium saccharin on hepatic and renal carcinogenesis in unilaterally nephrectomized rats given N-ethyl-N-hydroxyethylnitrosamine orally. *Carcinogenesis* **2**: 1299.

75. Pereira, M.A., S.L. Herren, A.L. Britt, and M.M. Khoury. 1982. Promotion by polychlorinated biphenyls of enzyme-altered foci in rat liver. *Cancer Lett.* **15**: 185.

76. Demi, E. and D. Oesterle. 1987. Dose-response of promotion by polychlorinated biphenyls and chloroform in rat liver foci bioassay. *Arch. Toxicol.* **60**: 209.

77. Preston, B.D., J.P. VanMiller, R.W. Moore, and J.R. Allen. 1981. Promoting effects of polychlorinated biphenyls (Aroclor 1254) and free Aroclor 1254 on diethylnitrosamine-induced tumorigenesis in the rat. *J. Natl. Cancer Inst.* **66**: 509.

78. Tsushimoto, G., C.C. Chang, J.E. Trosko, and F. Matsumura. 1983. Cytotoxic, mutagenic and cell-cell communication inhibitory properties of DDT, Lindane and chlordane on Chinese hamster cells in vitro. *Arch. Environ. Contam. Toxicol.* **12**: 721.

79. Warngard, L., S. Flodstrom, S. Ljungquist, and U.G. Ahlborg. 1985. Inhibition of metabolic cooperation in Chinese hamster lung fibroblast cells (V79) in culture by various DDT-analogs. *Arch. Environ. Contam. Toxicol.* **14**: 541.

80. Kurata, M., K. Hirose, and M. Umeda. 1982. Inhibition of metabolic cooperation in Chinese hamster cells by organochlorine pesticides. *Gann* **73**: 217.

81. Williams, G.M., S. Telang, and C. Tong. 1981. Inhibition of intercellular communication between liver cells by the liver tumor promoter 1,1,1-trichloro2,2-bis(p-chlorophenyl)ethane. *Cancer Lett.* **11**: 339.

82. Telang, S., C. Tong, and G.M. Williams. 1982. Epigenetic membrane effects of a possible tumor promoting type on cultured liver cells by the nongenotoxic organochlorine pesticides chlordane and heptachlor. *Carcinogenesis* **3**: 1175.

83. Xiang, L.Z., T. Kavanagh, J.E. Trosko, and C.C. Chang. 1986. Inhibition of gap junctional intercellular communication in human teratocarcinoma cells by organochlorine pesticides. *Toxicol. Appl. Pharmacol.* **83**: 10.

84. Peraino, C., R.J.M. Fry, E. Staffeldt, and J.P. Christopher. 1975. Comparative enhancing effects of phenobarbital, amobarbital, diphenylhydantoin, and dichlorodiphenyltrichloroethane on s-acetylaminofluorene-induced hepatic tumorigenesis in the rat. *Cancer Res.* **35**: 2884.

85. Williams, G.M. and S. Numoto. 1984. Promotion of mouse liver neoplasms by the organochlorine pesticides chlordane and heptachlor in comparison to dichlorodiphenyl-trichloroethane. *Carcinogenesis* **5**: 1689.

86. Ito, N., M. Tatematsu, K. Nakanishi, R. Husegawa, T. Takano, K. Imaida, and T. Ogiso. 1980. The effects of various chemicals on the development of hyperplastic liver nodules in hepatectomized rats treated with N-nitrosodiethylamine or N-2-fluorenylacetamide. *Gann* **71**: 832.

87. Scribner, J.D. and N.K. Mottet. 1981. DDT acceleration of mammary gland tumor induced in the male Sprague-Dawley rat by 2-acetamidophenanthrene. *Carcinogenesis* **2**: 1235.

88. IARC (International Agency for Research on Cancer). 1983. Miscellaneous pesticides. *IARC Monogr. Eval. Carcinog. Chem. Hum.* **30**: 73.

89. Trosko, J.E., C. Jone, and C.C. Chang. 1987. Inhibition of gap junctional-mediated intercellular communication in vitro by aldrin, dieldrin and toxaphene: A possible cellular mechanism for their tumor-promoting and neurotoxic effects. *Mol. Toxicol.* **1**: 83.

90. Tennekes, H.A., L. Edler, and H.W. Kunz. 1982. Dose-response analysis of the enhancement of the liver tumor formation in CF-1 mice by dieldrin. *Carcinogenesis* **3**: 941.

91. Reuber, M.D. 1979. Carcinogenicity of toxaphene: A review. *J. Toxicol. Environ. Health* **5**: 729.

92. Pereira, M.A., S.L. Herren, A.L. Britt, and M.M. Khoury. 1982. Sex differences in enhancement of GGTase-positive foci by hexachlorobenzene and lindane in rat liver. *Cancer Lett.* **15**: 95.

93. Hiasa, Y., Y. Kitahori, N. Konishi, N. Enoki, T. Shimoyama, and A. Miyashiro. 1984. Trisodium nitrilotriacetate monohydrate: Promoting effects on the development of renal tubular cell tumors in rats treated with N-ethyl-N-hydroxyethylnitrosamine. *J. Natl. Cancer Inst.* **72**: 483.

94. Tsushimoto, G., J.E. Trosko, C.C. Chang, and F. Matsumura. 1982. Inhibition of intercellular communication by chlordecone (Kepone) and Mirex in Chinese hamster V79 cells in vitro. *Toxicol. Appl. Pharmacol.* **64**: 550.

95. Guzelian, P.S. 1982. Comparative toxicology of chlordecone (kepone) in humans and experimental animals. *Annu. Rev. Pharmacol. Toxicol.* **22**: 89.

96. Sugar, J., K. Toth, E. Czuka, E. Gati, and S. Somfai-Relle. 1979. Role of pesticides in hepatocarcinogenesis. *J. Toxicol. Environ. Health* **5**: 183.

97. Reuber, M.D. 1979. The carcinogenicity of kepone. *J. Environ. Pathol. Toxicol.* **2**: 671.

98. Ulland, B.M., N.P. Page, R.A. Squire, E.K. Weisburger, and R.L. Cypher. 1977. A carcinogenicity assay of mirex in Charles River CD rats. *J. Natl. Cancer Inst.* **58**: 133.

99. Warren, S.T., D.J. Doolittle, C.C. Chang, J.I. Goodman, and J.E. Trosko. 1982. Evaluation of the carcinogenic potential of 2,4-dinitrofluorobenzene and its implication regarding mutagenicity testing. *Carcinogenesis* **3**: 139.

100. Bock, F.G., A. Fielde, H.W. Fox, and E. Klein. 1969. Tumor promotion by 1-fluoro-2,4-dinitrobenzene, a potent skin sensitizer. *Cancer Res.* **27**: 179.

101. Welsch, F. and D.B. Stedman. 1984. Inhibition of metabolic cooperation between Chinese hamster V79 cells by structurally diverse teratogens. *Teratog. Carcinog. Mutagen.* **4**: 285.

102. Kleinebrecht, J. 1982. Zur teratogenitat von cumarin-derivaten. *Dtsch. Med. Wochenschr.* **107**: 1932.

103. Malcolm, A.R., L.J. Mills, and E.J. McKenna. 1983. Inhibition of metabolic cooperation between Chinese hamster V79 cells by tumor promoters and other chemicals. *Ann. N.Y. Acad. Sci.* **407**: 488.

104. Ward, J.M., M. Ohshima, P. Lynch, and C. Riggs. 1984. Di(2-ethylhexyl)phthalate but not phenobarbital promotes N-nitrosodiethylamine-initiated hepatocellular proliferative lesions after short-term exposure in male B6C3F1 mice. *Cancer Lett.* **24**: 49.

105. Ward, J.M., J.M. Rice, D. Creasia, P. Lynch, and C. Riggs. 1983. Dissimilar patterns of promotion by di(2-ethylhexyl)phthalate and phenobarbital of hepatocellular neoplasia initiated by diethyl-nitrosamine in B6C3F1 mice. *Carcinogenesis* **8**: 1021.

106. Malcolm, A.R., L.J. Mills, and E.J. McKenna. 1985. Effects of phorbolmyrisate acetate, phorbol dibutyrate, ethanol, dimethylsulfoxide, phenol, and seven metabolites of phenol on metabolic cooperation between Chinese hamster V79 lung fibroblasts. *Cell Biol. Toxicol.* **1**: 269.

107. Chen, T.H., T.J. Kavanagh, C.C. Chang, and J.E. Trosko. 1984. Inhibition of metabolic cooperation in Chinese hamster V79 cells by various organic solvents and simple compounds. *Cell. Biol. Toxicol.* **1**: 155.

108. Boutwell, R.K. and D.K. Bosch. 1959. The tumor-promoting action of phenol and related compounds for mouse skin. *Cancer Res.* **19**: 413.

109. Hecht, S.S., S. Carmella, H. Mori, and D. Hoffmann. 1981. A study of tobacco carcinogenesis. XX. Role of catechol as a major cocarcinogen in the weakly acidic fraction of smoke condensate. *J. Natl. Cancer Inst.* **66**: 163.

110. Slaga, J., A.J. Klein-Szantos, L.L. Triplett, L.P. Yotti, and J.E. Trosko. 1981. Skin-tumor-promoting activity of benzoyl peroxide, a widely used free radical-generating compound. *Science* **213**: 1023.

111. Lawrence, N.J., E.K. Parkinson, and A. Emmerson. 1984. Benzoyl peroxide interferes with metabolic cooperation between cultured human epidermal keratinocytes. *Carcinogenesis* **5**: 419.

(*Continued on next page*)

112. Loch-Caruso, R., J.E. Trosko, and I.A. Corcos. 1984. Interruption of cell-cell communication in Chinese hamster V79 cells by various alkyl glycol ethers: Implications for teratogenicity. *Environ. Health Perspect.* **57**: 119.

113. Anonymous. 1982. The toxicology of ethylene glycol monoalkyl ethers and its relevance to man. European Chemical Industry Ecology and Toxicology Center, Belgium, Brussels, Technical Report No. 4, p. 55.

114. Hardin, B.D. 1982. Antifertility effects in rodents following treatment with alkylethers of ethylene glycol. *Arch. Androl.* **9**: 49.

115. Nagano, K., E. Nakayama, H. Oobayashi, T. Yamada, H. Adachi, T. Nishizama, H. Ozawa, M. Nakaichi, H. Okuda, K. Minami, and K. Yamazaki. 1981. Embryotoxic effects of ethylene glycol monomethylether in mice. *Toxicology* **20**: 335.

116. Hardin, B.D., R.W. Niemeier, R.J. Smith, M.H. Kuczuk, P.R. Mathinos, and T.F. Weaver. 1982. Teratogenicity of 2-ethoxyethanol by dermal application. *Drug. Chem. Toxicol.* **5**: 277.

117. Nelson, B.K., W.S. Brightwell, J.V. Setzer, B.J. Taylor, and R.W. Hothung. 1981. Ethoxyethanol behavioral teratology in rats. *Neurotoxicology* **2**: 231.

118. Driver, H.E. and A.E.M. McLeon. 1986. Dose-response relationship for initiation of rat liver tumors by diethylnitrosamine and promotion by phenobarbitone or alcohol. *Food Chem. Toxicol.* **24**: 241.

119. Trosko, J.E., C. Jone, C. Aylsworth, and G. Tsushimoto. 1982. Elimination of metabolic cooperation is associated with the tumor promoters, oleic acid and anthalin. *Carcinogenesis* **3**: 1101.

120. VanDuuren, B.L., G. Witz, and B.M. Goldschmidt. 1978. Structure–activity relationships of tumor promoters and cocarcinogens and interaction of phorbol myristate acetate and related esters with plasma membranes. In *Carcinogenesis—A comprehensive survey* (ed. T.J. Slaga et al.), vol. 2, p. 491. Raven Press, New York.

121. Hartman, T.G. and J.D. Rosen. 1983. Inhibition of metabolic cooperation by cigarette smoke condensate and its fractions in V79 Chinese hamster lung fibroblasts. *Proc. Natl. Acad. Sci.* **80**: 5305.

122. VanDuuren, B.L., A. Sivak, C. Katz, and S. Melchionne. 1971. Cigarette smoke carcinogenesis: Importance of tumor promoters. *J. Natl. Cancer Inst.* **47**: 235.

123. McGregor, J.F. 1982. Enhancement of skin tumorigenesis by cigarette smoke condensate following β-irradiation in rats. *J. Natl. Cancer Inst.* **68**: 605.

124. Saez, J.C., M.V.L. Bennett, and D.C. Spray. 1987. Carbon tetrachloride at hepatotoxic levels blocks reversibly gap junctions between rat hepatocytes. *Science* **236**: 967.

125. Solt, D.B., E. Cayama, H. Tsuda, K. Enomoto, G. Lee, and E. Farber. 1983. Promotion of liver cancer development by brief exposure to dietary 2-acetylamino-fluorene plus partial hepatectomy or carbon tetrachloride. *Cancer Res.* **43**: 188.

126. Lankas, G.R., C.S. Baxter, and R.T. Christian. 1978. Effect of alkane tumor promoting agents on chemically induced mutagenesis in cultured V79 Chinese hamster cells. *J. Toxicol. Environ. Health* **4**: 37.

127. VanDuuren, B.L. and B.M. Goldschmidt. 1976. Cocarcinogenic and tumor-promoting agents in tobacco carcinogenesis. *J. Natl. Cancer Inst.* **56**: 1237.

128. Rubinstein, C., C. Jone, J.E. Trosko, and C.C. Chang. 1984. Inhibition of intercellular communication in cultures of Chinese hamster V79 cells by 2,4-Dichlorophenoxyacetic acid and 2,4,5-Trichlorophenoxy acetic acid. *Fundam. Appl. Toxicol.* **4**: 731.

129. Caruso, R.L., I.A. Corcos, and J.E. Trosko. Inhibition of metabolic cooperation by soluble metal compounds. (Submitted).

130. Shirai, T., M. Ohshima, A. Masuda, S. Tamano, and N. Ito. 1984. Promotion of 2-(ethylnitrosamino)ethanol-induced renal carcinogenesis in rats by nephrotoxic compounds: Positive responses with folic acid, basic lead acetate and N-(3-5-dichlorophenyl)seccinimide but not with 2,3-dibromo-1-propenol phosphate. *J. Natl. Cancer Inst.* **72**: 477.

131. Sinnhuber, R.O., D.J. Lee, J.H. Wales, and J.L. Ayres. 1968. Dietary factors and hepatoma in rainbow trout. II. Cocarcinogenesis by cyclopropenoid fatty acids and the effect of gossypol and altered lipids on aflatoxin-induced liver cancer. *J. Natl. Cancer. Inst.* **41**: 1293.

132. Burghardt, R.C., D. Gaddy-Kurten, R.L. Burghardt, R.C. Kurten, and P.A. Mitchell. 1987. Gap junction modulation in rat uterus. *Biol. Reprod.* **36**: 741.

133. Herbst, A.L., D.C. Paskanzer, S.J. Robboy, L. Friedlander, and R.E. Scully. 1975. Prenatal exposure to diethylstilbesterol: A prospective comparison of exposed female offspring with unexposed controls. *N. Engl. J. Med.* **292**: 334.

134. Siegfried, J.M., K.G. Nelson, J.L. Martin, and D.G. Kaufman. 1984. Promotion effect of diethylstilbesterol on human endometrial stromal cells pretreated with a direct-acting carcinogen. *Carcinogenesis* **5**: 641.

135. Elmore E. Pers. comm.

136. Lapin, V. 1978. Effects of reserpine on the incidence of 9,10, dimethyl-1,2 benzanthracane induced tumors in pinealectomized and thymectomizal rats. *Oncology* **35**: 132.

Commentary

W. GARY FLAMM
U.S. Environmental Protection Agency
Washington, D.C.

Flamm: The first question is: Why is the application of molecular data to quantitative risk analysis perceived as a useful exercise to anyone? I am going to give a simple answer to that: it is because the usual, ordinary quantitative risk assessment (QRA) is believed by many people to vastly overstate the real risk in most situations with most compounds.

Why is that believed? It is obviously not believed by everyone, but I am giving you simple answers to simple questions. The simple answer to why it is believed to greatly overstate the risk is because of the many conservative scientific assumptions that are made, such as the use of the most-sensitive sex and the most-sensitive species or the most-sensitive strain, the use of upper confidence limits, the use of upper bound estimates of exposure, and assumptions about lifetime exposure. Also, QRA is often thought to overestimate because the dose response is often not believed to be linear throughout the entire range of its extrapolation from high dose to low dose. In some cases, the belief that there is a secondary mechanism of carcinogenesis that, if it can be properly shown mechanistically, will be found to involve some sort of biological event at threshold, so that there would be zero risk at doses above zero but below the threshold.

Some recent good examples of chemicals on which molecular data have been developed for QRA purposes include: saccharin and bladder cancer, formaldehyde and cancer of the nasal turbinates, methylene chloride and cancer of liver and lung, and butylated hydroxyanisole (BHA), which produces cancer of the forestomach.

If you apply traditional risk assessment to these four compounds, for saccharin you would have a calculated risk of about 10^{-4} under normal use conditions; for formaldehyde in an occupational setting, the risk would be 10^{-2}; methylene chloride, under the worst occupational conditions, perhaps 10^{-2}. These are the risks derived from using the traditional, if I can call it traditional, standard QRA, which has embedded in it all of these conservative scientific assumptions and essentially the use of a linearized extrapolation model, or, at least, a model that has a linear component that begins soon after you get away from the observable data. BHA, under normal use conditions, would have a risk of about 10^{-4}.

Banbury Report 31: Carcinogen Risk Assessment: New Directions in the Qualitative and Quantitative Aspects © Cold Spring Harbor Laboratory. 0-87969-231-6/88. $1.00 + .00

Starting with BHA, the contention on the part of those who believe BHA is safe is, first, built around the fact that it has an exceedingly steep dose-response curve. At 2% in the diet, it produces 100% carcinomas and papillomas of the squamous lining of the forestomach. At a quarter of that dose, 0.5%, it produces no tumors at all. This is quite a reproducible observation. So, there can be no question that the slope of the dose-response curve is extraordinarily steep.

Dr. Clayson has done extensive work on this subject. I think he has a considerable amount of evidence that relates certain early changes that may serve as a threshold for the late occurring events of tumors and papillomas and that has excellent correlations between the doses that produce the early changes with the doses that result subsequently in tumors and papillomas.

I believe that, if ever there was a compound where the evidence was in strong support of some kind of obligatory toxic mechanism that is necessary and partially responsible for the development of tumors and cancers, BHA is certainly an excellent case example and may be, in fact, the best that we have to offer.

Relative to saccharin, many mechanistic studies have been done. None of them have succeeded in establishing a link between the cancer that forms ultimately in chronic study and the various physiological, or perhaps pathological, changes that occurred early in the experiment.

The one thing that has been established with saccharin is it too has a moderately steep dose-response. In a study done two or three years ago at IRDC, a typical carcinogenicity experiment was run with an untypical design. This was a design where there were a few animals in high dose where enough cancer was being seen that the confidence intervals were quite good. However, at the lower doses, they went up to nearly 1000 animals in a single group. They were able to establish from this unbalanced design that saccharin, indeed, has a moderately steep dose-response curve.

The reason for the moderately steep dose-response curve, however, is not understood. The reason for saccharin's carcinogenicity is not understood. After hearing James (Trosko), a question that I have, which perhaps he could answer, is the following: Has anyone looked at what saccharin does to gap junctions?

Trosko: It was on the list. It is positive. It has a high threshold. You have to use tons of it to break it.

Flamm: However, you have to use tons of it to produce cancer, as well. I don't know what the possibilities are for looking at saccharin's effect in the urothelium of the bladder in vivo, but if that could be done, it would certainly be of great interest.

The one thing that I would point out about saccharin is that, although it does have a moderately steep dose-response curve, it is clear from work done at NCTR with an initiated bladder that it does act as a promoting agent and will promote at concentrations that are far below the concentrations of saccharin required to produce cancer when it is given by itself. There again, it may raise some interesting speculation and hypotheses about what might be occurring in that combination or that regimen, as opposed to saccharin alone with respect to gap junction closing and opening.

Formaldehyde is, I think, an absolutely fascinating chemical. Again, it has been studied extensively, principally at CIIT. It is apparent that it, too, has a very steep dose-response curve. Its adducts and cross-links have been studied as has its repair and the significance of cell turnover to eventual cancer outcome. There are a number of critical questions and issues that relate to which is most important in terms of cancer induction, the concentration of formaldehyde or the total dose of formaldehyde.

I think formaldehyde is a good example of a compound where, if sensitive enough techniques existed, it might be possible to look down the dose response curve and get a much better idea when it would leave its free-falling dose response and begin to enter a more linearized area.

Singer: Formaldehyde is a reversible reaction. You do not get adducts. It's a different mechanism.

Flamm: They have isolated cross-links.

Singer: Cross-links, methyl-O cross-links, yes, but it does not form adducts.

Flamm: We'll discuss the cross-links. For methylene chloride, the whole thrust to obtain relief from the very high risk values derived from quantitative risk assessment has been on physiologically based pharmacokinetics. The entire issue is premised on knowing the mechanism, or believing that you know the mechanism, by which methylene chloride induces cancer of the liver and lung in mice. The idea is that the glutathione transferase pathway is the critical pathway for generating a glutathione methylene chloride mustard-type compound that then can alkylate DNA. The mixed function oxidase pathway is envisaged as one that simply inactivates and detoxifies methylene chloride. So, the question, then, in part at least, concerns the competition between these two pathways and what happens to that competition as you go down to lower and lower dosages. Also at issue is the difference between the ratio of those two pathways.

I think probably the most important thing to say on all this is that we are entering a new era, where a far more complicated and involved science is beginning to affect the judgments that regulatory agencies are going to have to make. Right now, we don't really have a good process or a good system for doing that.

I think we can all expect that this is going to be a very dynamic period. It is going to be incumbent upon the regulatory agencies to recognize the difference between theories and hypotheses and data and substance that meets their own standard, whatever that standard may be.

Setlow: We do have a number of panelists who will speak to very different aspects of these subjects.

Panel Discussion

MURRAY S. COHN
U.S. Consumer Product Safety Commission, Washington, D.C.

FREDERICK A. BELAND
National Center for Toxicological Research, Arkansas

KENNETH KRAEMER
National Cancer Institute, Maryland

RAYMOND W. TENNANT
National Institute of Environmental Health Sciences, North Carolina

Cohn: I always look at dose-response curves and high-to-low-dose extrapolation. I am going to try to restrict my comments to those subjects. When one looks at initiators, our job has been a little easier because we can work under a hypothesis that the amount of an initiator that is present is somehow related to carcinogenic response.

The multistage theory that we have utilized, right or wrong as it may be, usually regards initiation as one of the original steps. There have been some theories now that direct DNA damage may occur later on in the carcinogenic process as well.

In the NTP and NCI and other type bioassays, when animals are treated with high doses, the chemicals can have multiple actions. There can be initiation. At a high enough dose, promotional events may also be caused. At such a high dose, chemicals may cause a second initiative event. However, at those very, very high doses, a lot of things are occurring. Some might say that's a detraction of the bioassay. It's also a strength, because it can detect the types of actions that might not be detectable at low doses.

So, the problem is what happens when you consider humans at low doses? Well, humans, unfortunately, live in a sea of promotion, a sea of initiation. Probably a large number of my cells are already in some transformed state. However, within that background, the chemical doesn't have to do everything that it did in the bioassay to affect the carcinogenic process. If, at low doses, the effect of an exogenous chemical initiator is much lower than the effect of the entire background process that is ongoing, then you can understand why we believe in linearity at low dose. For a very small effect added into this process, if it is doubled the ultimate risk is doubled, because the much larger background process will transform to a final carcinogenic state with a constant probability with respect to the small effect. The chemical itself

Banbury Report 31: Carcinogen Risk Assessment: New Directions in the Qualitative and Quantitative Aspects © Cold Spring Harbor Laboratory. 0-87969-231-6/88. $1.00 + .00
   175

might only have to cause the initiative event, and background does the rest.

To reflect this, we have either just been using straight lines at low dose or trying to get an idea of the amount of active metabolite at low dose using pharmacokinetic models and the like, to try to get at the relationship between an important initiator and an important response in this case at a specific active site or at multiple active sites.

For "nongenotoxic" or "epigenetic" activities of chemicals, the issue is much more difficult. I will use an example and assume that gap junction inhibitors are important in the carcinogenic process, which I think is a very possible situation. Looking at a dose-response relationship, was Dr. Trosko's gap junction inhibition linear?

Trosko: It's not. All of the chemicals that were tested all have no-effect, i.e., a threshold.

Cohn: All right. If it's definitely not linear or threshold, then there is an immediate complication because of the interaction of the dose-response curve with an area-under-the-curve type of analysis for the active species. The latter is necessary because we don't usually deal with constant exposure in the human situation. We usually deal with intermittent exposures. There might be an exposure for one hour, then an exposure for another hour the next day. There might be some of the chemical left in the body after 24 hours or the chemical might be totally cleared out of the system. Thus, what is needed to reach a threshold may change as exposures continue, depending on the situation. Mathematically, you must superimpose an area under the curve analysis for the biologically active concentration on top of the nonlinear dose-response curve, which leads to the complication I referred to if a threshold applies.

Another consideration is the length of time to see an effect at a specific point on the dose-response curve. If the gap junction inhibitor is in the air or food supply, there would be constant exposure. Even though the reaction might be reversible, the chemical is there at all times, so eventually you may observe an effect that would not occur from a short duration of exposure. That is, at a given dose for an hour, there may be no clonal expansion or other effect caused by inhibiting the gap junction communication. You might get the effect after long exposure to that dose. Another consideration is are there background processes causing gap junction inhibition that are additive to that of the specific chemical?

So, there are at least three different mathematical functions interacting with one another. This is a formidable task in order to account for gap junction inhibition in the risk assessment process. However, I think that the research community has the ability to provide the necessary data to accomplish this task.

One interesting research idea in this area would be to ascertain the potency of gap junction inhibitors as inhibitors versus their carcinogenic potencies in bioassays. Some sort of a correlation like that would be very interesting to see.

Wilson: Given what you have just said about high-dose processes being multivariant and probably nonlinear, how can you apply a linear extrapolation from these high-dose nonlinear processes?

Cohn: Easily. I'll use formaldehyde as an example because it's the most nonlinear one that I know of. This can be shown mathematically. If cancer is due to a multistage process, where formaldehyde is causing a number of things to occur, as there is an increase in a three-, four-, five-stage process in each step.

Wilson: Wait a minute. It's not multistage. They are going on simultaneously. They're not sequential, in the sense of the mathematics from which they are derived.

Cohn: That's true. However, as you increase the probability that each stage will occur, and you multiply those out, you have a nonlinear expectation on the total probability that the event will occur. For high-dose data, I don't take a straight line from such data and draw it down to the origin. I draw the line once the dose is below the high-dose nonlinearity. This is what Kenny Crump's models do, waiting until high-dose nonlinearity ends before imposing linear terms. So, the model is consistent with the high-dose data. Then, you force linearity to account for background additivity when you get below nontested doses. As far as I'm concerned, that's consistent.

Setlow: Jim Trosko, what do your data say? Is there a threshold for these gap junction effects?

Trosko: Absolutely. It's not a one-hit event. Every cell has multiple gap junctions. In the case, for example, with calcium-modifying gap junctions, you have to use a chemical, like an iontophore of some sort, at a certain level before you change the calcium level high enough to close the gap junction. There's a biochemical basis for its nonlinearity.

Cohn: We were talking about initiators. Gap junction inhibition would require the type of analysis I described.

Setlow: If the net effect was the product of a number of these curves, then it's a very simple process if one has a threshold.

Hart: There's only one problem that bothers me about Jim's (Trosko) statement. You say that there is a threshold, but in a whole animal system, not in a cell culture, gap junctions—dysjunctions, actually—are continuously occurring. In other words, you have a certain degree of dysjunctions that normally occur within the whole animal. So, really, you are overlaying an induced change, which would be from your promoters, onto a normally occurring change. In other words, a background level in vivo. The questions are: Where do you really in vivo, not in vitro, have this intersect, and do you actually see a threshold in the situation in vivo as opposed to in vitro?

Trosko: That can be tested. I'm glad you brought this up. Samuel Cohen has studied gap junctions in bladder tumors but in a complete carcinogen model. He can easily do that with saccharin, for example.

Hart: I don't know of anyone who has done that.

Trosko: Nobody has done that.

Hart: So, really, when you say, "Yes, there is definitely a threshold," you are talking about in vitro and not in vivo.

Trosko: That's right.

Cohn: That affects the interaction with background we talked about originally.

Setlow: There is also a background of initiation.

Hart: Exactly.

Setlow: Do you have a simple statement?

Perera: I hope it's simple. It really relates to something that Dr. Flamm said, as well as Murray (Cohn). Dr. Flamm mentioned that the conventional risk assessment methods are generally viewed as significantly overestimating human risk. Yet, we have been hearing, as you, Dr. Setlow, mentioned, the problem of the very important interindividual variation in response to exposures and differences in susceptibility between individuals. That is not accounted for in the conventional models. Correct me if I'm wrong, Dr. Flamm.

The other thing that also isn't plugged into the conventional risk assessment model is the fact that you might have greater than additive effects. The model does account for additivity on background, but not necessarily for a multiplicity of synergistic or antagonistic effects. In that sense, I am not sure that we can be so sanguine, but that we are always overestimating risk using this approach.

Setlow: We don't really want to take up this question. Suppose we put it on hold for the moment, whether we are overestimating or underestimating, until some of the models appear. That would then be appropriate.

I want to go on to some data. I think Fred Beland has some data.

* * *

Beland: Yesterday, Murray Cohn asked me how I would apply DNA adduct measurements to humans. My reply was rather pessimistic. Today I would like to tell you why.

The basic problem is that we have not studied animal models adequately. We have not studied adduct formation under chronic administration using conditions that result in tumor induction. The basic reason for that is that in the past we have had to use radiolabeled carcinogens, which restricted us to administering single or at most a few doses. In the last few years alternate methods of DNA adduct detection have been developed based upon immunoassays and ^{32}P-postlabeling. With these techniques it is now possible to administer carcinogens chronically and relate adduct formation and removal to a tumorigenic response. These results should then allow us to use human DNA adduct data to make some type of a risk estimation.

Today I would like to show you the results from our first dose-response experiment, where we chronically administered a carcinogen. The animal we used was the BALB/c mouse and the carcinogen was 2-acetylaminofluorene. We have used an antibody to detect adduct formation. This antibody was developed by Miriam Poirier, with whom I have collaborated in this and other studies, and it is specific for the major, if not only, adduct detected in mice.

There have been very few experiments conducted where tumor induction has been examined over a wide dose range. One was conducted by Peto using diethylnitrosamine, and recently Swenberg has examined the DNA adduct concentrations under a similar dose regimen. Another study was the EDO1 experiment, which was conducted at the National Center for Toxicological Research some years ago. In that study, 2-

acetylaminofluorene was administered over the lifespan of female BALB/c mice at doses up to 150 ppm in the diet. Under these conditions, liver tumor induction was linearly related to dose. This was not the case with bladder tumors where an apparent threshold was observed at low doses.

One interpretation of these data is that as you decrease the dose you reach a point at which the liver effectively detoxifies all the 2-acetylaminofluorene that is ingested. Thus, activated 2-acetylaminofluorene metabolites would not get to the bladder. This can be tested quite readily by examining the concentration of the DNA adducts.

In our experiment, we used the same doses used in the EDO1 study. The animals were fed for only one month, but from other experiments we know that steady-state conditions are reached by this time. What we observed in the liver was a linear relationship between the administered dose and the adduct concentration. Therefore, the adduct concentrations in the liver are quite predictive of the eventual tumor incidence in this organ. Interestingly, we also obtained a linear relationship between the administered dose and the adduct concentrations in the bladder. Furthermore, the adduct concentrations were fourfold higher in the bladder. Since there was an apparent threshold for bladder tumor induction, the relationship between adduct concentration and tumor incidence is not straightforward for this tissue.

Our interpretation of these data at present is that in the liver the limiting factor for tumors is the formation of DNA adducts. That is, there is a sufficient promotional stimulus for liver tumor induction in the mouse if the cells become initiated as a result of adduct formation. This is not the case in the bladder. Based on the adduct levels observed in the liver, you should have a very high incidence in the bladder. What appears to be limiting in the bladder is a promotional stimulus.

I believe this work relates to what Dr. Clayson mentioned earlier about BHA. 2-Acetylaminofluorene (2-AAF) is normally hepatocarcinogenic in the rat. However, if you coadminister BHA you diminish or abolish liver tumors, but now you start to get bladder tumors. If I remember correctly, you also start getting cell proliferation in the bladder. Perhaps if a tumor promoter could be found for mouse bladder, a linear relationship throughout the entire dose range would then be observed between the concentration of adducts and the tumor incidence.

Munro: Could I raise a point here? There was an elegant piece of work done by Willy Butler, published about a month ago in the *British Journal of Cancer*. What was shown was that there was no correspondence or correlation between the extent of adduct formation and the dose-response for carcinogenesis. The correlation does exist, however, between the repair process and the rate of adduct removal.

Beland: What was the agent?

Munro: This was with diethylnitrosamine in the infant rat. If you look at the curve for DNA adduct formation, it is linear, as you have demonstrated for 2-AAF. However, if you look at the dose-response curve for carcinogenesis in the infant rat, it is not linear and mirrors the repair process.

Neal: You referred to Jim Swenberg's data on DEN in rat liver as well, and he gets similar data used in the Peto incidence data, that adducts go down linearly, but that tumor incidence does play off at some lower dose. The adducts do not match the carcinogenesis.

Beland: I think it is going to depend upon the tissue.

Clayson: Have you tried to fit the two sets of data together using an assumption that maybe the liver required one hit on a vital region of the DNA and in the bladder you may require more than one target in the same region?

Beland: No, I haven't tried that.

Pfitzer: I'm not really quibbling with your interpretation, just with your use of the word linear. When you plot, as you did, adducts versus dose, you really had a log scale.

Beland: I agree.

Pfitzer: It's really a power function, not a linear relationship. It can look linear at certain levels. The same here with your log-probit plot. I just mention that because the term linear sometimes means something different to the mathematician than to the biologist.

Setlow: The biologists look upon it as a straight line, no matter what kind of a plot.

Singer: Repair is not uniform, Fred, and repair in different segments of the genome can be very different. Therefore, your adduct and your carcinogenesis data do not have to match at all.

Beland: I agree. We have looked at the removal of adducts in different regions of rat liver chromatin. This experiment was just completed within the last month.

Singer: What I'm trying to say is that this is apples and oranges again. You have initiated some cells that become tumorigenic, but other cells in which you are still measuring your total adducts are those in which repair takes place differently. You have a total repair picture, and you have only a few initiated cells that are represented there. That's why the two have no relationship to each other at long doses, by the time you get to your tumors.

Setlow: That's one way out of the dilemma.

Crump: I think another way to interpret the bladder response is that it, too, is linear at low doses. If you look at the lowest four or five doses, that applies very well. Then, there is something additional happening at the higher doses that makes it increase above the slope you get for the lower doses.

Wilson: It's a very nice quadratic curve.

Michejda: It's really remarkable, though, because from the 0 to 120 . . .

Setlow: There is no zero.

Michejda: Well, more or less. I can extrapolate pretty well. From the 0 slope there to 120, there is nothing in terms of an increase in tumors; and then, you go up to 180 and you jump tenfold. That's an incredible result.

Setlow: The next speaker will put in another complication, Ken Kraemer from NCI.

* * *

Kraemer: I'll be talking about ultraviolet (UV) photoproducts and studies with a new assay, the shuttle vector plasmid. UV causes skin cancer. Skin cancers are the most common cancers in Caucasians. About half a million people in the U.S. each year get skin cancers and the rate is increasing.

The types of photoproducts formed by UV include the cyclobutane dimers shown here. This is the TC cyclobutane dimer. Alternatively, this same TC can form a TC 6-4 photoproduct after UV radiation. In order of frequency, the TT cyclobutane dimer is the most frequent, followed by the TC, and then less frequently CT and CC dimers. 6-4 lesions are generally only TC or CC, and are very rarely formed at TT or CT.

I will explain the shuttle vector system we have used and how we have analyzed the survival of the plasmid, assessed mutagenesis in the plasmid at specific sites, and correlate that with the photoproduct frequencies. The shuttle vector was designed and constructed by Dr. Michael Seidman. It has a SV40 portion to permit growth in mammalian cells and a plasmid portion containing the ampicillin resistance gene for growth in bacteria and analysis of mutations. The marker for mutations is the suppressor tRNA, the *supF* gene. This is not essential for survival of the plasmid. The plasmid is called a "shuttle vector" because it shuttles between bacteria and mammalian cells. The protocol follows: We irradiate the plasmid in vitro, producing various photoproducts. We can measure the products at this stage, or we can alter the DNA of the plasmid at this stage by using some agent, such as photoreactivating enzyme, to selectively remove certain of the photoproducts, the cyclobutane dimers, and leave others. Then we transfect the plasmid into the mammalian cells. We used human cells for these studies but monkey cells can also be used. In the cells, the cellular enzymes repair the plasmid and facilitate plasmid mutation or replication. Thus, this is a host-cell reactivation assay. After 48 hours, we harvest the replicated plasmid and use it to transform an indicator strain of bacteria that has a β-galactosidase mutation that can be suppressed by the suppressor tRNA. We then count the number of ampicillin-resistant colonies to get an indication of plasmid survival, look at the color of the colonies to tell whether they contain mutated plasmids, and then sequence the plasmids generated from the mutated colonies.

We have a patient with xeroderma pigmentosum complementation group A whose cells we used for the study. She has had more than 100 skin cancers on her face. We irradiated the plasmid, transfected it into her cells, harvested it, and transformed the indicator strain of bacteria. We count the total number of colonies to get survival. Certain colonies were nonmutated. Other colonies indicate that there was a mutation that occurred inactivating the action of the marker gene, the suppressor transfer RNA, so β-galactosidase is not formed. Thus, merely by counting the number of colonies, we get indication of survival, and by looking at the selected colonies, we get an indication of the mutation frequency. After in vitro treatment of the plasmid, these changes are introduced by the human cells.

As an indication of survival, we measured UV dose to plasmid versus the relative number of bacterial colonies. With the normal cells in this dose range, we have virtually no inhibition of plasmid survival. In the xeroderma group *A* cells, that are very repair-deficient, we have a marked inhibition of the number of colonies, indicating that they are very sensitive to the UV damage.

If we selectively remove cyclobutane dimers leaving nondimer photoproducts, we can determine the effects that are due to the cyclobutane dimers versus those due to the nondimer photoproducts. Survival increases after photoreactivation, indicating that the cyclobutane dimers in the repair-deficient cell are very important to lethality. However, the nondimer photoproducts are also important because the curve does not go up to normal. Thus, both cyclobutane dimers and nondimer photoproducts are important in survival in this system.

Similar mutagenesis studies were performed by looking at the mutant colonies formed as a proportion of the total number of colonies and as a function of UV dose. In the normal cells, we measured the dose-response. In the XP cells, with UV treatment, without photoreactivation, there is a steep mutagenic induction. If we photoreactivate, we reduce a large proportion of the mutations, indicating that the cyclobutane dimers are mutagenic in this system. However, we don't come down all the way to normal. Thus, noncyclobutane dimers are also mutagenic.

We were able to assay the base sequences of the mutations induced. In the normal, we had 81 independent plasmid sequences. In the xeroderma, we had 71 plasmid sequences. The vast majority in both cases, without photoreactivation and even with photoreactivation, showed transition mutations. The G:C base pairs changed to A:T, in 93% with the xeroderma, and in 73% with the normal. This means that the major photoproduct that I mentioned before involving thymine, the TT dimer, is not mutagenic. It is not the major mutagenic lesion, since the C is involved in the mutation and not the T.

How can we explain this finding? An "A rule" was proposed many years ago by Drake and Tessman, and more recently by Strauss and Loeb and Kunkle, in that polymerases, if they see a noninstructional lesion, put in an A opposite. In other words, "When in doubt, put in an A." With the major photoproduct, the TT dimer, when the polymerase does not know what to do, it puts an A opposite. Since this is the appropriate base, this is not mutagenic. In the case of the TC or the CC, where we see most of our mutations, inserting As results in a G:C to A:T transition. Thus, the TTs would mutate much less frequently than the other photoproducts.

Our data is most consistent with this theory. We mapped the sequence of the tRNA. There were hot spots generated in the xeroderma and in the normal cells. After photoreactivation, the same hot spots were seen indicating that the dimers were mutagenic and the nondimer photoproducts were also mutagenic even at the same base pairs.

Furthermore, we can do Maxam-Gilbert type sequencing and photoproduct frequency measurements, as done by Dr. Douglas Brash. There are three TC cyclobutane dimers in a short stretch. They have a different frequency of formation just in a short stretch of DNA. In addition to the cyclobutane dimers, 6-4 photoproducts are also formed at these sites. When we photoreactivate, we completely remove the cyclobutane dimers. We were able to measure the frequency of the 6-4 photoproducts and the cyclobutane dimers at nearly 60 sites in the marker gene.

Since we also had our mutagenesis data both in the normal and in the xeroderma cells, we asked the question: Is there a correlation between the frequency of the formation of these photoproducts and the frequency of mutations induced at these particular base pairs in the human cells? We measured the proportion of cyclobutane dimers versus the number of mutants in both the normal and the xeroderma, and then the same for the 6-4 photoproducts versus the number of mutants in the normal and the xeroderma. What is apparent is that there is a scattering. There is certainly no linear relationship between one or the other. Thus, there does not appear to be a simple, direct correlation between the photoproduct frequency and the mutation frequency at these sites in the xeroderma cells or in the normal cells.

These experiments lead to the following conclusions: (1) cyclobutane dimers and 6-4 photoproducts are mutagenic; (2) the major UV photoproduct, the TT dimer, is weakly mutagenic; (3) mutation frequency does not correlate with photoproduct frequency at individual base pair sites that we know to be mutagenic.

Singer: Do you know that Jim Cleaver has an XP strain that repairs 6-4 lesions and does not repair the dimers?

Kraemer: Yes. We have given him some of these same plasmids to use in his system. My interpretation of his data is that the plasmids are measuring specific repair systems. There is another set of plasmids that we use to measure repair rather than the mutation. With his revertant, the plasmid shows the xeroderma response rather than the normal response. What Cleaver has are xeroderma cells that have good UV survival, but poor repair of cyclobutane dimers and good repair of nondimer photoproducts. The plasmid assay apparently reflects the cellular handling of dimers. Cleaver has also done a few experiments with the mutagenesis plasmid, and it also does not revert.

Setlow: What does that mean?

Kraemer: My interpretation of that data is there are a number of repair pathways, and the chemically-induced xeroderma revertant (his was transformed by EMS) may have yet another pathway activated, not necessarily the normal functioning pathway.

Our suspicion as to why we find a lack of correlation between photo-product frequency and mutagenic frequency is that just because you know the name of the photoproduct or of the lesion, you don't know whether it will be mutagenic. The effect it has on the particular sequence of DNA in which it lies and how it will interact with polymerases and other enzymes that are necessary to function may be of paramount importance. For example, two TC dinucleotides, just a few bases apart, might have profoundly different implications in terms of mutagenesis, in terms of blocking polymerases, and in terms of causing mutations. I think it's a new ballgame.

Michejda: Is there any information on the location of the photo dimers and the other photo adducts, in terms of, say, the linker region versus nucleosomal DNA. I mean, the physical characteristics of all these regions of DNA can be quite different.

Kraemer: There may very well be. Bohr and Hanawalt's experiments have shown differential repair in certain regions with active genes having greater repair than inactive genes. They are working at levels of kb, whereas we are working at individual bases. We find 80-fold variation between frequencies of photoproducts in one region, versus another in a 150-base pair region.

Beland: What about the sequence of the hot spots? Are they similar from one of your hot spots to the other?

Kraemer: There are common hot spots, and then there are different hot spots. The xeroderma and the normal have a common hot spot. There are additional hot spots in the xeroderma that are not seen in the normal. This indicates that cell polymerases or other enzymes differ in their action on the same damaged DNA. The xeroderma cells are repair-deficient cells. This particular one is one of the lowest we have, less than 2% of normal repair. So, repair isn't playing a role in the mutations that we found in the xeroderma. The lack of correlation between mutations and photoproducts is seen to a similar extent in the xeroderma and the normal, but you can't just say, "Oh, those lesions are being repaired."

Farland: Dick, you have some data that relate to the dimer content and carcinogenicity, some of the work that was done a few years ago. Is there a way to relate that to what we have heard here?

Setlow: I'll pass that question to Dr. Hart.

Hart: I think that when you get the photoreversals through photoreactivation, you never can totally reverse tumor induction or transformation. In the original paper, there were two explanations provided: that there might be other photoproducts that were not being affected, and that repair was not total because of photoreactivation. I think this is carrying that work on further. It's nice to see this type of evolution. It's really a very impressive piece of work.

Setlow: In all biological systems looked at, the amount of biological photoreactivation is never as great as the amount of physical removal of pyrimidine dimers. So, one describes this by saying that the photoreactable sector is less than 100%. Even in *Escherichia coli*, it's somewhere in the neighborhood of 80–90%. That automatically leaves you 10–20% of something else.

Hart: And it's amazing to me how close the correlations are, in fact, that you see.

Farland: Just one other comment. When I was at Brookhaven, we started a few experiments looking at the accessibility of those lesions to the photoreactivating enzyme that was put into the cells, and you could see a difference, depending on whether you started to break up the nucleosomal structure or not, both in the test tube and in the nuclii.

Setlow: In these particular cases, though, the treatment was in vitro, so that is not a problem.

Hart: I was wondering, if you remember the paper that Wilkins and I did in *Nature* looking at preferential DNA repair. Have Doug or yourself gone back and looked at some of that relative to these other photoproducts to see if there is differential repair between linker and nonlinker regions?

Kraemer: No, but Bohr and Hanawalt have looked in the xeroderma group C and found uniformly reduced repair.

Hart: So, it's the same as you would see with the TT analogs?

Kraemer: However, they didn't compare linker to nonlinker. They looked at active versus inactive gene.

Setlow: Essential versus nonessential genes.

Hart: Right. However, the same proportion appears between the cyclobutane-type pyrimidine dimer and the photoproducts that you described?

Setlow: They were only looking at pyrimidine dimers.

Kraemer: They were doing that. We would distinguish among the cyclobutane dimers. Certainly, the TT cyclobutane dimer is the most common one. Presumably, polymerases have evolved to deal with them because, before the ozone layer appeared, UV radiation from sunlight formed these photoproducts. Polymerases evolved to deal with them, and thus, you end up having other photoproducts being more mutagenic, even though they are less frequent.

Setlow: The ultimate, of course, in a risk assessment problem is how fluorocarbons affect the ozone and therefore affect skin cancer. This is something that EPA has done. It has international repercussions.

    The next panelist of this session is Ray Tennant from NIEHS. He has the privilege, if he wishes, to reply to Jim Trosko.

*   *   *

Tennant: Dr. Trosko was correct in describing the overall results of the study that we recently published (*Science* **236:**933[1987]). Most of you may know that it involved an evaluation of a group of carcinogens and noncarcinogens characterized by The National Toxicology Program. It was an objective comparison of the ability of in vitro or genetic toxicity assays to predict either carcinogenicity or noncarcinogenicity, that is, the relative sensitivity and specificity of these assays.

    An interesting result was the relatively high proportion of nonmutagenic carcinogens in this sample, relative to what had been reported previously by Ames and others. Whereas they found a concordance of approximately 90%, our systems showed approximately a 60% concordance between carcinogenicity and in vitro genetic toxicity.

    Our logical questions, then, would be: Is there something wrong with either our protocols, our reagents, or our methods? Have we systematically employed inadequate S-9, or something to that effect?

    In an attempt to address the issue of to what extent we are able, in vitro, to identify intrinsically mutagenic substances, we collaborated with Dr. John Ashby of Imperial Chemical Industries England and chose a larger group of chemicals. There are over 200 substances that have been tested in the same rodent species by NCI or the National Toxicology Program. Independently, Dr. Ashby evaluated those chemicals for structural alerts that would indicate intrinsic electrophilic potential, direct or indirect, and compared that to the results of *Salmonella* mutagenicity assays conducted under code on the same compounds. We found that the relationship between structural features of these chemicals and results obtained in *Salmonella* show a remarkably high degree of concordance, indicating that the *Salmonella* assay does have the capacity to identify a vast majority of substances that are intrinsically mutagenic, based on electrophilic structures.

These results, therefore, tend to verify the fact that the substances that we are classifying as nonmutagenic lack intrinsic mutagenic potential, and may be acting by mechanisms or modes of action that are fundamentally different from the substances that are the mutagenic carcinogens.

However, we are not discounting the value of the mutagenicity results, and we believe that it is important to give some weight to those substances that are mutagenic. A basis for doing this is found in the in vitro genetic toxicity patterns of the substances that The International Agency for Research on Cancer has listed as its class 1 carcinogens. That means, those substances for which there is sufficient clinical or epidemiological data to identify them as etiologically linked to human cancers. The majority of those substances that have been adequately tested are mutagenic. In addition, the majority of those that have been tested adequately in rodents, or in other species, show activity in each of the species in which they are examined.

These results, and those obtained from the rodent studies referred to previously, indicate that once a mutagen is identified, it carries with it a high probability of tumorigenicity. Not only that, but there is a high probability of tumorigenicity at multiple sites in the rodents. The single-sex species or single-site carcinogens, however, include a higher proportion of the nonmutagenic carcinogens.

The primary conclusion of the study reported in *Science* was that among the four in vitro assays that we evaluated, there was no evidence of complementation. That is, in combination they would not help us to resolve between the substances that were mutagenic noncarcinogens or mutagenic carcinogens. Therefore, we have to continue to search for some means to actually complement the *Salmonella* assay. Our preliminary results do suggest that the use of in vivo cytogenetic assays, for example, for chromosome aberrations or micronucleus induction, may provide the precision to help us to segregate the hazardous mutagens from the nonhazardous mutagens. In order to do this, we must evaluate the same characteristics of sensitivity and specificity that we have applied to these other four assays. Therefore, over the next two years, we will be evaluating the same group of chemicals, under code, in the appropriate in vivo bone marrow cytogenetic and micronucleus assays.

I believe that the same methodology is going to have to be applied to any system that is proposed to distinguish between nonmutagenic carcinogens and nonmutagenic noncarcinogens. That is, the data base is going to have to be composed of substances that are both tumorigenic and nontumorigenic, promoter and nonpromoter, mutagen and non-mutagen. It is only through clearly defining the sensitivity and specificity characteristics of any proposed assay system that it really has any potential utility.

In terms of classifying nonmutagenic carcinogens as promoters, Dr. Trosko described to you two of the most potent substances, on a dose basis, identified among the 73 chemicals we evaluated that have been shown to act as tumor promoters in two-stage model systems. The two chemicals were 2,3,7,8-tetrachlorodibenzo-*p*-dioxin (TCDD) and poly-brominated biphenyl (PBB). Concomitantly, they are both car-cinogenic, and when applied under a prolonged dose rate, they demon-strate the ability to induce tumors in the absence of any sort of chemical initiation. It is possible to invoke a variety of ambient environmental initiators to explain the origin of spontaneous tumors. However, PBB-induced cholangiocarcinomas are very rare tumors that must have some obscure basis for initiation, if PBB is not acting as a carcinogen.

I think that we are faced to some degree with a semantic paradox. In some cases it may be only dose rate that separates a complete car-cinogen from a tumor promoter. Until we have evaluated a sufficient number of substances that have been shown to be two-stage promoters under the same methodology by which we identify carcinogens (chronic exposures at a maximum tolerated dose), we are not going to know whether or not tumor promoters are tumorigenic on their own or not. We simply have to generate the data. There are experimental designs that can be used in chronic toxicity studies to concomitantly learn a great deal more about those chemicals, for example, the requirement for persistence of the chemical for progression of neoplastic lesions, and so on. However, there is no simple answer.

I would, however, very briefly like to offer, for those of you who dislike the use of the terms epigenetic and genotoxic, an entirely differ-ent semantic paradox. The majority of substances that are the non-mutagenic carcinogens do require prolonged exposures. Relatively few substances can be identified as tumorigenic after a single-dose exposure, and most are mutagenic. I suggest considering substances that are nonmutagenic and that require long term exposures as "adaptive car-cinogens," rather than classifying them as either promoters or complete carcinogens. This would distinguish them from mutagenic carcinogens that could be called inductive carcinogens.

Setlow: Thank you, Ray. Did I hear an objection from the back?

Wilson: I don't object to it. I think that's a great idea, if we can agree on terminology. The problem, as you observed, is partly one of semantics. The public thinks of carcinogens as basically those things that are extremely dangerous on small exposure. It's a good idea to identify all these things that we call here nonmutagenic or adaptive carcinogens. I like them both. They imply to us in the field that they may well carry a much lower threat, especially in single doses. That is a perfectly good idea. What I have a problem with is that I didn't understand what it is you expect to learn from redoing your extremely nice study of the mutagens with these other tests.

Tennant: I brushed over that very quickly. We believe that it is valuable in two ways. First of all, there are some substances that are not adequately metabolized in vitro. Benzene would be one of the best examples, but benzene is clearly a clastogenic compound in vivo that does not produce those effects in most in vitro systems, as they are currently conducted. Therefore, the use of an in vivo cytogenetic assay may help us to identify prospectively such chemicals. Other chemicals that may fall into that category would be furan and furfural, recently reported as carcinogens, that have not registered in the in vitro systems.

The second purpose is to help us prospectively distinguish those chemicals that are going to be rapidly metabolized, quickly excreted, or efficiently detoxified, that they do not get effective access to DNA in the whole animal. They are the mutagenic noncarcinogens. Such results would be a complementation to the *Salmonella* assay.

Michejda: I missed that last point. Mutagenic noncarcinogens because they are excreted rapidly? Give me an example of something that is excreted so rapidly that it doesn't register in the animal bioassay.

Tennant: There are several substances that are clearly mutagenic but that do not induce tumors when administered to B6C3F1 mice or Fischer-344 rats.

Michejda: However, you also superimposed a mechanistic explanation.

Tennant: I don't mean to offer it in a mechanistic way. There are simply substances that are metabolized differently, conjugated rapidly, and so on, that do register in vitro, but that may not register in the whole animal. There is at least some preliminary evidence that would suggest that is the case. A few examples are 2-chloromethylpyridine, 2,6-toluenediamine or 4-nitro-O-phenylenediamine.

Weisburger: Sodium azide is a mutagenic compound in insects, but it doesn't seem to be carcinogenic.

Tennant: That's a good one.

Lijinsky: There are several. Hydroxylamine and nitrous acid, as examples.

Trosko: Ray (Tennant) and I have discussed this before, but I think there are two points that should be brought up to the people who don't do mutation studies or mutation assays. We all realize that the definition of a mutagen is that which brings about a qualitative and quantitative change in genetic information in the host, which is to say there are different kinds of mechanisms that lead to gene mutations as well as chromosomal mutations, and within each category there are different mechanisms that lead to deletion mutations as opposed to base substitutions, for example.

   However, the point I want to make is regarding the distinction between gene mutations and the clastogens, that many of the chemicals that affect membranes will lead to clastogenic changes. Therefore, what you are looking at as the end point, the clastogenic change, may be an irrelevant one to something that already happened to the membrane, for example. That gets me back to gap junction.

   Secondly, many of the short-term assays used to pick up mutations are not all equivalent; i.e., the sister chromatid exchange is, unfortunately, used equivalently to a point mutation. We know there are all kinds of artifacts in every one of these short-term assays.

   For example, the TK$^-$ system, the thymidine kinase negative phenotype, can in fact be brought about by a point mutation, a deletion mutation, and an event that turns off the gene that codes for that enzyme. So, when you isolate that clone that is TK$^-$, it resists bromodeoxyuridine, it could be due to a mutagenic, as well as an epigenetic, phenomenon. There is no way you can distinguish those two from just looking at the clone.

   Regarding sister chromatid exchanges, you are using an indirect measure, you are using a tracer, bromodeoxyuridine or whatever, and if you have a chemical that affects transport of the tracer or affects the nucleotide pools, what you are going to get is a false positive. In fact, we know from the literature that has been done with these assays that these assays seem to be supersensitive, and they picked up too many false positives.

   Although people know that these are artifacts, they never seem to take into account the possibility that the positive results, particularly false positives, may involve that artifactual component.

Hart: Just one observation, really. At the Williamsburg meeting, there was a discussion about the need for the study that you are about to conduct.

That is the problem of predictabilitiy of in vitro and in vivo mutagenesis. I think that is the main justification for the study. I think it is going to be a very important study because we need to bridge this gap between the in vitro and in vivo mutagenicities. I think that is going to be an important study. So, when people ask questions why, it is because we need to make that bridge or that connection.

Travis: I would just like to comment on that, just as an outside observer. It seems to me that there has been a lot of attention towards mutagenicity. Everybody recognizes, as Trosko has pointed out, that promotion is also an important aspect. I see the mutagenicity people proposing a test, they try it, it doesn't correlate well with carcinogenicity, so they say, "Well, it's not measuring it correctly, let's get a better test." They get a better test, and there's still no correlation, and they say, "We need a battery of tests." The battery of tests still doesn't correlate, so they say, "We've got to go in vivo." When are you going to move over to promotion and start getting some short-term tests for promotion?

Tennant Our Board of Scientific Counselers also raises that issue consistently, and we struggle with it. I would put it this way: If you've got a good system and you're willing to accept a large number of chemicals under code, we'll attempt to support the evaluation of it in any way we can.

Now, the problem is, what is a promoter? Is it a substance that will not induce tumors by a low-dose rate but may be tumorigenic by a protracted dose rate, or one that sometimes requires an initiator? I don't know what definition to work under.

Setlow: We just have to set up the definitions.

Farland: Ray, would you mention the recent work on the B6 mouse with the oncogenes and nongenotoxic and genotoxic chemicals?

Tennant: That's why I mentioned the furan and the furfural results. I'm not sure that they have identified unique mutations induced by non-mutagens. I think the structure of furan is amenable to metabolism in vivo, just like benzene. So, at this stage Marshall Anderson's program hasn't really looked at clear-cut, nonmutagenic carcinogens for their effect on oncogene expression. I think it's an essential way to go. It is the most logical target for some nonmutagenic carcinogens, and I am sure that Dr. Anderson is pursuing this issue.

Setlow: The last word will be had by the first speaker.

Singer: I would only like to make a comment that needs no reply, that being that the word epigenetic is a pseudonym for a word that is used when one doesn't know mechanism.

Approaches Toward Integration

Is It Possible to Predict the Carcinogenic Potency of a Chemical in Humans Using Animal Data?

BRUCE ALLEN, KENNY CRUMP, AND ANNETTE SHIPP
Clement Associates
Ruston, Louisiana 71270

OVERVIEW

Quantitative comparisons of carcinogenic potency in animals and in humans are made for 23 chemicals for which suitable animal and human data exist. These comparisons are based upon estimates of transforming doses (TD_{25}), defined as the average daily dose per body weight of a chemical that would result in an extra cancer risk of 25%.

TD_{25} obtained from animal and human data are found to be strongly correlated. The knowledge that this correlation exists should strengthen the scientific basis for risk assessment and cause increased confidence to be placed in estimates of human cancer risk from animal data.

Better predictors of human TD_{25} are obtained by using statistical lower confidence bounds for animal TD_{25} rather than maximum likelihood estimators and by using the median of lower bounds of animal TD_{25} obtained from different studies, species or sex groups, rather than using the smallest lower bounds. The analysis approaches applied to the animal data that best predict the results from human data also utilize data from several routes of exposure and employ the assumption that animals and humans were equally sensitive to a carcinogen when dose was measured in units of mg/kg body weight/day.

INTRODUCTION

In addition to gaining a better understanding of basic biological mechanisms as they relate to cancer, a basic reason for carcinogenicity testing in animals is to evaluate whether the tested chemicals present carcinogenic hazards to humans. Not only have animal tests been used to detect carcinogens, they have also been used to determine acceptable levels of exposure in humans. This practice makes a fundamental assumption that, not only are animal carcinogens likely to be carcinogenic in humans, but that the carcinogenic potency of a chemical measured in animal studies is related in a specific manner to its potency in humans. This study judges the validity of that assumption by comparing carcinogenic potencies estimated for animal and

Banbury Report 31: Carcinogen Risk Assessment: New Directions in the Qualitative and Quantitative Aspects © Cold Spring Harbor Laboratory. 0-87969-231-6/88. $1.00 + .00

human data for 23 chemicals. In the process, a number of approaches for estimating human risk from animal data are evaluated.

RESULTS

There are two requirements that a chemical needed to satisfy in order to be included in the study:

1. There has to be reasonably strong evidence of carcinogenicity in either animal or human data (but not necessarily both);
2. Suitable data from both animal and human studies needed to exist for quantifying carcinogenic potency.

Chemicals found to satisfy these requirements are listed in Table 1 along with the International Agency for Research on Cancer (IARC 1982) evaluations of the evidence for carcinogenicity in animals and in humans. Included in this study are 13 industrial chemicals, 7 drugs, a food contaminant (aflatoxin), a food additive (saccharin), and tobacco smoke.

It is considered important not to exclude from the analysis animal carcinogens such as saccharin and trichloroethylene, which are not confirmed human carcinogens. The correlation between animal and human data could be overstated if the study is limited to chemicals that are known to be carcinogenic in both animals and humans. A similar study by the National Academy of Sciences (National Academy of Sciences Executive Committee 1975) was limited to six chemicals that were carcinogenic in both animals and humans; however, the potential for bias in this approach was acknowledged.

The human data for some of the chemicals in the study are limited, particularly in the area of exposure data. It is considered important for the purpose of this study to include as many chemicals as reasonably possible rather than to include only a few of the chemicals having the very best data. The minimal requirements for human data are a usable measure of risk (generally a relative risk) in an exposed cohort and a usable measure of dose for that cohort (generally in terms of cumulative dose such as ppm-years or mg-total-intake). Dose-response data involving multiple exposure groups are utilized whenever available.

In many cases, there is considerable uncertainty regarding human exposures and, an attempt is made to quantify that uncertainty. In addition to obtaining best estimates of exposure, upper and lower bounds for exposures are also estimated. These are made by a single investigator (B. Allen, unpubl.) using criteria set out in advance. Cross-checks between chemicals are made to ensure all chemicals are treated evenly. All evaluations of the human data are made blind, i.e., without knowledge of the results from the animal data.

Table 1
Chemicals for Which Minimal Human and Animal Data Exist for Quantifying Carcinogenic Potency

Chemical	IARC classification		Chemical	IARC classification	
	human	animal		human	animal
Aflatoxin (AF)	L	S	Estrogens (ES)	S	I
Arsenic (AS)	S	I	Ethylene oxide (EO)	I	L
Asbestos (AB)	S	S	Isoniazid (IS)	I	L
Benzene (BN)	S	L	Melphalan (ML)	S	S
Benzidine (BZ)	S	S	Methylene chloride (MC)	I	S
Cadmium (CD)	L	S	Nickel (NC)	L	S
Chlorambucil (CB)	S	S	PCBs (PC)	I	S
Chromium (CR)	S	S	Phenacetin (PH)	S	L
Cigarette smoke (CS)	—	—	Reserpine (RS)	I	L
Diethylstilbestrol (DS)	S	S	Saccharin (SC)	I	L
Epichlorohydrin (EC)	I	S	Trichloroethylene (TC)	I	L
			Vinyl chloride (VC)	S	S

S = sufficient; L = limited; I = inadequate.

The animal data are entered into a computerized data base in a form that permits a wide range of calculations to be performed automatically. The extent of the data base is indicated by Tables 2 and 3. The data base includes mainly rodent species, but contains some data on other species such as dogs and primates. Routes of exposure are primarily oral, gavage, and inhalation, although limited data are included on other routes, including implantation, instillation, and injection. The data on individual chemicals are highly variable in terms of both quantity and quality. As an example, the number of animal data sets available for a given chemical ranged from 1 (for melphalan) to 64 (for asbestos).

Potency is basically "risk per unit dose." Recognizing that the potency of a chemical can be dose-dependent if the dose-response curve is nonlinear, the end point selected for comparing animal and human results is the dose rate (labeled TD_{25}) in units of mg intake/kg body weight/day that would cause 25% of subjects to get cancer (who would otherwise be free of the cancer of interest) if exposed daily for a major fraction of their normal life span (from age 20 to age 65 in humans and from weaning onward in animals). A life table approach is used to estimate TD_{25} from human data, based on a linear dose-response model. The multistage dose-response model (Crump and Crockett 1985) is applied to the animal data. A 25% reference risk was selected because this risk value is normally in the experimental range of response in animal studies. Its use requires an extrapolation to higher risk values for most, but not all, human studies. It is presumed that the analysis

Table 2
Summary of Animal Database

(a) Number of chemicals with given type of data				
	Rat	Mouse	Other species	
	21	19	11	
Oral	Gavage	Inhalation	Other route	
17	9	11	17	

(b) Number of data sets in animal database				
Oral	Gavage	Inhalation	Other	Total
126	44	108	110	388
	Rat	Mouse	Other	Total
	214	119	55	388

Table 3
Results from Selected Prediction Analyses

No.	Description[a]	Correlation	Normalized loss	Bias removal factor[b]	Residual error[c]
	(a) Analyses that employ mg/m²/day as surrogate dose				
0	Base case	0.78	1.2	1.8	4.7
0	Base case using minimum lower bound TD_{25} (intended to mimic USEPA)		2.1	12.0	16.2
7	Malignant tumors only	0.76	1.7	2.4	4.8
11c	Rat data only	0.79	1.0	1.6	3.8
11d	Mouse data only	0.76	1.2	4.0	2.5
	(b) Analyses that employ mg/kg/day as surrogate dose				
30	Any exposure route	0.91	0.39	1.4	2.0
43	Total tumor-bearing animals, any exposure route	0.74	0.28	0.23	2.8
45	Average TD_{25} from males and females, any exposure route	0.91	0.27	1.4	1.7

[a] Description gives manner in which analysis differs from base case. All analyses used the median lower bound (L_{20}) as the animal estimator except for the exception noted.
[b] Average amount by which animal TD_{25} underestimate human TD_{25}.
[c] Average relative discrepancy between animal and human TD_{25} not explained by uncertainty in the human TD_{25}.

results are insensitive both to the choice of the multistage model (note that no extrapolation to low doses is involved) and to the choice of a reference risk of 25%. However, thus far no formal investigation of the effects of these choices has been undertaken.

For each set of animal or human dose-response data from each chemical, a best estimate of the TD_{25} is obtained as well as corresponding upper and lower bounds. For animal data the upper and lower bounds are 95% statistical confidence bounds. For human data the bounds reflect both statistical variation and the uncertainty ranges estimated for human doses.

Frequently, more than one TD_{25} for a given chemical is calculated owing to the fact that more than a single data set is available upon which to base the calculation. For human data a single TD_{25}, with related bounds, is selected from among those calculated to use for comparing to animal results. For each chemical, the TD_{25} selected is that thought to best represent the preponderance of the human evidence. For example, the human TD_{25} selected for vinyl chloride is based upon data from liver tumors because that response is most firmly linked to vinyl chloride exposure. On the other hand, the data on isoniazid do not conclusively demonstrate carcinogenicity in humans and do not indicate a particular site of action. Consequently, the response selected is all malignant neoplasms and the TD_{25} selected is one having an associated infinite upper bound, which is consistent with no carcinogenic effect.

A number of different methods for estimating TD_{25} from the animal data are evaluated using a computerized approach to data analysis. Most are closely related to a standard method called the "base case," which involves the following choices:

1. Data from longer studies and those involving larger numbers of animals are given preference;
2. Data from studies in which statistically significant carcinogenic effects were obtained are given preference;
3. Data are incorporated from studies involving the following exposure routes: inhalation, gavage, and in food or drinking water, or by the route most similar to that of humans if different from one of these;
4. Mg intake/m^2 body surface area/day is used as the surrogate dose (i.e., the dose measure assumed to provide equivalent risks in animals and humans);
5. Data on either benign or malignant tumors or both are utilized;
6. The tumor type selected for risk assessment from an experimental group of animals is the individual site found to provide the strongest evidence of a carcinogenic effect;
7. TD_{25} calculated from separate sexes within a study, studies in different species, and separate species are not averaged but used separately.

This base case analysis method is intended to mimic the risk assessment method employed by the United States Environmental Protection Agency (USEPA). Additional details on these and other methods, as well as additional results, may be found in Allen et al. (1987 and in prep.).

Correlation analyses are used to determine whether TD_{25} calculated from animal data are correlated with those calculated from human data. Note that the choices listed above for the base case method for estimating a single TD_{25} do not determine a unique TD_{25} for a chemical but rather determine a separate TD_{25} for each animal data set analyzed. In the correlation analyses a unique TD_{25} is defined for each chemical by the median of the TD_{25} available. Similarly, unique upper and lower bounds are defined by the median of the upper and lower 95% confidence bounds for the TD_{25} obtained from the multistage model.

Figure 1 depicts graphically a correlation analysis of one method for estimating TD_{25}. The method used for calculating a single animal TD_{25} differs from the base case only in that data involving injection, implantation, and instillation exposure routes were allowed. Inclusion of these routes allows all

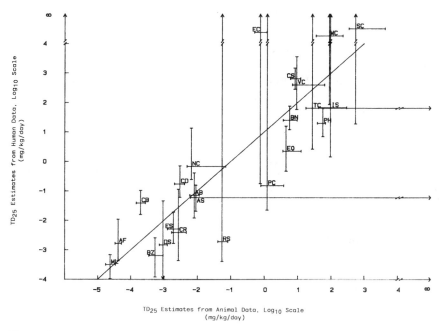

Figure 1

Human TD_{25} estimates versus animal TD_{25} estimates (variant of the base case).

23 chemicals to enter the analysis, as data involving only routes of exposure used in the base case were not available for three of the chemicals. For each chemical the estimated human TD_{25} (vertical axis) is plotted against the corresponding animal TD_{25} (horizontal axis). The horizontal lines through the TD_{25} points indicate the upper and lower bounds for the animal TD_{25} and the vertical lines indicate the corresponding bounds for the human TD_{25}. The semi-infinite vertical lines correspond to chemicals that are not proven human carcinogens, as the upper bound on the human TD_{25} for these chemicals is infinite. The slanted line represents the line of unit slope that provides the best fit to these data (best in the sense of minimizing the distance from the line to the rectangles defined by the data for each chemical).

Figure 1 shows that chemicals that are more potent human carcinogens (i.e., those having smaller human TD_{25}) also tend to be more potent animal carcinogens. A Spearman-type correlation of 0.90 was calculated for these data, which is highly statistically significant ($p < 0.0001$).

For the base case analysis, the correlation is 0.78, which is also highly significant ($p = 0.0001$). More than 100 different correlation analyses have been conducted to date. These analyses represent systematic modifications of the choices described earlier for the base case. A positive correlation was found in all of these analyses; in the majority of cases the estimated correlation was in excess of 0.7 and was statistically significant ($p < 0.01$).

Having demonstrated that TD_{25} calculated from animal data are strongly correlated with TD_{25} calculated from human data, we now turn to analyses conducted to determine which methods applied to the animal data provide the best predictions of the human results. As with the correlation analyses, many methods for calculating TD_{25} from animal data are evaluated; again these methods are defined by systematically modifying the choices used to define the base case method. Unlike the correlation analyses, in these prediction analyses a single TD_{25} is defined from the animal data for each chemical.

The results of one such prediction analysis are illustrated graphically in Figure 2. Note that in this figure a unique animal TD_{25} is defined for each chemical rather than having a best estimate and related upper and lower bounds as in the correlation analysis illustrated in Figure 1. The straight line fit to the data in Figure 2 is determined by minimizing a statistical squared error loss function defined as the average squared distance from the line to the vertical intervals representing the human TD_{25} for each chemical (if the line intersects an interval, the distance is taken to be zero). This minimal average squared distance is a measure of how well the animal TD_{25} predict the human TD_{25}, with lower values indicating better predictions. Two other such loss functions are also used to evaluate the predictions of the animal TD_{25} (see Allen et al. 1987 for a definition of these).

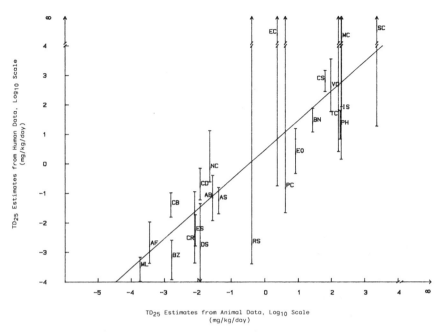

Figure 2

TD$_{25}$ plot for analysis 45 (all routes, average over sex).

Four methods of combining TD$_{25}$ calculated from individual animal data sets into a single predictor for a chemical are evaluated. These are MLE$_{2Q}$, the median of the point estimates (maximum likelihood estimates) calculated from the multistage model; MLE$_M$, the minimum of the point estimates; L$_{2Q}$, the median of the 95% lower bounds calculated from the multistage model; and L$_M$, the minimum of these lower bounds. Of these four methods for combining TD$_{25}$, L$_{2Q}$ is clearly superior to the others in terms of providing lower values of the loss functions. For example, of 20 analysis methods defined by modifying the base case described earlier, based on the squared error loss function, L$_{2Q}$ gives a smaller loss than L$_M$ in every case; with a second loss function, L$_{2Q}$ gives the smallest loss of any of the four methods of combining TD$_{25}$ in 18 of 20 analysis methods; and with a third loss function, L$_{2Q}$ gives the smallest loss of any of the four in 15 analysis methods.

Table 3 provides a summary of results for eight analysis methods. These eight were selected from over 100 evaluated as being of general interest or as appearing to be good predictors of the TD$_{25}$ from human data. The description provided of each method explains how the method differs from the base case. In every case except the one indicated, L_{2O} was the method used for combining TD_{25} from animal data.

Four summary statistics are provided in Table 3 for each analysis method: the correlation, the normalized loss, the residual error, and the bias removal factor. The normalized loss is a summary loss measure synthesized from all three loss functions. The residual error is defined exactly as the squared error loss function except that the distance itself is used in place of the squared distance. The residual error represents roughly the average multiplicative error in estimating human TD_{25} from the animal data that is not explainable by the uncertainty in the human TD_{25} (this uncertainty being expressed as the ranges calculated for the TD_{25} derived from the human data). The bias removal factor is 10^c, where c is the y-intercept from the fitted line of the log-log plot of the animal and human TD_{25} as exemplified by Figure 2. This factor represents the average factor by which animal TD_{25} overestimate or underestimate a single, human TD_{25}, with values greater than one indicating a tendency for animal TD_{25} to underestimate human TD_{25} and vice-versa.

The base case analysis method using the L_M method for combining animal TD_{25}, which was intended to mimic the risk assessment approach used by the USEPA, performs poorest of all of those represented in Table 3. Not only does the method provide a higher normalized loss and residual error than the other methods, but TD_{25} derived from this method also underestimate TD_{25} calculated from human data on average by a factor of 12. However, it should be noted that the computerized approach applied here to selecting and applying data may not adequately represent the approach applied by the USEPA.

There seems to be no particular advantage to restricting analyses to malignant tumors only, and analyses restricted to either mouse or rat data do not predict human results better than analysis methods that combine data from both species. The analysis based on all tumor-bearing animals provides the lowest correlation of all of the methods summarized in Table 3 despite the fact that it provides a relatively small normalized loss.

Analysis methods 30 and 45 appear to perform best overall. These two methods provide higher correlations than any of the other analysis methods and also provide small normalized losses, residual errors, and bias correction factors. Both have a bias correction factor of 1.4, indicating that TD_{25} from animal data calculated using these methods underestimate the corresponding TD_{25} from human data by a factor of 1.4 on average. Method 30 differs from the base case analysis in that all routes of exposure are used and mg/kg/day is used as the surrogate dose rather than $mg/m^2/day$. Method 45 differs in these ways and also in the fact that TD_{25} calculated from a male and female data from the same study were averaged.

DISCUSSION

The very small p-value obtained from the data in Figure 1 implies that the observed correlation of 0.90 is highly unlikely to be due to chance. We believe that it is also unlikely to be due to bias. All potency estimates obtained from the human data were made blind, without knowledge of the animal results. The animal calculations were made by computer and no chemical-specific decisions were involved. With this approach, limitations in the data bases should weaken observed correlations but not create spurious correlations.

We conclude from these results that carcinogenic potencies in animals and humans are highly correlated for the 23 chemicals contained in this study. This correlation strengthens the scientific basis for the use of animal data in risk assessment.

The data used in this study are crude in many respects. As an example, the dose measures used reflected only external exposure. Much research is currently being directed toward measuring and developing predictive models for more biologically relevant indicators of exposure, such as amounts of particulates deposited in various regions of the lungs or the amount of material metabolized into an ultimate carcinogen in various organs. Use of such dose measures should provide better correlations between animal and human data. We hope to be able to incorporate such dose measures into our analyses in the future.

Humans differ from experimental animals in many ways. For example, there are differences in cell structure, distribution of cell types within the lung airways, and metabolism. Other more obvious differences involve size and life span. These latter differences seem particularly important in view of the possibility that cancer may originate in a single cell and in view of the long latency of many cancers.

In addition to these and other physiological and biochemical differences, human and animal carcinogenic end points are usually quite different. A human carcinogenic response is generally clinically observable and generally involves a malignant tumor. Most of the epidemiological studies included in this analysis are mortality studies and a cancer had to cause death in order to contribute. On the other hand, an animal response could be either a benign or malignant tumor and could be a microscopic lesion discovered only at final sacrifice. Animals and humans also differ in regard to "background carcinogenic stress." Whereas laboratory animals live in carefully controlled environments, humans are exposed environmentally to many potentially carcinogenic substances.

Given these many differences between animals and humans, it seems highly unlikely that it will be possible in the near future to account for all of them theoretically in a validated model. However, work aimed towards better understanding of the animal and human differences and how to account for them quantitatively should be encouraged. Current research aimed at better understanding the differences in distribution and metabolism of zenobiotics should be immediately useful in risk assessment. For the time being, however, approaches for effecting an overall extrapolation from quantitative estimates from animal data to estimates pertaining to humans can best be evaluated using an empirical approach such as is applied herein. Specifically, analysis methods can be developed that both seem reasonable biologically and that provide the best quantitative correlation between animals and humans. These methods, having been shown to provide good predictions of human results (subject to the uncertainty in the human results themselves) from animal data for 23 chemicals of diverse types and potentially diverse carcinogenic mechanisms, can be applied on a provisional basis to other chemicals not in the data base and for which only animal data are available.

REFERENCES

Allen, B., A. Shipp, K. Crump, B. Kilian, M. Hogg, J. Tudor, and B. Keller. 1987. *Investigation of cancer risk assessment methods.* Prepared for U.S. Environmental Protection Agency under contract to Research Triangle Institute, contract no. 68-01-6807.

Crump, K. and P. Crockett. 1985. Improved confidence limits for low-dose carcinogenic risk assessment from animal data. *J. Hazard. Mater.* **10:** 419.

International Agency for Research on Cancer (IARC). 1982. Chemical, industrial processes, and industries associated with cancer in humans. *IARC Monogr. Eval. Carcinog. Risk Chem. Hum.* (Suppl. 4): 1.

National Academy of Sciences (NAS) Executive Committee. 1975. *Pest control: An assessment of present and alternative technologies,* vol. 1. National Academy of Sciences Printing and Publishing Office, Washington, D.C.

COMMENTS

Neal: Kenny, could this be applied to compounds that are not carcinogenic in experimental animals that have been tested properly? Could this whole exercise be done with noncarcinogens, theoretically?

Crump: In the animals?

Neal: Yes.

Crump: Yes. In fact, some of our animal data were negative in this analysis.

Neal: What's the correlation between compounds that are negative in the animal and the correlation with humans where there is no evidence of human carcinogenicity? Is there a good correlation there?

Crump: We didn't look at that specifically, but I could show you on a graph where those negative chemicals come out. Basically, they are indicated by a line that goes out infinitely in this direction. However, in all cases lower limits for the TD_{25} were not too far from that line that best fit the data for all of the chemicals. So, subject to the statistical uncertainty, the negative chemicals were not too far off the general trend of all the data.

Neal: So, there is a reasonable correlation between compounds that are negative for carcinogenicity in animals and predicted carcinogenicity in humans?

Crump: I would say, subject to the sensitivity of the animal system, the chemicals that are negative in animals are not inconsistent with the positive correlation. Certainly, if they are truly negative, they are totally inconsistent with the positive carcinogenicity in humans. However, every assay has a sensitivity associated with it, even though we classify them as positive or negatives. When we indicate negative, we mean negative up to the sensitivity of the system. That's true in every system.

Let's just take the potency here. The estimated potency is zero, but, subject to the sensitivity of the system, it is consistent with some positive potency. We estimated statistically how high the potency could have been and not been detected. Then, when we drew our best-fitting regression line, it turned out for every chemical that the range of potencies consistent with the chemical did not miss the regression line by much.

If they are truly noncarcinogenic in animals, then they are certainly inconsistent with the human results. However, subject to what we know, we can't say for sure that they're inconsistent, taking into account the sensitivity of the assay.

Qualitative Factors in Carcinogen Classification

IAN CRAIG MUNRO
Canadian Centre for Toxicology
Guelph, Ontario N1G 1Y3

OVERVIEW

The assessment of the carcinogenicity of chemicals in animal studies forms a critical aspect of research and regulatory programs designed to reduce human exposure to potentially carcinogenic substances. The premarket evaluation of the safety of many of the new chemical products and the evaluation of environmental chemicals and industrial wastes in water and food is predicated on the belief that laboratory tests in animals are an accurate surrogate for humans. This thesis rests in large part on accumulated knowledge that most, if not all, human carcinogens produce cancer in one or another species of animals, often with similar site specificity (Tomatis 1979). The converse argument, namely that test results from animals are predictive of what might be expected in humans, is now widely accepted by regulatory agencies and international organizations. Thus, industry or others wishing to market newly discovered drugs, food additives, or other chemicals often will be required to undertake tests of carcinogenicity in the course of obtaining regulatory approval for their products.

The techniques used to determine whether or not an agent is carcinogenic in animal systems have been the subject of many recent reviews and need not be reiterated in detail. In general, however, these procedures involve daily administration of graded doses of the test chemical to groups of rodents, by an appropriate route, over the major portion of their lifespan. These essential features of the animal bioassay obviously limit routine testing of smaller, short-lived species such as rats and mice. The statistical power of tests to detect carcinogenic responses increases with increasing number of animals employed (Krewski and Van Ryzin 1981), which adds further to the practical necessity of confining testing to rodent species. The dose levels of the test substance, which usually number two to four, may be selected to represent multiples of human exposure but also include a high dose, defined as the maximum tolerated dose, which is considered to reflect the extreme upper limit of exposure that the animals will tolerate and yet survive for sufficient time to be "at risk" for tumor development. Most health authorities endorse the high-dose testing concept because it is considered to maximize the potential for detecting carcinogens in the usual group sizes used in the standard carcinogen bioassay.

Banbury Report 31: Carcinogen Risk Assessment: New Directions in the Qualitative and Quantitative Aspects © Cold Spring Harbor Laboratory. 0-87969-231-6/88. $1.00 + .00

The use of high dose levels in cancer testing is nevertheless a contentious issue. Often it is claimed that high-dose testing, which may involve the administration of chemicals to animals at several orders of magnitude above any potential human exposure, may produce a highly artificial situation of questionable relevance to the human population. Furthermore, it may be argued that high doses of chemicals produce marked derangements in endogenous metabolism and physiology that predispose animals to chronic toxic effects including cancer. This state of affairs has resulted in great controversy over the predictive value of animal tests, particularly when the nature and level of human exposure to the test substance differs greatly from the conditions of the animal bioassay. The purpose of this paper is to examine this controversy in the light of contemporary programs designed to regulate carcinogens and to propose some criteria for determining the weight of evidence for carcinogenicity and for assessing the relevance of animal findings to the human population.

Classification Systems for Carcinogens

It has long been recognized by students of oncology, that the assessment of animal data on carcinogenicity and its extrapolation to humans is a complex and difficult process involving considerable uncertainty. Because of this, regulatory agencies and international organizations have expended considerable effort in the development of criteria and guidelines for the interpretation of animal cancer bioassays. The fruits of these endeavors may be found in reports from the U.S. Environmental Protection Agency (1986), the U.S. Food and Drug Administration (1982), the National Toxicology Program (1984), the Office of Science and Technology Policy (1985), agencies of other governments and international agencies such as the International Agency for Research on Cancer (IARC) (1987) and the World Health Organization (1987), to name but a few sources. These activities are driven by the need to standardize the interpretation of cancer bioassays in the manner designed to produce consistent interpretations. In addition, the advent of these interpretative guidelines has given rise to classification systems in which the weight of evidence for carcinogenicity in animals is assessed and subsequently translated to humans. Most regulatory scientists are familiar with the phrase included in the preamble to the IARC monographs (IARC 1987) which states, "In the absence of adequate data on humans, it is reasonable, for practical purposes, to regard chemicals for which there is 'sufficient' evidence of carcinogenicity in animals as if they presented a carcinogenic risk to humans." Clearly, the basic assumption is that oncogenic effects observed in animals are predictive of what might be expected to occur in man. Although classification systems tend to simplify the task of the regulator in assessing evidence for carcinogenicity, they also tend to oversimplify the complexities of carcinogen hazard assessment, because they fail to incorporate the broad array of data that constitutes a detailed scientific assessment of chemical carcinogenesis. In addition, they often fail to incorporate appropriate scientific criteria for assessing the relevance of animal bioassays to humans.

The use of cancer bioassay data for assessing potential carcinogenicity in man involves two distinct activities. The first of these involves the assessment of the weight of evidence for carcinogenicity in animals, whereas the second involves extrapolation of findings to the human population. It is of fundamental scientific and regulatory importance that these two functions be viewed separately and conclusions not be drawn ipso facto that evidence of carcinogenicity in animals is predictive of human hazard.

Weight of Evidence for Carcinogenicity in Animals

Although in some instances the evidence for carcinogenic activity in animals will be unequivocal, this is not usually the case. In weighing the evidence, it is necessary to include data from other relevant end points, such as structure/ activity relationships, metabolism, and pharmacokinetic studies, the results of in vivo and in vitro tests for genetic activity and biochemical studies to assess reactivity with DNA and other target molecules (e.g., adduct formation). Such studies are of immense value in gaining an appreciation of the possible mode of action of carcinogens and in making a final determination of the strength of evidence for carcinogenic potential (OSTP 1985; Weisburger 1985).

The weight accorded specific animal studies depends to a significant extent on the quality of the experimental data. Factors such as the design and conduct of carcinogenicity studies have an important bearing on their interpretation and subsequent value in hazard evaluation (International Life Sciences Institute 1984). Confidence in the results of carcinogenicity studies will be greater when experiments are carried out in accordance with generally accepted criteria for the design, conduct, and interpretation of such studies (Organization for Economic Co-operation and Development 1981; NTP 1984). In evaluating negative evidence for carcinogenic potential, more weight should be given to adequately designed and conducted negative studies than to more limited experiments demonstrating marginally positive or equivocal results (Clayson and Krewski 1986). The strength of evidence for a negative association between treatment and response will be enhanced by pharmacokinetic, biochemical, and other ancillary studies that also indicate a lack of evidence for carcinogenic potential. As has been pointed out previously (IARC 1983), the assessment of experimental evidence requires an evaluation of both qualitative and quantitative aspects of the available data. This assessment should encompass the totality of evidence bearing on the question of carcinogenic potential. The criteria listed below, when considered collectively, form the basis for a weight of evidence approach to the evaluation of data. Thus, in conducting an evaluation of experimental data, it is necessary to take into consideration the degree to which:

1. The composition of the test substance and its stability in the dosing media, as well as its bioavailability from such matrices, has been documented. Complex mixtures must be sufficiently well characterized to ensure that they are representative of material to which man may be exposed.

2. The carcinogenicity tests were of appropriate statistical resolving power in terms of numbers of animals per group, duration of the test, survival of test animals, and extent of observations to minimize the possibility that increased tumor incidence was due to chance.

3. The doses selected and route of exposure were appropriate and the rationale for dose selection was stated. (Dose selection should involve range-finding studies coupled with adequate subchronic studies describing the pharmacokinetic, biochemical, and toxicological profile of the test substance.)

4. The experiments were conducted in accordance with generally accepted principles of scientific investigation. The diet used was consistent in quality and nutritionally complete for the species of animal used. Constituents that could interfere with the outcome of the study such as toxic fungal products, antioxidants, heavy metals, pesticides, and other contaminants were identified and quantified. Appropriate clinical examinations were performed to evaluate animal health and, if possible, the onset of clinically detectable tumors.

5. The species and strain of animals used were adequately characterized in regard to their response to carcinogens and adequate historical control data relating to disease processes, longevity, and tumor incidence were available and used for comparison with the animals in the study.

6. Appropriate statistical criteria were applied to account for intermittent mortality, high background tumor incidence, and other factors affecting the apparent tumor incidence.

7. There was a demonstrated consistency and reproducibility of results as judged by statistical and biological criteria in multiple independent studies involving different species and strains.

8. The level and extent of pathological examination were comparable in control and treated groups and the description of the pathological findings was consistent with generally accepted criteria for tumor nomencla-

ture. The pathological report described the full spectrum of toxic, preneoplastic, and neoplastic lesions, preferably including the results of
interim sacrifices.

9. The classification of pathological end points was confirmed by peer
   review.
10. A dose-response relationship was observed and confirmed statistically by
    the application of appropriate methods.
11. Factors such as microbial status of the test animals, various forms of
    stress, immune modulation, hormonal status, diurnal rhythms, and dis-
    ease processes that may have caused or contributed to the increased
    tumor incidence were considered.
12. There was positive evidence for genetic activity in appropriate, well
    validated, short-term tests and biochemical investigations demonstrated
    the formation of chemically reactive intermediates along with DNA
    adduct formation in target organs.

The weight of evidence for carcinogenicity would be decreased in instances
where:

1. Impurities, chemical breakdown, or reaction products not expected to be
   associated with human exposure pathways were judged to be responsible
   in whole, or in part, for the observed carcinogenic response.
2. The results were confounded by the use of doses that caused a marked
   alteration in physiological homeostasis, nutritional status, hormone balance, reduced ability of the test animals to metabolize and eliminate the
   chemical, clinical or pathological evidence of stress, toxicity, intercurrent
   disease, or poor survival. Such confounding variables may invoke mechanisms that lead secondarily to tumor formation that may not be relevant to
   humans.
3. An inappropriate experimental design or dosing regime was used.
4. No dose response was observed.
5. Only benign tumors, with no evidence of progression towards malignancy,
   were induced.
6. An unusual pattern of tumor incidence was reported (e.g., less than the
   expected incidence or no tumors in controls), raising questions regarding
   the validity of the pathological diagnosis.
7. If the compound was administered parenterally, tumors were observed
   only at the injection site.
8. There were serious flaws in the design and/or conduct of the study, as
   judged by recognized principles of good laboratory practice, that were
   likely to have affected the results of the study.

Under such circumstances, the evidence for carcinogenicity may be considered as marginal or limited.

Relevance of Animal Bioassays to Humans

The second step in the evaluation of data on carcinogenesis involves the assessment of the relevance of animal studies to humans. There is now substantial evidence to indicate that, for certain types of carcinogens and carcinogenic responses, animal evidence is unlikely to be predictive of probable human response. Table 1 lists a series of animal carcinogens, many of which would be classified as having "sufficient" evidence for carcinogenicity according to existing criteria. A fundamental question, however, is whether, given the nature of human exposure conditions, they pose any potential hazard at all. In assessing the relevance of such findings to humans, clearly one must recognize that the doses used in testing these chemicals exceed human exposure levels by several orders of magnitude. This, of course, provides for a very large margin of safety between animals and man, but there are other factors operative in these studies that cast doubt on the relevance of the findings to humans. Most importantly, in nearly every instance, tumors are associated with persistent, chronic toxicity and repeated tissue injury, a phenomena that could not conceivably occur under usual conditions of human exposure. Furthermore, tumors fail to occur in groups of animals exposed at doses that do not produce evidence of tissue toxicity, further suggesting that the tumor response in animals is closely linked to chronic proliferative tissue damage. In effect, all these substances appear to demonstrate thresholds in terms of carcinogenic action.

In assessing the relevance to humans of animal studies such as these, it is clear that mechanistic-type investigations form a critical aspect of the evaluation. The administration of carcinogens in different dose/time combination experiments may provide important clues as to whether a substance is acting primarily as an initiating agent, primarily displays enhancing activity, or both. In addition, it may be apparent from dose-response studies that the agent demonstrates practical thresholds. For example, the induction of tumors may be related to specific metabolic aberrations resulting from chronic toxicity or

Table 1

Example Animal Carcinogens of Questionable Relevance to Humans

Chemical	Tumor Site
Butylated hydroxyanisole	forestomach
Ethyl acrylate	forestomach
Ethylenethiourea	thyroid gland
Melamine	bladder
Potassium bromate	forestomach
Xylitol	adrenal gland/bladder

physical processes such as chronic inflammation and fibrosis that would not be expected to occur at low doses (Grasso and Goldberg 1966; Shank and Barrows 1981; Jensen et al. 1983; Nutrition Foundation 1983; Ghanayem et al. 1986). Experimental data that can be used to assess the effect of chemicals on the integrity of genetic material (Radman et al. 1977), gene expression (Razin and Friedman 1981), DNA damage repair (Larsen et al. 1982), or the application of techniques that make it possible to detect and measure altered DNA bases or specific DNA adducts (Randerath et al. 1985) have an important bearing on the qualitative assessment of hazard as well as in the extrapolation from high to low dose. In addition, metabolic and pharmacokinetic studies may be used to identify metabolites, to gain an understanding of relationships between increasing dose and absorption, distribution, metabolism, and excretion, and to assess physiologic/metabolic thresholds that may have an important bearing on the relevance of experimental studies to man (Ramsey and Gehring 1980; Reitz et al. 1980; Wolf 1980).

These observations lead to the conclusion that, in the hazard identification process, it is becoming increasingly important to develop rigorous criteria by which to judge the relevance of animal cancer bioassays to humans. There is obvious need to assess the relevance of animal studies against such criteria before making any conclusions regarding the human risk. In keeping with this concept, I have elaborated a number of criteria that may be applied in assessing the relevance of animal studies to humans. The predictive value of studies in animals, even those studies demonstrating sufficient evidence of carcinogenicity, may be diminished or questioned in instances where:

1. The test chemical or complex mixture was not representative of that to which humans are exposed.
2. The nature (route) of human exposure differs markedly from that used in the animal tests.
3. The tumor response was limited to an increase in tumors that occur with a high spontaneous incidence in the test animals.
4. The doses producing evidence of carcinogenicity were sufficiently high that they induced toxicity incompatible with normal physiological function, *and* no tumors were observed at doses immediately below those that produced evidence of toxicity.
5. Tumors were limited to specific anatomical sites or tissues not shared by humans.
6. Mechanistic studies demonstrated that tumor induction was closely linked with chronic physical irritation, physiological perturbations, or marked derangements in endogenous metabolism.

7. Pharmacokinetic studies and structure/activity relationship investigations strongly suggested that the parent compound was either not metabolized (inert) or metabolized rapidly to innocuous end products. Pharmacokinetic studies demonstrated marked differences in disposition between test animals and man or between high and low doses in test animals.
8. Epidemiological evidence exists, which, while not definitive, weighs against the possibility that the chemical or complex mixture is carcinogenic in humans under the usual conditions of exposure.

If these criteria are applied to the substances listed in Table 1, it is evident that the relevance to humans of these findings of carcinogenicity is questionable. For example, in the case of butylated hydroxyanisole (BHA) the existing studies demonstrate the presence of forestomach tumors in rats only at very high doses and no tumors at dietary levels as high as 1.0% (Ito et al. 1986). In effect, the tumor response demonstrates a threshold. Furthermore, mechanistic studies demonstrate that chronic irritative hyperplasia, which is accompanied metabolically by increased thymidine uptake in the forestomach epithelium, is a prerequisite for tumor development and that these effects, as well, demonstrate clearly defined thresholds (Altmann and Grunow 1986; Clayson et al. 1986). Importantly, no such effects are noted in species possessing only a glandular stomach such as monkeys or pigs, suggesting this response is limited to those species having a forestomach (Iverson et al. 1986; Würtzen and Olsen 1986). Finally, there is no evidence that BHA or its major metabolic products possess genotoxic activity (Williams 1986). As another example, xylitol is one of several commercially used polyols. Xylitol produces adrenal pheochromocytoma in rats and bladder tumors in mice (FAO/WHO 1978, 1983; Roe and Bär 1985; Life Sciences Research Office 1986). Both these effects are noted only at the high dose levels and demonstrate thresholds. Mechanistic studies demonstrate that xylitol, when fed at dietary levels of 20%, produces cecal enlargement in rodents, a phenomena which is often accompanied by alterations in mineral metabolism (LSRO 1986). In this regard, xylitol administered at high levels, leads to increased calcium uptake from the gastrointestinal tract, as well as increased water uptake (Bär 1986). These effects are closely related, in the case of xylitol, as well as with many other substances, to the development of adrenal medullary hyperplasia in rats, which in some animals proceeds chronically to pheochromocytoma (LSRO 1986). In mice, high doses of xylitol, which overwhelm the normal metabolism through the pentose phosphate shunt, lead to increased oxalate excretion, a precursor of urinary bladder stone formation. The relationship between bladder stone formation and bladder tumors is well known (Ball et al. 1964). Dose-response studies have demonstrated that all these effects have thresholds (Bär 1983). There is no evidence that xylitol is genotoxic (LSRO

1986). Finally, the adrenal medullary effects observed with xylitol are common to many other dietary polyols and indeed even have been observed with lactose (FAO/WHO 1983; LSRO 1986).

The application of these criteria are therefore important in making a determination of the possible relevance of animals studies to humans. If it is judged that animal carcinogenicity data are not relevant to human exposure conditions or if the analysis leads to serious questions regarding relevance of experimental studies to man, then such data should not be used as a basis for human risk assessment.

On the other hand, there are many substances that demonstrate all the hallmarks of classical carcinogenic action. These chemicals may be metabolized to reactive intermediates that form stable, identifiable DNA adducts in target tissues (Randerath et al. 1985; Rajewsky 1986), induce DNA repair mechanisms (McQueen and Williams 1985), and produce consistent evidence of carcinogenicity, when administered at low doses, in multiple species and strains. Substances possessing these properties cannot be equated for purposes of hazard assessment with chemicals that only cause an increase in the yield of common tumors, reduce the latent period, or cause tumors through secondary mechanisms at maximum tolerable exposures. For most of these substances, the relevance to humans is clearly implied by the data, particularly in instances where:

1. There is strong evidence, over a range of doses, for carcinogenicity in multiple species or strains.
2. The route of exposure and the experimental design used in the animal studies appropriately represented the nature of human exposure.
3. The chemical or complex mixture tested was chemically identical to that to which humans are exposed.
4. Tumor induction was not due to secondary or confounding factors unique to the test system that would not be expected, for reasons of dose or otherwise, to occur in humans under the usual conditions of exposure.

Confidence in the predictive value for humans of experimental studies of carcinogenesis may be further enhanced when:

1. Metabolic studies in test animals and man in vivo and/or in vitro indicated similar patterns of metabolites and pharmacokinetics.
2. Mechanistic studies were consistent with the substance acting as a typical carcinogen.
3. There was positive evidence for genetic activity in appropriate, well validated, short-term tests, and biochemical investigations demonstrated the formation of chemically reactive intermediates along with DNA adduct formation in target organs.

In applying these criteria in practice, it must be recognized that the characterization of human hazard based upon experimental studies requires that judgment be applied in assessing the weight of evidence for carcinogenic potential in man. No procedure exists that can routinely be applied to this exercise. Each bioassay is unique, both in terms of its design and the results it produces. Each substance, therefore, must be evaluated on a case-by-case basis in accordance with recognized scientific principles.

CONCLUSIONS

Animal bioassays are an important component of research and regulatory programs to reduce human exposure to carcinogenic substances. The assessment of the weight of evidence for carcinogenicity in animals requires a critical evaluation of all data bearing on the question of carcinogenesis. It is considered essential that factors such as the appropriateness of experimental design, route and level of exposure, statistical power of tests, histopathological criteria, the susceptibility of the species and strains used for bioassay, and the consistency and reproducibility of findings in multiple independent experiments be carefully considered in evaluating evidence for carcinogenicity.

The assessment of the relevance of animal studies to humans likewise requires a careful evaluation of the predictive value of animal bioassay results on a case-by-case basis. There are now numerous examples of chemicals that will produce evidence for carcinogenicity in animals under specific laboratory conditions; however, the relevance of these findings to humans is limited or questionable. Criteria to assess the relevance of experimental findings to humans include the appropriateness of experimental designs relative to human exposure conditions, the characteristics of the strains and species of animals used, the nature of tumor response, dose-response relationships, mechanistic considerations, and other auxiliary studies.

It is considered essential that the assessment of carcinogenicity in animals be viewed separately from the evaluation of the relevance of animal findings to humans. Existing carcinogen classification systems would be improved by the addition of objective criteria by which to judge the relevance of animal tests to humans.

REFERENCES

Altmann, H.J. and W. Grunow. 1986. Effects of BHA and related phenols on the forestomach of rats. *Food Chem. Toxicol.* **24:** 1183.

Ball, J.K., W.E.H. Field, F.J.C. Roe, and M. Walters. 1964. The carcinogenic and co-carcinogenic effects of paraffin wax pellets and glass beads in the mouse bladder. *Br. J. Urol.* **36:** 225.

Bär, A. 1983. *Modulating factors in xylitol-induced urolithiasis: Comparison of NMRI vs. Fuellinsdorf-Albino mice and comparison of different xylitol grades.* Report of F. Hoffmann-La-Roche and Company, Limited, Basle, Switzerland. Docket no. 121.1114. Dockets Management Branch, Food and Drug Administration, Rockville, Maryland.

———. 1986. *Adrenomedullary tumours in xylitol-fed rats: Dietary levels of calcium as a determinant factor.* Research report no. B-44112, prepared by Xyrofin UK Limited, United Kingdom.

Clayson, D.B. and D. Krewski. 1986. The concept of negativity in experimental carcinogenesis. *Mutat. Res.* **167**: 233.

Clayson, D.B., F. Iverson, E. Nera, E. Lok, C. Rogers, and C. Rodrigues. 1986. Histopathological and radioautographical studies on the forestomach of F344 rats treated with butylated hydroxyanisole and related chemicals. *Food Chem. Toxicol.* **24**: 1171.

Food and Agriculture Organization/World Health Organization (FAO/WHO). 1978. *Summary of toxicological data of certain food additives and contaminants.* Twenty-second report of the Joint FAO/WHO Expert Committee on Food Additives. WHO technical report series no. 631. Geneva, Switzerland.

———. 1983. *Evaluation of certain food additives and contaminants.* Twenty-seventh report of the joint FAO/WHO Expert Committee on food additives. WHO technical report series no. 696. Geneva, Switzerland.

Ghanayem, B.I., R.R. Marapot, and H.B. Matthews. 1986. Ethyl acrylate induced gastric toxicity. III. Development and recovery of lesions. *Toxicol. Appl. Pharmacol.* **83**: 576.

Grasso, P. and L. Golberg. 1966. Subcutaneous sarcoma as an index of carcinogenic potency. *Food Cosmet. Toxicol.* **4**: 297.

International Agency for Research on Cancer (IARC). 1983. *Approaches to classifying chemical carcinogens according to mechanism of action.* IARC technical report 83/001. International Agency for Research on Cancer, Lyon, France.

———. 1987. *IARC Monogr. Eval. Carcinog. Risk. Chem. Hum.* IARC Internal technical report 87/001. Lyon, France.

International Life Sciences Institute (ILSI). 1984. *Current issues in toxicology* (ed. H.C. Grice). Springer-Verlag, New York.

Ito, N., M. Hirose, H. Fukushima, H. Tsuda, T. Shirai, and M. Tatematsu. 1986. Studies on antioxidants: Their carcinogenic and modifying effects on chemical carcinogenesis. *Food Chem. Toxicol.* **24**: 1071.

Iverson, H., J. Truelove, E. Nera, D.B. Clayson, and J. Wong. 1986. A 12-week study of BHA in the cynomolgus monkey. *Food Chem. Toxicol.* **24**: 1197.

Jensen, R.K., S.D. Sleight, S.D. Aust, J.I. Goodman, and J.E. Troskos. 1983. Hepatic tumor-promoting ability of 3,3',4,4',5,5'-hexabromobiphenyl: The interrelationship between toxicity, induction of hepatic microsomal drug metabolizing enzymes, and tumor-promoting ability. *Toxicol. Appl. Pharmacol.* **71**: 163.

Krewski, D. and J. Van Ryzin. 1981. Dose response models for quantal toxicity data. In *Statistics and related topics* (ed. M. Czorgo et al.), p. 201. North Holland, Amsterdam.

Larsen, K.H., D. Brash, J.E. Cleaver, R.W. Hart, V.M. Maher, R.B. Painter, and G.A. Sega. 1982. DNA repair assays as tests for environmental mutagens. A report of the U.S. EPA Gene-Tox program. *Mutat. Res.* **98:** 287.

Life Sciences Research Office (LSRO). 1986. *Health aspects of sugar alcohols and lactose.* Life Sciences Research Office, Bethesda, Maryland.

McQueen, C.A. and G.M. Williams. 1985. Mammalian cell DNA repair assays for carcinogens. *Adv. Environ. Toxicol.* **11:** 129.

National Toxicology Program (NTP). 1984. *Report of the NTP ad hoc panel on chemical carcinogenesis testing and evaluation.* U.S. Department of Health and Human Services, Washington, D.C.

Nutrition Foundation. 1983. *A report of the International Expert Advisory Committee to the Nutrition Foundation. The relevance of mouse liver hepatoma to human carcinogenic risk.* Nutrition Foundation, Washington, D.C.

Office of Science and Technology Policy (OSTP). 1985. *Chemical carcinogens: A review of the science and associated principles.* Office of Science and Technology Policy. *Fed Reg.* **50:** 10372.

Organization for Economic Co-operation and Development (OECD). 1981. *Guidelines for testing chemicals.* Organization for Economic Co-operation and Development, Paris, France.

Radman, M., G. Villani, S. Boiteux, M. Defais, P. Caillet-Fauquet, and S. Spadari. 1977. On the mechanism and genetic control of mutagenesis induced by carcinogenic mutagens. *Cold Spring Harbor Confr. Cell Proliferation* **4(B):** 903.

Rajewsky, M. 1986. Immunoanalysis of structural DNA modifications induced by N-nitroso compounds. In *Proceedings of the Toxicology Forum Meeting,* p. 159. Toxicology Forum, Inc., Washington, D.C.

Ramsey, J.C. and P.J. Gehring. 1980. Application of pharmacokinetic principles in practice. *Fed. Proc.* **39:** 60.

Randerath, K., E. Randerath, H. Agrawal, R. Gupta, M. Schurdak, and M. Reddy. 1985. Postlabeling methods for carcinogen-DNA adduct analysis. *Environ. Health Perspect.* **62:** 57.

Razin, A. and J. Friedman. 1981. DNA methylation and its possible biological roles. *Prog. Nucleic Acid Res. Mol. Biol.* **25:** 33.

Reitz, R.H., J.F. Quast, A.M. Schumann, P.G. Watanabe, and P.J. Gehring. 1980. Non-linear pharmacokinetic parameters need to be considered in high dose/low dose extrapolations. *Arch. Toxicol. Suppl.* **3:** 79.

Roe, F.J.C. and A. Bär. 1985. Enzootic and epizotic adrenal medullary proliferative disease of rats: Influence of dietary factors which affect calcium absorption. *Hum. Toxicol.* **4:** 27.

Shank, R.C. and L.R. Barrows. 1981. Toxicity-dependent DNA methylation: Significance to risk assessment. In *Health risk analyses* (ed. C.R. Richmond et al.), p. 225. Franklin Institute Press, Philadelphia.

Tomatis, L. 1979. The predictive value of rodent carcinogenicity tests in the evaluation of human risks. *Annu. Rev. Pharmacol. Toxicol.* **19:** 511.

U.S. Environmental Protection Agency (USEPA). 1986. Guidelines for carcinogen risk assessment. *Fed. Reg.* **51:** 33992.

U.S. Food and Drug Administration (USFDA). 1982. *Toxicological principles for the safety assessment of direct food additives and color additives used in food.* U.S. Food and Drug Administration Bureau of Foods, Washington, D.C.

Weisburger, J.H. 1985. Definition of a carcinogen as a potential human cancer risk. *Jpn. J. Cancer Res.* **76:** 1244.

World Health Organization (WHO). 1987. *Principles for the safety assessment of food additives and contaminants in food.* Environmental Health Criteria 70, World Health Organization, Geneva, Switzerland.

Williams, G.M. 1986. Epigenetic promoting effects of butylated hydroxyanisole. *Food Chem. Toxicol.* **24:** 1163.

Wolf, F.J. 1980. Effect of overloading pathways on toxicity. *J. Environ. Pathol. Toxicol.* **3:** 113.

Würtzen, G. and P. Olsen. 1986. BHA study in pigs. *Food Chem. Toxicol.* **24:** 1229.

COMMENTS

Michejda: The trouble with these kinds of factors that decrease relevance is that you used a couple of "straw men," namely xylitol and perhaps BHA. The point is that the study of tumors in organs such as the forestomach, has been used by various organizations to discount uncomfortable bioassay data, sometimes quite incorrectly. One that I remember quite recently was an EPA panel discussion on methacrylates. One of the representatives of the methacrylate makers was upset that only forestomach tumors were observed, since man doesn't have a forestomach. He thought it was crazy to use that type of criteria, but I don't.

Munro: I don't think it is either.

Michejda: Likewise, using the Zymbal's gland is not crazy.

Munro: You cannot predict site specificity from animals to man, I don't think.

Michejda: That's right. That's the point.

Munro: That's an accepted point. I didn't say that it was that criteria, producing tumors in the forestomach, that I would not consider relevant to man. There is a whole series of other data surrounding BHA, relating to its metabolism, its tissue-binding characteristics or lack of tissue-binding characteristics, that leads one to the conclusion that it's not relevant to humans. Clearly, there are carcinogens that produce forestomach tumors or Zymbal's gland tumors, and I think everyone in this room would agree that would be of great significance to man. The reason I raise this as an issue is that it is important to structure our discussion so that all of the relevant information that is necessary to make a determination of relevance is considered.

Wilson: I don't think that BHA is a straw man. Certainly, from the regulatory point of view, it's a very important and difficult decision.

Munro: In dealing with assessing relevance for carcinogenicity from experimental studies and extrapolating to humans, it is easy to deal with what Willy (Lijinsky) would call the strong carcinogens. On the other end of the spectrum, we have the BHAs or xylitols, and I did use those as examples, and to that extent they are straw men.

    The difficulty arises with the gray areas in between, some of which were discussed this morning: PBB, dioxin, and others.

Pfitzer: I think Chris' (Michejda) point is a very important one for us to keep in mind. There is always in the back of our mind, when we look at these kinds of factors and select which ones become relevant to a particular decision, that we are explaining away something that may be very important. Our problem, I think, is that risk assessors have to evaluate the scientific evidence on all the factors and not throw out something because it's in the forestomach, because it's a natural product, or for whatever reason. I think the point you have raised is one that creates a lot of controversy in our discussions because of the fear that we may be just trying to whitewash a given bioassay, as opposed to using good science and considering all the factors relevant to extrapolation.

Weisburger: Could I ask you a question about the xylitol experiment? Was anything seen at the 5% dose level?

Munro: Nothing.

Weisburger: Then, if it had been done at the 5% dose level, according to current NTP guidelines . . .

Munro: You wouldn't have detected it.

Weisburger: You wouldn't have seen anything?

Munro: Nothing.

Pfitzer: Maybe I should respond to that since I was personally responsible for designing that study.

Munro: I didn't realize that.

Pfitzer: I've gotten a lot of grief from my associates, for having designed that experiment at 20% in the diet. We talked about saccharin at 5% and higher and the ton quantities required. I can tell you that, in doing a two-year mouse study, a two-year rat study, a two-year dog study, a three-generation/two-litter rat reproduction study, and a rabbit teratology study, that it took four tons of xylitol, about the first year's manufacturing from the plant.

I can also tell you that in the 13-week studies that we did in preparation for the 2-year studies, we went to 50%. The only thing that happened was massive diarrhea, and some animals died of diarrhea. Even doing studies at 20%, you have to adapt the animals to prevent diarrhea. The guidelines recommending a maximum dose level of 5% or 10% were designed for a nonnutrient. With xylitol we are talking about a nutrient, and so we are talking about a situation that is not necessarily creating a major problem.

Just to maybe wrap this up, the point is, that what FDA said was, "Explain these tumors. Here you have a natural product, present in prunes to a high concentration, part of our endogenous metabolism in the normal cycle of events. Nobody would expect it to be a problem. There were no genotoxicity problems."

Initially, nobody believed the calcium oxalate stones in the bladder. Nobody believed that calcium oxalate stones caused the bladder cancer. That seemed to be rather accepted. It took a lot of work to show that at these very high concentrations you did invoke now the pentose-phosphate shunt and you did produce some oxalate which, along with excess absorption of calcium, caused calcium oxalate stone. The phaeochromocytomas were a very different story and not completely answered.

Michejda: However, that's a tumor in an aging rat anyway.

Pfitzer: Absolutely.

Munro: You see them in the controls, but in the xylitol animals you see a very high incidence. I've forgotten the numbers.

Pfitzer: Many pathologists do not consider phaeochromocytomas to be a problem in rats. A lot of drugs that are on the market cause phaeochromocytomas, and we say they're just not relevant to humans. It's a very different tumor in the animal. In Finland, people have been exposed to xylitol for two years in their diet, where all the sugar was replaced, so that the xylitol concentration was upwards of 10% of the total diet. There were births that took place with no problems of any kind.

However, the question that is unanswered is the scientific documentation that explains the adrenal gland phaeochromocytomas. The hypothesis is that a major upset in calcium metabolism which clearly takes place (and which also takes place with lactose and other polyols, such as sorbitol) can in some way interfere with homeostasis of the adrenal gland, leading to enlargement and an increase in tumors. That experiment has not been fully completed.

I think the question for a scientific body is: What would be a definitive experiment that would allow the scientific community to say, "Yes, those phaeochromocytomas are specific to upset calcium homeostatis and should not be extrapolated to humans?" It's that with which the risk assessors have to deal.

Munro: As I recall, there was some data to demonstrate that with the increased calcium uptake there is an increase in either adrenal medullary levels or circulating EPIs. If you block that, you can reduce the calcium level in the body. That may have some mechanistic implications.

Pfitzer: Yes. By reducing the calcium in the diet, you can show that with either lactose or xylitol given at high concentrations, even with a low amount in the diet, you increase the absorption sufficiently to maintain adequate calcium in the body. That is an excellent experiment for somebody to do.

Perera: You state that a lack of genetic toxicity data would cause you to be far less concerned about the potential of human cancer risk. You list that as one of your criteria. Yet, I find that a bit speculative in light of the fact that several of the most potent animal carcinogens do not manifest genetic toxicity. To my knowledge, we do not know the shape of the dose-response curve for the so-called nongenotoxic carcinogens at the low end of the curve. So, on what is this based? I realize that we had some discussion earlier about experimental thresholds, Jim Trosko mentioned those, but I think that it is very different talking about human thresholds.

Munro: That is an extremely important point. Maybe you misinterpreted. I was very careful not to include that as a criteria, that the lack of genotoxicity would reduce relevance. What I said was that where there was evidence for genotoxicity that would increase my level of concern, but I was very careful not to include that lack of evidence for genotoxicity or mutagenicity as a criteria. Of course, as pointed out by Dr. Trosko and others, there are many, many carcinogens that do not produce evidence of mutagenicity, and one cannot use the negative test as a criteria to say that you would not be concerned about it.

Pfitzer: Just to expand on that, I think in the case of xylitol we would include that in Ray's (Tennant) list as an adaptive carcinogen. That is, there is a mechanism of adaptation in the animal that causes tumors in the absence of any known genotoxicity.

Neal: Related to your comment about no data on low-dose or thresholds for promoters, I think Henry Pitot's data on the promotion of DEN by phenobarbital was done at low enough concentrations to suggest there really was a threshold. If not, it's very close to one. I think Butwell did the same thing on TPA in the skin papillomas. I think that the data bases are available, and it's a matter of whether you interpret that it was done at low enough doses with no effect to call it a threshold.

Perera: I'm not denying that there are experimental thresholds; those have been shown for various compounds under certain test conditions. What I am saying is that it's difficult to leap from there to the human situation and to say that we understand the shape of the dose-response curve in the humans.

Munro: You are absolutely right.

Wilson: I would observe that there is no information that I have seen supporting any choice of any dose-response at sufficiently low dose. The toxicologists typically assume that something like a probit curve or one of the similar S-shaped saturation curves apply. However, the practical matter of statistics at doses below 5%, let alone 1% of 10^{-4}, are such that I am not optimistic that you can ever define what that shape will be. It's a lot easier in my mind if the consensus of experts suggests that what applies in animals ought to apply in humans, rather than to try to determine what in fact the dose-response curve looks like at very low incidence.

Michejda: This is for promoters?

Wilson: That's for anything.

Michejda: There are some excellent data for diethylnitrosamine.

Wilson: That's not at 10^{-4} incidence.

Michejda: That data are at very low doses.

Wilson: No, that's not at very low doses but at very low incidence.

Michejda: Well, he just pulled 10^{-4} out of the hat.

Lijinsky: Unless you're going to use 10,000 animals per group, you can only really get down to about 2%, using a reasonable number of animals. Even if you use 500 animals, you're going to require 2% incidence to be statistically significant.

Michejda: However, one does know what the shape of that curve is beginning to look like in the end.

Wilson: You cannot distinguish between several different models.

Munro: I think that's the whole problem. Even the recent studies that were done by Pitot on DMN or DEN . . .

Lijinsky: He didn't have 50 animals per group.

Munro: Why 50 animals per group? You cannot really predict what is going to happen at a risk of 10^{-5} or 10^{-6}.

Lijinsky: You can guess, but then it's a guess.

Munro: In fact, the most recent data in the paper by Willy Butler that I quoted earlier suggested, even with a chemical as potent as dimethylnitrosamine, there is a suggestion of a threshold in the dose-response curve. Realistically, at that level, I don't know if it makes any difference for a regulatory point of view, practically speaking.

Trosko: To follow up on Dr. Perera's point, for example, if one just assumed for the moment that blockage of cell communication plays on mechanistic role in tumor promotion, we and others now have shown that with the five known mechanisms to block cell communication. If you interact two chemicals by themselves, that are not at a concentration high enough to activate PKC, for example, a low level of TPA that just pickles the enzyme and a low level of DET, you get no effect on the blockage of cell communication and, presumably, no effect on tumor promotion. However, if you add both of them together at these two low levels, you synergize the reaction and produce block communication.

So, this goes from the experimental situation to the real life situation. We can measure single chemical effects on a mechanism and make predictions. However, in the real life, as with that example, you have this interaction going on. We have always had endogenous chemicals that can modulate cell communication and will always be exposed to exogenous ones. The real question is can we ever predict, from a single cell analysis in an experimental system, what is going on in your stomach right now because of what you ate for dessert today.

Pfitzer: There is another question in that regard, and that is, if you have a plausible mechanism, whether it's cell-cell communication or some other reason to suggest a promotion, the question always is: Well, perhaps that mechanism does exist, but will the chemical also, in addition, produce some genotoxic or other effect? I don't know how one answers that question other than by utilizing the battery of tests that we use. That is a problem that certain risk assessors always bring up.

Neal: Not an absolute answer, but you get a preponderance of evidence that it is acting by a promotional mechanism or whatever you choose to call it.

Pfitzer: That, I think, is what Ian's (Munro) paper is about, the preponderance of weighted evidence and how you use it. One thing that is clear for those of us who work a bit on the international circuit is that the weights given to all these things are very different in Europe than they are in the United States.

Munro: Absolutely. They differ everywhere.

Expert Scientific Judgment in Quantitative Risk Assessment

JOHN D. GRAHAM,* NEIL C. HAWKINS,† AND MARC J. ROBERTS*
*Department of Health Policy and Management and
†Department of Environmental Science and Physiology
Harvard School of Public Health
Boston, Massachusetts 02115

INTRODUCTION

The birthdate of quantitative cancer risk assessment varies depending on your perspective. The pathbreaking academic papers were published beginning in the 1950s (Armitage and Doll 1954, 1961; Mantel and Bryan 1961; Mantel et al. 1975; Crump et al. 1976; Hoel et al. 1983). The use of the tool by federal regulatory agencies began with the Food and Drug Administration in 1973 (Hutt 1985) and the Environmental Protection Agency (EPA) in 1977 (Albert et al. 1977). The Occupational Safety and Health Administration (OSHA) resisted risk assessment until Supreme Court Justice John Paul Stevens wrote the plurality opinion in the famous benzene case (IUD 1980). The Carcinogen Assessment Group of EPA has been very influential in promoting the application of a particular analytical approach to cancer risk assessment (Anderson et al. 1983).

For better or for worse, quantitative cancer risk assessment is here to stay. The powerful sustaining forces include at least the following:

1. Regulators find the carcinogen versus noncarcinogen distinction unhelpful; they want to know something about the magnitude of risk in order to chart priorities and to set standards (Graham et al. 1988).
2. Courts demand that regulators show some quantitative indication of risk in order to satisfy the threshold tests of substantial evidence of significant risk of cancer (Graham 1987).
3. Professional economists at federal agencies and the Office of Management and Budget need numerical risk estimates in order to conduct their now mandatory cost-benefit analyses (Haigh et al. 1984).
4. Many industrial interests have difficulty arguing against the technique(s) (despite profound reservations), since they were such aggressive proponents of them in the 1970s.
5. Many environmental and labor activists, although suspicious of the tools, seem resigned to working with them or around them rather than against them in their campaigns for regulation of toxic substances.

Banbury Report 31: Carcinogen Risk Assessment: New Directions in the Qualitative and Quantitative Aspects © Cold Spring Harbor Laboratory. 0-87969-231-6/88. $1.00 + .00

6. A literal industry of academic research and professional consulting has been built around this tool (and such industries tend to be self-perpetuating).

The only resistance to quantitative risk assessment, and the resistance is in some cases significant, lies in the scientific community (Graham et al. 1988).

The natural inclination of many first-rate toxicologists, biologists, chemists, and epidemiologists is to stay away from quantitative risk assessment. As we shall note below, the reasons for this inclination are quite understandable. Quantitative cancer risk assessment is not yet scientific, in our view. The dilemma is, however, that nonparticipation by practicing scientists is not a neutral policy position, even though it may seem so at first glance. Since regulators face legal and political demands to quantify risk before regulating, scientists who choose not to participate have taken a profoundly (however unintentional) antiregulation position. It is quite possible that the practicing scientists who do participate in cancer risk assessment are not a random draw of the best scientific talent in the world. On the other hand, the scientists who currently participate in risk assessment may have more proregulation inclinations than those who do not participate. In any event, we believe that it is crucial for the competency and legitimacy of the regulatory process to increase the rate of scientific participation in risk assessment (Graham et al. 1988).

AN EVALUATION OF PREVAILING ANALYTICAL PRACTICE

The prevailing practice of quantitative cancer risk assessment is probably best represented by EPA's recent carcinogen assessment guidelines (United States Environmental Protection Agency 1986). When the mush words and qualifiers are set aside, the normal procedure for assessing potency is as follows:

1. Since good human data are rarely available, choose the data set from animal studies that shows the greatest sensitivity.
2. Count both benign and malignant tumors when calculating incidence.
3. Fit the data to the "linearized multistage model" as embodied in computer programs such as GLOBAL79, GLOBAL82, and RISK81, which assume (among other things) that the added effect of exposure to a carcinogen at low doses is virtually linear.
4. Define dose as cumulative lifetime exposure (or average daily dose) to the substance of question.
5. Use relative surface area as a standardized scaling factor for interspecies conversions.

These guidelines are accompanied by instruction to "do otherwise" if compelling scientific evidence contradicts any of the normal procedures. Risk assessors are encouraged to make assumptions explicit and to convey the degree of uncertainty in risk estimates when possible.

A classification system adapted from the International Agency for Research in Cancer is also used by EPA to convey the weight of evidence for carcinogenicity from human and animal studies. Published risk numbers are supposed to be accompanied by a weight-of-the-evidence classification on a scale from A to E.

Strengths

Most decision makers desire some information about worst-case scenarios and the EPA potency factors can be interpreted as an upper bound on the true yet unknown carcinogenic potency. The multiple conservative assumptions seem likely to result in an overstatement of human risk (Nichols and Zeckhauser 1985) even though factors such as highly sensitive human subpopulations are not explicitly taken into account (Finkel 1984). Although it is far from clear how conservative the EPA potency estimate is for any specific chemical, it seems very unlikely that the true potency at low doses will exceed the EPA estimate in most cases (Crump 1981).

Another strength of the current procedure is that in principle it can be applied to a large number of substances at relatively low cost. The classification system is fairly easy to apply, and the software is available to crank the numbers when bioassay data are available (Crump and Watson 1979; Kovar and Krewski 1981; Howe and Crump 1982). Indeed, the widespread use of EPA's potency estimates in the public and private sectors is an indication of the practicality of the procedure.

And for those who are inclined to inquire, the assumptions of the EPA procedure are explicit and open to criticism. The explicitness of the assumptions also makes the risk assessment process fairly predictable for outsiders who learn the game. In an adversarial regulatory process, explicitness and predictability are often considered to be virtues (Graham et al. 1988).

Weaknesses

The fundamental weakness of the EPA procedure is that it is unscientific. Risk estimates based on the EPA potency factors are typically unverifiable. Practical constraints on the size of human and animal studies prevent validation of EPA potency factors in the low-dose range, where regulatory policy is usually made. Note that this criticism is not unique to the EPA procedure; it applies to any procedure currently available for generating low-dose risk estimates. Although laudable attempts are underway to verify animal-based risk estimates for known human carcinogens (e.g., see DuMouchel and Harris 1983), the extrapolation problem will persist at doses below the range of doses observed by epidemiology. Moreover, most animal carcinogens have not yet been shown to cause cancer in humans.

Another key weakness of the standard EPA procedure is that it censors much of the available experimental, biological, and "soft" information. The drive to be conservative, which is a strength of the procedure, causes alternative bioassays, nonlinear dose-response hypotheses, and pharmacokinetic data and judgments to be set aside. Any procedure that excludes so much information is bound to have acceptance problems, let alone concerns about technical accuracy.

If the upper bound produced by the EPA procedure were accompanied by a quantitative treatment of uncertainty, resistance to the approach might be lessened (Lave 1982). Unfortunately, the prevailing treatment of uncertainty suffers from the twin evils of false precision and false imprecision. When the EPA potency factor is reported by itself, it conveys a false sense of precision. Even though it is intended solely as an upper bound, the absence of other numbers causes people to focus on the single number that is reported. When EPA reports that the true risk could be anywhere from zero to the upper bound, it is conveying a false sense of imprecision since each value between zero and the upper bound is not usually considered equally likely. The EPA procedure has no basis for conveying the relative plausibility of risk numbers between zero and the upper bound. The increasingly popular practice of reporting the maximum likelihood estimate (MLE) of risk in addition to the upper bound derived from the multistage model is a step in the right direction. However, the MLE is itself based on the choice of a mathematical model and the choice of a particular experimental data set. These choices are themselves often a contributor to the concealment of uncertainty.

Finally, the EPA procedure is arbitrary and, therefore, causes interests who dislike its output in particular cases to feel unjustly victimized. Although the procedure is probably conservative in most cases, the extent of conservatism built into the procedure is arbitrary. It is very easy to imagine other procedures that would be more or less conservative. For instance, a more conservative practice would be to compute the highest risk estimate for each substance that is not contradicted by published epidemiology (regardless of what the data from animal experiments suggest). The EPA procedure is especially frustrating to interest groups because EPA officials, when criticized, are naturally inclined to respond that "the Guidelines made me do it" or "GLOBAL82 made me do it." Interest groups are more likely to accept an unfavorable result if it is imposed by credible scientists than if it is imposed by seemingly arbitrary guidelines and computer programs.

FUTURE RESEARCH STRATEGIES FOR RISK ASSESSMENT

Current risk assessment practice can be improved by research. Research efforts can be usefully subdivided into three strategies: mechanistic and pharmacokinetic research, statistical modeling, and expert scientific judgment.

The first research strategy entails discovery of the mechanisms of cancer and the distribution and fate of chemicals in the body. It will lead to improved understanding of biological mechanisms and markers of dose more directly correlated with health effects. Basic pharmacokinetic research on chemical carcinogens in both animal and human models may lead to improved bases for extrapolation. Another basic strategy is development of dosimetric methods for epidemiological studies. The use of carefully developed human biomarkers may improve the link between animal models and epidemiology and also may lead to more powerful epidemiology. The fruits of such research would guide risk assessors in extrapolation from rodent to man, in properly defining dose, and in extrapolating from high to low doses.

The second strategy, improved statistical modeling, is needed to better utilize available bioassay data and to begin linking models to biology. A good example of where statisticians are making better use of available data is time-to-tumor analysis (Krewski et al. 1983). Another line of work seeks to modify statistical models in response to advancing biological knowledge (Watanabe et al. 1977; Anderson et al. 1980; Starr and Buck 1984).

Lastly, research aimed at incorporating expert scientific judgement into cancer risk assessment is needed. Risk assessors generally are not practicing scientists. They often lack the intuition and laboratory experience that is needed to interpret the complex array of data available for risk assessments. The judgments of practicing scientists should go beyond "peer review" and help guide the use of data, help build models more related to the biology of a given substance, and help convey plausible ranges of uncertainty.

Although all three strategies need to be pursued in order to improve risk assessment practice, our view is that the first priority in terms of allocating limited research resources must be given to original scientific research. This priority reflects the fact that this area could lead to the greatest breakthroughs, despite the high costs of such research. With improved knowledge of biological mechanisms of carcinogenesis, advances in statistical modeling and in elicitation of expert judgment may become less important. In the short run, breakthroughs in biology may not emerge, necessitating improved statistical modeling and incorporation of expert scientific judgment. Even if breakthroughs do occur, statistical modeling and expert judgment will be necessary to manipulate and interpret results. The focus of the remainder of this paper is on the research strategy that we believe is most neglected: incorporation of scientific judgment into cancer risk assessment.

HOW SCIENTIFIC JUDGMENT CAN HELP RISK ASSESSORS

Since practicing scientists are familiar with laboratory methods and have a wealth of experience to draw upon, they can be of significant assistance to risk assessors. As an example, practicing scientists can review available experimental data as to their quality and recommend which experimental results (if several are available) are most appropriate for risk assessment. Additionally, judgments about pooling results from different studies or species could be elicited, or judgments about benign tumors and their possible progression to malignancy would be valuable.

When a choice of statistical models is available, expert judgment may be the only course. The expert scientists may provide judgments about which mathematical model is most likely to reflect the biological mechanisms acting for a given chemical. Additionally, scientific judgment could provide a basis for departing from traditional modeling to physiological pharmacokinetic modeling. Once a model is chosen and used to analyze data, a practicing scientist could intuitively provide plausibility assessments of the assumed model and its predictions. These plausibility assessments could also be helpful in reducing the problems caused by falsely imprecise and falsely precise reporting of risk estimates, as discussed in an earlier section.

Lastly, expert judgments are needed to guide future research efforts on a given substance. When conflicting experimental results leave the risk assessment with great uncertainty, expert judgments about what research is needed to reduce uncertainty would be very helpful. Practicing scientists could recommend a research agenda, predict a reasonable time frame for seeing results, and estimate the total costs of the proposed effort. Given these judgments, the regulatory agency could rationally decide if the additional research is worth its cost in terms of reducing uncertainty about risk and improving regulatory decisions arising out of the risk assessment.

IMPLEMENTING EXPERT SCIENTIFIC JUDGMENT

Although expert judgments might assist risk assessors, how to elicit these judgments and from whom are critical issues that must be addressed. The form of the elicited judgments must also be carefully considered to ensure the usefulness of the judgments. The following sections highlight some of the issues in expert judgment research that need to be explored.

Selection of Experts

There are many approaches that might be employed to select experts for providing judgments. Obviously, the ideal approach would be the one that ultimately produces the correct scientific information. However, since no one is in a position today to judge which approach accomplishes that ideal, more process-oriented criteria must govern the selection process.

We believe that approaches to expert selection should be evaluated according to at least the following criteria:

1. *Relevant expertise.* The extent to which the approach generates experts with the specific kinds of scientific skills, knowledge, and experience relevant to the problems.
2. *Explicitness.* The extent to which outsiders can discern how and why participating scientists were selected.
3. *Reproducibility.* The extent to which a credible effort could be made to generate the same group of experts by a repetition of the same approach assuming such a repetition were desired.
4. *Ease of execution.* The amount of time, money, good will, and administrative resources expended.
5. *Sponsor control.* The extent to which the sponsor (often a regulatory agency) can control which particular scientists are selected.
6. *Balance.* The extent to which the approach achieves diversity in disciplinary, institutional, and political perspective.

In the context of regulatory decision making, we believe that, other things equal, approaches to expert selection should be used that achieve more explicitness, greater potential for reproducibility, more ease of execution, more relevant expertise, less sponsor control, and more balance than would result from a purely ad hoc or informal approach.

Methods for Elicitation of Expert Judgment

Elicitation of expert judgment can proceed by several methods: personal interviews, groups or panels, conferences, or a combination thereof. When expert panels or groups are convened to review scientific data, they are often asked to develop a consensus within their ranks (if possible) about the quality of the data and suitability for their use in the regulatory environment. In this framework, dominant personalities can guide the formation of the consensus, and opinions of less vocal members may not emerge. A reported consensus may be genuine or superficial (Graham et al. 1988).

The personal interview approach, which we prefer, attempts to preserve the unique perspective of each expert. In keeping with the need to express uncertainty, preservation of individual opinion is considered very important so that a full range of expert judgments can be reported. This approach accommodates consensus where it emerges but does not strive to foster or manufacture it. However, this approach may sacrifice some mutual education among experts.

Form of Elicited Judgments

Judgments can be reported either in a consensus form or with opinions of individuals preserved. As mentioned previously, we believe that forcing a consensus may be inappropriate with judgments about carcinogenicity and biological data. Forcing a consensus mutes the opinions of those experts on the ends of the spectrum, but, as experts, their opinions must also be considered by regulators. The full range of judgments reflects the range of possibilities deemed scientifically plausible by a group of experts.

For individual judgments, several forms of reporting might be useful. Verbal descriptions of plausible ways to use data would be helpful, or a ranking of preferred treatments of data could be elicited. Plausibility or quality weights could be elicited for various data sets and risk assessment options, or subjective probabilities could be elicited about mutually exclusive dose-response hypotheses.

Obstacles to Using Expert Scientific Judgment

Although expert judgments are clearly needed and sometimes used informally, there are several obstacles operating against their explicit incorporation in risk assessment. First, governmental, industrial, and consulting risk assessors may be reluctant to have their turf invaded. The participation of practicing scientists in risk assessment may shift the balance of power away from those practicing it currently, creating a shared power situation between risk assessors and practicing scientists. Second, expert scientists are themselves often reluctant to participate in a speculative, unscientific exercise, namely, providing judgments. Lastly, there is probably a perception among some that judgment is often not needed at all because uniform guidelines for risk assessment are already in place at federal agencies (National Academy of Sciences 1983). We contend that judgment is needed to augment or replace the guidelines when data and hypotheses conflicting with them are presented for consideration in cancer risk assessment.

Work in Progress

In an ongoing research program funded by the Risk Science Institute, the Alfred P. Sloan Foundation, and the Richard King Mellon Foundation, we are exploring on a pilot scale the use of expert scientific judgment in risk assessment. For our pilot study, we have chosen several issues in formaldehyde risk assessment. A great deal of experimental and biological research is available for formaldehyde as well as a long history of regulatory deliberation and risk assessments. Because of this, formaldehyde provides an ideal but challenging case study for expert judgment methods.

We are now in the process of analyzing two separate formaldehyde issues for our pilot study:

1. How should risk assessors utilize information about benign tumors in rats when making cancer risk estimates?
2. How should risk assessors utilize pharmacokinetic information when making cancer risk estimates?

These two issues were selected because of the availability of unusual formaldehyde data on these issues and also because a history of the treatment of these data by risk assessors is available to compare with expert judgments about how the data should have been used.

Formal methods for expert selection were developed and implemented for the pilot project. For the benign tumor question, experts were identified by a literature search method, and the experts in Table 1 were chosen for personal interviews. For the pharmacokinetic issues, a peer nomination process was utilized and the experts in Table 2 were chosen for personal interviews. We seek comment from the readers of this paper on how well these groups satisfy the criteria cited above.

All interviews have been completed and results are now being analyzed. The judgments on the scientific issues provided by the two sets of experts will be compared to how agencies handled the data in actual risk assessments. Each expert's judgment will also be compared to his or her colleagues, but each expert's perspective will be preserved. No attempt has been made to foster or force a consensus view. The results of the pilot are now being compiled into two papers, one on the benign tumor issues and the other on the pharmacokinetic issues. Our goal is to demonstrate some credible methods for applying expert scientific judgment to cancer risk assessment.

Table 1
Participating Experts in Benign Tumors (Alphabetical Order)

Benign tumor issue	
Dr. Stuart Aaronson	National Cancer Institute
Dr. Emmanuel Farber	University of Toronto
Dr. Curtis Harris	National Cancer Institute
Dr. William Lijinsky	National Cancer Institute
Dr. Paul Nettesheim	National Institute for Environmental Health Sciences
Dr. Henry Pitot	University of Wisconsin
Dr. I.B. Weinstein	Columbia University
Dr. Stuart Yuspa	National Cancer Institute

Table 2
Participating Experts in Pharmacokinetics (Alphabetical Order)

Pharmacokinetics issue	
Dr. Melvin E. Andersen	United States Air Force
Dr. Fred Beland	National Center For Toxicological Research
Dr. Robert L. Dedrick	National Institutes of Health
Dr. Frederica Perera	Columbia University School of Public Health
Dr. Miriam Poirier	National Institutes of Health
Dr. Richard Reitz	Dow Chemical Company
Dr. James Swenberg	Chemical Industry Institute of Toxicology
Dr. Steven Tannenbaum	Massachusetts Institute of Technology

WHY MORE EXPERT JUDGMENT?

We conclude with a pitch for more reliance on the judgments of practicing scientists in risk assessments. Our case boils down to three contentions. First, risk assessment with expert scientific judgment will be more competent (i.e., more likely to be accurate) than are traditional procedures. Second, expert judgment can be used as the basis for a nonarbitrary reporting of uncertainty in risk assessments, since differences among experts would translate into alternative risk estimates. Third, the use of more expert judgment will increase the legitimacy of regulation by assuring affected parties that risk estimates reflect the best judgments of scientists about evidence, not simply arbitrary guidelines and computer programs. We acknowledge that the first contention must rest on faith since it cannot yet be validated with evidence.

ACKNOWLEDGMENTS

This work was funded by the Risk Science Institute, the Richard King Mellon Foundation, and the Alfred P. Sloan Foundation. N.C.H. also received support from the Occupational Safety and Health Educational Resource Center NIOSH grant award 5-T15-OHO7096 at the Harvard School of Public Health. Dr. Susan Kennedy and Scott Wolff provided essential technical support during initial stages of this research.

REFERENCES

Albert, R.E., R.E. Train, and E. Anderson. 1977. Rationale developed by the Environmental Protection Agency for the assessment of carcinogenic risks. *J. Natl. Cancer Inst.* **58:** 1537.

Anderson, E.L. and Carcinogen Assessment Group. 1983. Quantitative approaches in use to assess cancer risk. *Risk Anal.* **3:** 277.

Anderson, M.W., D.H. Hoel, and N.L. Kaplan. 1980. A general scheme for the incorporation of pharmacokinetics in low-dose risk estimation for chemical carcinogenensis. *Toxicol. Appl. Pharmacol.* **55:** 154.

Armitage, P. and R. Doll. 1954. The age distribution of cancer and a multistage theory of carcinogenesis. *Br. J. Cancer* **18:** 1.

———. 1961. Stochastic models for carcinogenesis. *Proc. Berkeley Symp. Math. Stat. Probab.* **4:** 19.

Crump, K.S. 1981. An improved procedure for low-dose carcinogenic risk assessment from animal data. *J. Environ. Pathol. Toxicol.* **52:** 675.

Crump, K.S. and W.W. Watson. 1979. GLOBAL 79: A FORTRAN program to extrapolate dichotomous animal carcinogenicity data to low doses. National Institute for Environmental Health Sciences (NIEHS) contract no. 1-ES-2123.

Crump, K.S., D.G. Hoel, C.H. Langley, and R. Peto. 1976. Fundamental carcinogenic processes and their implications for low-dose risk assessment. *Cancer Res.* **36:** 2973.

DuMouchel, W.H. and J.E. Harris. 1983. Bayes methods for combining the results of cancer studies in humans and other species. *J. Am. Stat. Assoc.* **78:** 293.

Finkel, A.M. 1984. Heterogeneity in human susceptibility to environmental carcinogens: Public health, regulatory, and ethical implications. Working Paper E-84-08, John F. Kennedy School of Government, Harvard University, Cambridge, Massachusettes.

Graham, J.D. 1987. Cancer in the courtroom: Risk assessment in the post-BENZENE era. *J. Policy Anal. Management* **6:** 432.

Graham, J.D., L. Green, and M.J. Roberts. 1988. *Seeking safety: Science, cancer risk, and public policy.* Harvard University Press, Cambridge, Massachusetts. (In press.)

Haigh, J.A., D. Harrison, and A.L. Nichols. 1984. Benefit-cost analysis of environmental regulation: Case studies of hazardous air pollutants. *Harvard Environ. Law Rev.* **8:** 395.

Hoel, D.G., N.L. Kaplan, and M.W. Anderson. 1983. Implication of nonlinear kinetics on risk estimation in carcinogenesis. *Science* **219:** 1032.

Howe, R.B. and K.S. Crump. 1982. GLOBAL82: A computer program to extrapolate quantal animal toxicity data to low doses. Prepared for Occupational Safety and Health Administration (OSHA) under contract no. 41USC252C3.

Hutt, P.B. 1985. Use of quantitative risk assessment in regulatory decisionmaking under federal health and safety statutes. *Banbury Rep.* **19:** 15.

Industrial Union Department (IUD) 1980. AFL-CIO vs. American Petroleum Institute (API). 448 U.S. 607.

Kovar, J. and D. Krewski. 1981. User instructions for RISK81: A computer program for low-dose extrapolation for quantal response toxicity data. Department of Health and Welfare, Canada.

Krewski, D., K.S. Crump, J. Farmer, D.W. Gaylor, R. Howe, C. Portier, D. Salsburg, R.L. Sielken, and J. Van Ryzin. 1983. A comparison of statistical methods for low-dose extrapolation utilizing time-to-tumor data. *Fundam. Appl. Toxicol.* **3:** 140.

Lave, L.B., ed. 1982. *Quantitative risk assessment in regulation.* Brookings Institution, Washington, D.C.

Mantel, N. and W.R. Bryan. 1961. Safety testing of carcinogenic agents. *J. Natl. Cancer Inst.* **27**: 455.

Mantel, N., N.R. Bohidar, C.C. Brown, J.L. Ciminera, and J.W. Tukey. 1975. An improved Mantel-Bryan procedure for "safety" testing of carcinogens. *Cancer Res.* **35**: 865.

National Academy of Sciences (NAS). 1983. *Risk assessment in the Federal Government: Managing the process.* National Research Council, Washington, D.C.

Nichols, A.L. and R.J. Zeckhauser. 1985. The dangers of caution: Conservatism in assessment and the mismanagement of risk. Working Paper E-85-11, John F. Kennedy School of Government, Harvard University, Cambridge, Massachusetts.

Starr, T.B. and R.D. Buck. 1984. The importance of delivered dose in estimating low-dose cancer risk from inhalation exposure to formaldehyde. *Fundam. Appl. Toxicol.* **4**: 740.

United States Environmental Protection Agency (U.S.EPA). 1986. Guidelines for carcinogen risk assessment. *Fed. Reg.* **51**: 33991.

Watanabe, P.G., J.D. Young, and P.G. Gehring. 1977. The implications of non-linear (dose-dependent) pharmacokinetics on hazard assessment. *J. Environ. Pathol. Toxicol.* **1**: 147.

COMMENTS

Singer: You didn't recruit anybody in formaldehyde chemistry.

Graham: That's a good point. We had an explicit policy decision at the beginning, regarding whether we wanted compound-specific expertise or just experimental expertise on delivered dose type of experiments. We explicitly said in the recruitment letter, and maybe it was a mistake, that we did not require formaldehyde expertise.

Singer: This is one compound where the chemistry becomes important. Ask Swenberg, he'll tell you.

Graham: We did. We talked to him at length.

Singer: You need expertise in the chemistry?

Graham: Absolutely, because it's a very difficult one, particularly on measuring delivered dose, because of its metabolism rate.

St. Hilaire: The two questions that you chose in terms of formaldehyde, why did you choose those particular questions?

Graham: We thought in both cases there was a very interesting pattern and amount of data that arose in the case of formaldehyde that looked like it would call into question whether the standard approaches to risk assessment would be appropriate. So, in some sense, if we were to find through this process that the standard risk assessment process is sanctioned by at least these small numbers of experts, that would be a tremendous victory for the status quo. It's a very harsh test for the standard risk assessment practice, because the benign tumor data are very peculiar and the delivered dose information is unusual. There are many chemicals about which we have no such data.

St. Hilaire: So you don't have a best guess as to how this is going to come out?

Graham: We're writing it now. We are within weeks of sending it out.

St. Hilaire: However, when you chose the questions, did you choose them thinking that you were likely to get more of an agreement on one than the other? Did that enter into your decision in terms of selection?

Graham: I'll be honest because I'm a policy thinker. I thought the pharmacokinetic information might make the risk estimates look smaller, and in the case of benign tumors it might make the risk estimates look bigger. I wanted to have one issue on both sides at which to look. Admittedly, that's not a science call, that's a policy call.

Crump: I would question a couple of things. Rather than singling out these two issues, I really feel that the whole process needs to be looked at as a whole. Results could be quite different if the whole process is considered. Can you really tell how the whole process would be affected just by looking at these individual issues?

Graham: That's a good question. The one factor to keep in mind in this area is that because there are so many different types of scientific expertise, whether they be in mutagenicity, delivered dose, or in epidemiology, it's very hard to think of generalist experts. There are only a very small number of people who are really good on all those fronts. So, in principle, I would prefer a setting where I could go to a group of experts and say, "Just give me probability distributions on the overall risk of formaldehyde at various doses." However, we don't believe there are very many people who have the breadth of expertise necessary to answer the question that way. Instead, we are doing a classic decision analysis: break the problem down into parts and elicit expertise on the pieces before making an overall risk estimate. However, it's a good point. I would prefer to do it holistically if I felt there were people who could answer the big questions.

Crump: That's one thing that makes me concerned about this. You were more than fair in giving the strengths of the risk assessment process.

Wilson: I think he's right.

Crump: I would have a question about the procedure. If you look at the strengths that you gave, it's a workable process. I really feel that what is being proposed would detract from each one of those strengths.

Graham: It would detract from predictability. It would detract from the . . .

Crump: The cost and the timeliness.

Graham: That's right. So that's why I think the expert judgment approach has to be explored at a very small scale for now. It is not yet clear how unpredictable or how costly an expert judgment approach would be. On the other hand, the current process achieves predictability and ease of execution at a stiff price in diminished scientific credibility and perhaps inaccuracy. The consequences of these alternative approaches and the tradeoffs involved need to be carefully examined.

Quantitative Dose-response Models for Tumor Promoting Agents

TODD THORSLUND AND GAIL CHARNLEY
Clement Associates, Inc.
Fairfax, Virginia 22031-1207

OVERVIEW

A model based on a two-stage paradigm for carcinogenesis that can incorporate biological information on the proposed mechanism of action of tumor promoters is described here and applied to two putative promoting agents, 2,3,7,8-tetrachloro-dibenzo-p-dioxin (TCDD) and chlordane. Tumor rates predicted by this model fit observed bioassay rates extremely well. Moreover, estimates of human cancer risks provided by the model are at least two or three orders of magnitude lower than those provided by the linearized multistage model. Biologically based models for cancer risk assessment are more flexible than the linearized multistage model and provide risk estimates that are more defensible biologically than those provided by that model.

INTRODUCTION

Most quantitative dose-response models for carcinogens that are used to extrapolate cancer risk from animal bioassays to humans rely on an empirical curve-fitting procedure using the linearized multistage model. The basis for using this model is that a series of mutations are needed to produce a malignant cell from a normal cell and all carcinogens are mutagens. Dose-response models based on this assumption, however, are likely to be inappropriate for assessing the human cancer risk of tumor promoting agents, because there is very little evidence to suggest that these agents are mutagenic.

A mathematical model based on a two-stage theory for carcinogenesis has been developed by Moolgavkar, Venzon, and Knudson (Moolgavkar and Venzon 1979; Moolgavkar and Knudson 1981). According to the model (Fig. 1), only proliferating (stem) cells (those from which most other cells in an organ arise) are at risk, because once a stem cell differentiates, it no longer is susceptible to heritable alterations of its DNA. A normal, susceptible stem cell may divide into two daughter stem cells, terminally differentiate, die, or undergo a mutation that results in formation of a preneoplastic (intermediate) cell. A preneoplastic cell has undergone one of the changes necessary to become a cancer cell but is not yet cancerous. The preneoplastic cell may, in

Banbury Report 31: Carcinogen Risk Assessment: New Directions in the Qualitative and Quantitative Aspects © Cold Spring Harbor Laboratory. 0-87969-231-6/88. $1.00 + .00

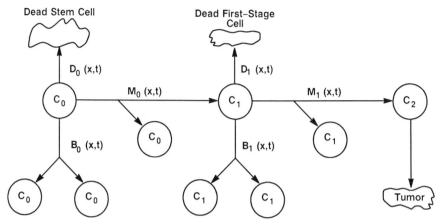

Figure 1
Basis of the Moolgavkar-Venzon-Knudson two-stage model: paradigm for the induction of a malignant tumor. C_0 is a normal, susceptible stem cell. C_1 is a preneoplastic, first-stage cell that can proliferate into a premalignant clone. C_2 is a cancerous cell that will eventually develop into a detectable tumor. $D_0(x,t)$, $B_0(x,t)$, and $M_0(x,t)$ are the exposure- and time-dependent death, birth, and transition or mutation rates for the normal stem cell. $D_1(x,t)$, $B_1(x,t)$, and $M_1(x,t)$ are the exposure- and time-dependent death, birth, and transition or mutation rates for the first-stage cell. x is the exposure level, which is assumed to be constant over time. t is the age of the subject. (Reprinted, with permission, from Thorslund et al. 1987.)

turn, divide into two daughter preneoplastic cells, differentiate, die, or undergo further mutation to produce a cancerous cell. The cancerous cell will, after a sufficient length of time, divide into enough cells that it becomes a detectable tumor. All of these processes can be described mathematically by postulating specific rates for the cell changes. Moolgavkar and Knudson (1981) showed that to a close approximation, the age-specific tumor rate at time t for their two-stage model may be expressed as:

$$I(t) = M_0 M_1 \int_0^t C_0(v) \exp([B - D][t - v]) \, dv$$

where:

$I(t)$ = Age-specific cancer incidence at age t;
M_0 = Transition rate from stem to preneoplastic cell;
M_1 = Transition rate from preneoplastic to cancerous cell;
$C_0(v)$ = Number of susceptible stem cells per individual target organ at age v;
B = Birth rate or rate of cell proliferation of preneoplastic cells; and
D = Death rate of preneoplastic cells.

The Moolgavkar-Knudson equation describes the progression from a normal stem cell to a cancerous cell with a combination of deterministic and stochastic components. The numbers of preneoplastic and fully malignant cells at any time are assumed to be random variables that are dependent upon these event rates, whereas the number of normal cells at risk of transformation at time t, denoted by $C_0(t)$, is assumed to be deterministic and known.

The biological processes described by Equation 1 can be affected by the level of exposure to carcinogenic agents, and are more likely to occur as the length of exposure increases; as a result, they are exposure and time dependent. Thorslund et al. (1987) have described an exposure- and time-dependent version of the model that can be used to predict the risk of agents that exert their effects in a number of different ways. In this discussion, we will focus on promoting agents that may increase the proliferation rate of preneoplastic cells (by increasing B or decreasing D).

TUMOR PROMOTER MODEL

In the context of the two-stage model, a specific dose-response model for tumor promoting agent can be generated based on the following assumptions:

1. The agent is not genotoxic and does not affect the transition rates between cell stages so that

$$M_0(x, t) = M_0 \text{ and } M_1(x, t) = M_1$$

2. The agent acts by increasing the proliferation (growth) rate of first stage, preneoplastic cells.
3. The rate of cell growth (clone development) is time independent so that for all values of t

$$G(x) = B_1(x, t) - D_1(x, t)$$

4. The number of susceptible stem cells in an adult animal is relatively stable so that $C_0(v) \sim C_0$, which is a time-independent constant.

Based upon these assumptions, a mathematical model for the probability that a tumor will develop by time t following constant exposure to a promoting agent at level x can be derived directly from Equation 1 by substituting the appropriate terms and integrating to yield the relationship

$$P(x, t) = 1 - \exp - \{M(\exp G[x]t - 1 - G[x]t)/G^2(x)\}$$

where $M = M_0M_1$.

In this model, the growth rate $G(x)$ may be expressed in the general form

$$G(x) = G(0) + (G[\infty] - G[0])R(x)$$

where:

$G(0)$ = Normal cell growth rate;
$G(\infty)$ = Upper bound on the agent-induced cell growth rate; and
$R(x)$ = The fraction of the maximal increase in the cell growth rate that is induced by a constant exposure to the agent at level x.

The functional form chosen for $R(x)$ is the single most critical element in determining cancer risk estimates for tumor promoters at environmental levels of exposure. Two functional forms of $R(x)$ that can be used to obtain specific dose-response models for promoting agents are the following:

1. The one-hit model

$$R(x) = 1 - \exp - Vx$$

which assumes the increase in preneoplastic cell growth rate resulted from a single irreversible event (such as the interaction of a single receptor protein complex with a single site on DNA), and

2. The log-logistic model

$$R(x) = (1 + \exp - [I + S\ln x])^{-1}$$

which assumes the increase in preneoplastic cell growth rate is proportional to the fraction of cells in which the agent receptor sites are saturated. In this equation, I is proportional to the binding constant of the agent, and S is the average number of receptors within a preneoplastic cell.

In summary, the complete tumor promoter dose-response model has the form

$$P(x, t) = 1 - \exp - \{M(\exp G[x]t - 1 - G[x]t)/G^2[x]\}$$

where:

$$G(x) = G(0) + (G[\infty] - G[0])R[x] ,$$

and

$$R(x) = 1 - \exp - Vx, \text{ or } (1 + \exp - [I + S\ln x])^{-1} .$$

To illustrate the advantages of using the two-stage model for carcinogenesis, it is applied to tumor bioassay data for TCDD and chlordane, two agents suspected to act as promoting agents but not as tumor initiators. Potential biological mechanisms of action for these agents are postulated and their associated effects on model parameters are described.

RESULTS

TCDD

There is little evidence that TCDD binds covalently to DNA or causes point mutations (Poland and Glover 1979), but it does interact with a cytosolic receptor protein, and the resulting TCDD-receptor complex can be translocated to the cell nucleus. The TCDD-receptor complex may increase tumor promotion by regulating levels of other enzymes such as ornithine decarboxylase, DT-diaphorase, and UDP-glucuronyl transferase, and by interfering with the ability of other sites on DNA to bind receptor complexes such as those of epidermal growth factor and glucocorticoids (Poland and Knudson 1982). Both effects may increase the number of stem cells, either by increasing cell proliferation rates or decreasing the number of cells that terminally differentiate, and hence may increase the likelihood of mutational events by tumor initiators or may permit clonal expansion of initiated cells.

The TCDD cancer dose-response model first was applied to data from a single sex and strain of rat. Model parameters were estimated (Table 1) using epidemiological data[1] and rat liver tumor data (Kociba et al. 1978). Both the

Table 1
Parameter Estimates for TCDD Dose-response Model

Symbols	Estimates		Source
$G(0)$	0.0533		typical human equivalent[a]
$G(\infty)$	0.0817		animal data
M	2.3798×10^{-6}		animal data
	one-hit	log-logistic	
V	109.51	—	animal data
I	—	-14.50	animal data
S	—	3.0	assumed

[a]Assumptions: (1) Age-specific cancer rates increase at a minimum to the third power of age. (2) The human lifetime is 70 years. (3) The rat lifetime is 104 weeks.

[1]Human age-specific liver cancer death rates were derived from Table 1–25, Section 1, Vol. II, Part A of the Vital Statistics of the United States 1980 and the 1980 U.S. census.

Table 2

Comparison of Observed and Predicted TCDD-induced Rat Liver Tumor Rates

Exposure (μg/kg/day)	Number of rats with tumors		
		predicted	
		cell growth rate model form	
	observed[a]	one-hit	log-logistic
0	16 (19%)	16.0 (19%)	16.0 (19%)
0.001	8 (16%)	10.8 (23%)	9.4 (20%)
0.01	27 (56%)	27.0 (56%)	27.0 (56%)
0.1	33 (82%)	33.0 (82%)	33.0 (82%)
χ^2		0.96	0.16
d.f.		1	1
p value		0.32	0.78

The difference between p values may be due to chance alone and should not be construed as an indication of better fit for the log-logistic model.
[a]Source: Kociba et al. (1978).

one-hit and log-logistic forms predict rat liver tumor rates extremely well (Table 2). As a further validation, the TCDD cancer dose-response model, adjusted only to account for differences in the background (spontaneous) tumor rates, was used to estimate responses observed in a different bioassay using both sexes of another strain of rat. Again, the one-hit form provided an accurate prediction of observed tumor rates (Table 3).

Table 3

Comparison of Observed and Predicted TCDD-induced Liver Tumor Rates

Exposure (μg/kg/day)	Number of animals exposed		Number of animals with tumors			
			observed[a]		predicted[b,c]	
	female	male	female	male	female	male
Historical control	970	975	21 (2.2%)	9 (0.9%)	—	—
0	75	74	5 (6.7%)	0	2.8 (3.7%)	0.3 (0.4%)
0.0014	49	50	1 (2.0%)	0	2.4 (4.9%)	0.2 (0.5%)
0.0071	50	50	3 (6.0%)	0	5.4 (10.8%)	0.6 (1.2%)
0.0714	49	50	14 (28.6%)	3 (6.0%)	13.2 (26.9%)	1.6 (3.2%)

[a]Source: National Cancer Institute (1980).
[b]Based on the one-hit model and previous model parameters except for the background mutation rate parameter M, which was changed to 4.30×10^{-7} (female) and 4.42×10^{-8} (male).
[c]$\chi^2 = 6.36$, d.f. = 6, $p = 0.49$.

Table 4
Parameters in Human Dose-response Model for TCDD

Symbols	Estimates	Source
$G(0)$	0.0938	human mortality data
$G(\infty)$	0.1438	proportional to rat tumor data in Kociba et al. (1978) study
M	1.44×10^{-8}	human mortality data

	one-hit	log-logistic	
V	589.16	—	$(V^a)(\sqrt[3]{\text{human body weight/rat body weight}})$
I	—	-19.55	$(I^a) + ([3 \log \sqrt[3]{\text{human body weight/rat body weight}}])$
S	—	3.0	assumed

[a]From Kociba et al. (1978) study.

Next a human dose-response model for TCDD was developed based on the rat model and certain assumptions (Table 4). Predictions of human cancer risk based on this promoter model were found to be at least two orders of magnitude less than those predicted using the 95% upper confidence limit of the linearized multistage model (Table 5).

Chlordane

Experimental evidence has demonstrated the ability of the termiticide chlordane to act as a tumor promoter in the mouse liver (Williams and Numoto 1984). Male B6C3F$_1$ mice exposed to diethylnitrosamine (DEN) for 14 weeks followed by 25 weeks on control diet developed a 40% incidence of liver

Table 5
Estimates of Low-dose Incremental Human Cancer Risk from TCDD

Dose (ng/kg/day)	Promotion model one-hit[a]	Promotion model log-logistic[a]	Linearized multistage model (95% upper confidence level used by EPA)
10^{-5}	1.7×10^{-8}	—	1.6×10^{-6}
10^{-4}	1.7×10^{-7}	—	1.6×10^{-5}
10^{-3}	1.7×10^{-6}	$<10^{-13}$	1.6×10^{-4}
10^{-2}	1.7×10^{-5}	8.8×10^{-10}	1.6×10^{-3}
10^{-1}	1.8×10^{-4}	8.8×10^{-7}	1.6×10^{-2}
1	2.4×10^{-3}	9.3×10^{-4}	1.6×10^{-1}

[a]Growth rate model.

neoplasms, whereas those given chlordane afterwards at 25 and 50 ppm in the diet had approximately an 80% incidence of liver neoplasms. Mice exposed to DEN also developed neoplasms of the forestomach and lung, but the incidences of these tumors were not increased by chlordane. None of the chemicals given alone for the last 25 weeks of the study increased the incidence of liver neoplasms, and none given before DEN produced a syncarcinogenic effect. Thus, chlordane yielded experimental results that are consistent with all the criteria that classify an agent as a tumor promoter. In view of these observations and its general lack of mutagenicity (Environmental Protection Agency 1986), it is reasonable to suggest that chlordane elicits hepatocellular tumors exclusively by its tumor promotional activity. This hypothesis is supported by observations in chronic bioassays of this agent, which have demonstrated a proliferative response in the livers of exposed animals. Such a response may result from chlordane-induced mitogenesis, expanding the population of preneoplastic initiated cells.

The dose-response model for tumor promoters described in the previous section was applied to tumor bioassay data obtained from chlordane in male mice (Table 6). The one-hit form was not consistent with the data, so only the results obtained from the log-logistic form are presented. The response for female mice was estimated using the parameter estimates (Table 7) obtained based on the data for male mice and adjusted solely for the differences in background tumor rates. Again, predicted hepatocellular carcinoma rates obtained from the model matched the observed rates very well, particularly for males.

Table 6

Comparison of Observed and Predicted Chlordane-induced Mouse Liver Tumor Rates

Exposure (ppm)	Number of mice with tumors			
	male		female	
	observed[a]	predicted	observed[a]	predicted
0	3/33 (9%)	3.0 (9%)	0/45 (0%)	2.5 (6%)
5	5/55 (9%)	5.8 (11%)	0/61 (0%)	3.9 (6%)
25	41/52 (79%)	41.0 (79%)	32/50 (64%)	30.4 (61%)
50	32/39 (82%)	32.0 (82%)	26/37 (70%)	23.8 (64%)
χ^2		0.08		7.60
d.f.		1		3
P value		0.78		0.06

[a]Source: IRDC (1973) as diagnosed by Reuber.

Table 7
Parameter Estimates for Chlordane Dose-response Model

Symbol	Source	Growth rate model one-hit	Growth rate model log-logistic
$G(0)$	human mortality data	0.06314	0.06314
M	males estimated from matched control tumor rates	2.8622×10^{-6}	2.8622×10^{-6}
	females estimated from entire experiment	—	1.722×10^{-6}
$G(\infty)$	animal data	0.11523	0.11527
I	animal data	—	-9.524
S	assumed by analogy from other logistic responses	—	4.0
V	animal data	0.1365	—

A human chlordane cancer dose response model was developed based on the mouse data. Predictions of human cancer risk from this model were at least three orders of magnitude lower than those using the Environmental Protection Agency's linearized multistage upper-bound procedure (Table 8).

DISCUSSION

Use of a biologically based model for cancer risk assessment that accounts for the proposed mechanisms of action of tumor promoters yields low-dose estimates of risk that are more defensible biologically than those obtained using the linearized multistage model. Moreover, these models also have immense flexibility, as they can be used to predict bioassay results in other experiments simply by adjusting for differences in background tumor rates. Additional efforts to develop parameter estimation techniques and to evaluate sensitivity of the low-dose estimates to the parameter values are ongoing.

Table 8
Estimates of Low-dose Cancer Risk From Chlordane

Dose (ppm)	Promotion model (male or female mice)	Linearized multistage model (95% upper confidence level used by EPA) male	Linearized multistage model (95% upper confidence level used by EPA) female
1	1.6×10^{-5}	4.8×10^{-2}	3.1×10^{-2}
0.1	1.2×10^{-9}	4.9×10^{-3}	3.1×10^{-3}
0.01	8.8×10^{-14}	4.9×10^{-4}	3.1×10^{-4}

REFERENCES

Environmental Protection Agency (EPA). 1986. *Carcinogenicity assessment of chlordane and heptachlor/heptachlor epoxide.* EPA Publ. no. OHEA-C-204.

International Research and Development Corporation (IRDC). 1973. Chlordane: Eighteen-month oral carcinogenic study in mice. Report to Velsicol Corporation, December 14, 1973.

Kociba, R.J., D.G. Keyes, J.E. Beyer, R.M. Carreon, C.E. Wade, D.A. Dittenber, R.P. Kalnins, L.E. Franson, C.N. Park, S.D. Barnard, R.A. Hummel, and C.G. Humiston. 1978. Results of a two-year chronic toxicity and oncogenicity study of 2,3,7,8-tetrachlorodibenzo-p-dioxin in rats. *Toxicol. Appl. Pharmacol.* 46: 279.

Moolgavkar, S.H. and A.G. Knudson, Jr. 1981. Mutation and cancer: A model for human carcinogenesis. *J. Natl. Cancer Inst.* 66: 1037.

Moolgavkar, S.H. and D.J. Venzon. 1979. Two-event models for carcinogenesis: Incidence curves for childhood and adult tumors. *Math. Biosci.* 47: 55.

National Cancer Institute (NCI). 1980. *Bioassay of 2,3,7,8-tetrachlorodibenzo-p-dioxin for possible carcinogenicity,* publ. no. 80-1765. U.S. Department of Health and Human Services, Washington, D.C.

Poland, A. and E. Glover. 1979. An estimate of the maximum *in vivo* covalent binding of 2,3,7,8-tetrachlorodibenzo-p-dioxin to rat liver protein, ribosomal RNA and DNA. *Cancer Res.* 39: 3341.

Poland, A. and J.C. Knudson. 1982. 2,3,7,8-tetrachlorodibenzo-p-dioxin and related halogenated aromatic hydrocarbons: Examination of the mechanisms of toxicity. *Annu. Rev. Pharmacol. Toxicol.* 22: 527.

Thorslund, T.W., C.C. Brown, and G. Charnley. 1987. Biologically motivated cancer risk models. *J. Risk Anal.* 7: 109.

Williams, G.M. and S. Numoto. 1984. Promotion of mouse liver neoplasms by the organochlorine pesticides chlordane and heptachlor in comparison to dichlorodiphenyltrichloroethane. *Carcinogenesis* 5: 1689.

COMMENTS

Kraemer: I've been learning about these models with interest, coming from a background of cancer-prone genetic diseases in humans. I wonder, on the one hand, if we are trying to protect the most sensitive humans in the population. If that is the case, then these patients might serve as sources of information for many of these model-building exercises. Cells from these patients can be obtained, and the data may be much easier to work with. First, I guess the question is: Are we aiming to protect everyone in the society?

Thorslund: That's not my area of expertise.

Anderson: I think it would be interesting to this audience if you would talk a little bit about the kinds of research data that you and your group have been proposing and link your proposals to the earlier papers presented in this workshop on pharmacokinetics and molecular biology. Linking these proposals and data to your model would be of real interest.

Thorslund: Of course, my model relates response to exposure at the organ that you think is going to be affected. Any information on pharmacokinetic data that provides an organ-specific dose would be the dose I would put into this model, not the external exposure, but the best surrogate exposure that we would have for the dose at the site of action. In the case of DNA adducts, for example, response might be more related to a certain type of DNA adduct level than to the external exposure level. The DNA adduct relative exposure level would then be put into the function X rather than the external exposure level itself.

There are a lot of things I have been thinking about regarding the kinds of information one might gather. I wouldn't really spring it on this august group because I would display my naivete. However, there are many things that can be done, and we are trying to get our ideas in order and talk with as many people as we can to expand and support our work in this area.

Pfitzer: Maybe in the general discussion we will have time for you to expand on that.

Quantitative Factors in Carcinogenic Risk Assessment

DANIEL KREWSKI AND DUNCAN MURDOCH
Health Protection Branch
Health and Welfare Canada
Ottawa, Ontario, Canada K1A OL2 and
Department of Mathematics and Statistics
Carleton University, Ottawa, Ontario
Canada K1S 5B6

OVERVIEW

Statistical methods for the quantitative assessment of carcinogenic risks based on toxicological data have undergone considerable refinement in recent years. In this paper, biologically motivated models for carcinogenesis are reviewed along with model-free approaches to low-dose risk assessment. Pharmacokinetic models for determining the dose delivered to the target tissue are examined, and the implications of using such models in extrapolating between doses, routes of exposure, and species considered. The estimation of risks with time-dependent exposure patterns is discussed, and conditions under which the use of time-weighted average dose is appropriately identified. Finally, the estimation of carcinogenic risks posed by exposure to complex mixtures is explored.

INTRODUCTION

The area of carcinogenic risk assessment has received considerable attention in recent years (Krewski and Brown 1981; Environmental Protection Agency 1986a), and continues to be a subject of much current debate (Office of Science and Technology Policy 1985). Information on carcinogenic risks may be obtained using epidemiological studies of human populations (Day 1985) and toxicological experiments conducted in the laboratory (Bickis and Krewski 1985). Whereas epidemiological investigations can provide information on adverse health effects directly in man, experimental studies using animal models have the advantage of being able to predict potential health hazards in advance of actual human exposure, and thus continue to be widely used for identifying substances with carcinogenic potential.

The main disadvantage of toxicological testing is the ultimate need to translate test results obtained in animals to the human situation. Because laboratory tests are conducted at relatively high dose levels to induce measur-

Banbury Report 31: Carcinogen Risk Assessment: New Directions in the Qualitative and Quantitative Aspects © Cold Spring Harbor Laboratory. 0-87969-231-6/88. $1.00 + .00

able rates of response in a small sample of experimental animals, it is often necessary to extrapolate these results to lower doses corresponding more closely to anticipated human exposure levels. Because the test species will not resemble the target species in all respects, it is also necessary to take into account interspecies difference when extrapolating between the animal model used and man. It may also be necessary to infer what would occur if the test compound were administered by a different route of exposure than that actually employed.

RESULTS

Estimating Risks at Low Doses

To estimate the level of risk associated with exposure to low doses of carcinogenic substances, it is necessary to extrapolate downward from the high doses used in laboratory studies using an assumed functional relationship between dose and response. Such extrapolations can depend strongly on the mathematical model of carcinogenesis employed (Krewski and Van Ryzin 1981) due to differences in the shape of the dose-response curve implied at low levels. If attention is restricted to models for which the dose-response curve is linear at low doses, however, such differences become slight (Krewski et al. 1984).

A number of arguments may be advanced in support of the hypothesis of low-dose linearity (Krewski et al. 1986; Murdoch et al. 1987). For example, the class of additive background models considered by Crump et al. (1976) predict low-dose linearity provided only that the response increases smoothly with dose. The assumption of low-dose linearity in carcinogenic risk assessment is supported by the U.S. Office of Science and Technology Policy, which stated that ". . .when data and information are limited, models or procedures that incorporate low-dose linearity are preferred (OSTP 1985)."

Given the assumption of low-dose linearity, the estimation of carcinogenic risks at low levels of exposure essentially involves estimating the slope of the dose-response curve at the origin. This may be done by fitting the multistage model to the available data and computing upper confidence limits on risk in the low-dose region (Crump 1984). Because these confidence limits are linear in the low-dose region, this is referred to as the linearized multistage model. This model is currently used by the Carcinogen Assessment Group of the Environmental Protection Agency for purposes of low-dose extrapolation (Anderson et al. 1983).

Krewski et al. (1986) have proposed a different approach to linear extrapolation that avoids the need for the specific parametric assumptions underlying the multistage model. In most cases, this model-free approach to linear extrapolation will provide results similar to these based on the linearized multistage model. However, this method of robust linear extrapolation can be advantageous in cases where the multistage model provides a poor fit to the experimental data, as may occur when the dose-response curve tends to rise sharply at low doses and then plateau at higher doses.

Pharmacokinetics

Pharmacokinetic models may be used to describe the fate of chemical substances upon entering the body (O'Flaherty 1981), thereby providing useful information on the formation of the reactive metabolites responsible for the induction of toxic effects in individual tissues. These models may be used to describe the relationship between the dose administered in toxicological tests and the dose delivered to the target tissue. The delivered dose may then be used in place of the administered dose in an attempt to obtain more accurate estimates of risk.

Mathematical pharmacokinetic models employed in these applications generally envisage biological systems as being comprised of a small number of compartments, with interactions among these compartments described by a corresponding set of differential equations (Gibaldi and Perrier 1975; Godfrey 1983). In contrast, physiological pharmacokinetic models in which the body is considered to be comprised of a larger number of relevant physiological compartments have also been employed in recent years (Bischoff 1987).

When one or more steps in the process of metabolic activation are saturable, the relationship between the dose d^* delivered to the target tissue and the administered dose d can be nonlinear (Hoel et al. 1983). To explore the effects of metabolic activation on estimates of low-dose risks, consider the simple pharmacokinetic model for metabolic activation of a particular toxicant shown in Figure 1 (Krewski et al. 1986). Here, exposure occurs at a

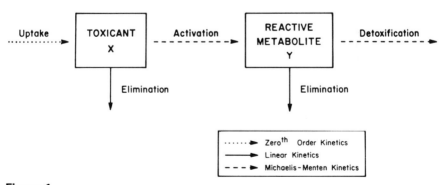

Figure 1
A simple pharmacokinetic model for metabolic activation.

constant rate d. Once absorbed into the body, the toxin X may be either eliminated or activated to its reactive form Y. The reactive metabolite may then be eliminated or detoxified.

It is assumed that the elimination both of X and Y follows first order linear kinetics, whereas activation and detoxification are assumed to be enzymatically mediated processes following saturable Michaelis-Menten kinetics. At steady state, the dose d^* of the reactive metabolite reaching the target tissue may be expressed as a function $d^*=f(d)$ of the administered dose.

This simple model may be used to illustrate the impact of saturation effects on the relationship between the dose d^* delivered to the target tissue and the administered dose d (Fig. 2). When both activation and detoxification follow linear kinetics, d^* is proportional to d. If the detoxification process is allowed to be saturable, d^* will still be proportional to d at low doses. Once the process saturates, however, the delivered dose d^* increases rapidly as a function of d. Conversely, if only the activation step is considered to be saturable, d^* levels off in relation to d as saturation occurs. A combination of both these effects can occur when both activation and detoxification are saturable.

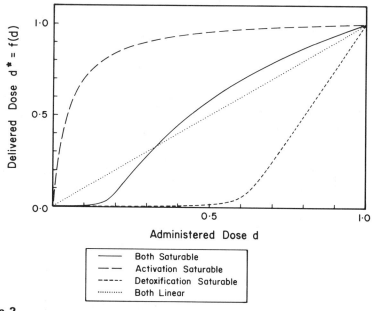

Figure 2

Relationship between the dose d^* delivered to the target tissue and the administered dose d with saturable activation and detoxification.

Using this simple mathematical pharmacokinetic model for metabolic activation in which the probability of tumor induction is proportional to the delivered dose, it can be shown using computer simulation that saturation effects in metabolic activation resulting in curvilinear dose response can impact estimates of low-dose risk obtained using linear extrapolation (Krewski et al. 1987). In particular, saturation of detoxification processes can result in appreciable overestimation of risk, whereas saturation of activation processes may lead to some underestimation of risk. The most accurate estimates of risk are obtained with a linear-dose response. Similar results were obtained by Whittemore et al. (1986), who also demonstrated that bias can be reduced by appropriate use of pharmacokinetic data.

Physiologically based pharmacokinetic (PBPK) models require information based on the anatomy and physiology of the test animal, the solubility of the test chemical in various organs, and biochemical constants for tissue binding and metabolism in specific organs. Three types of information are essential. First, partition coefficients are required to express the relative solubility of the compound in blood and various tissues in the model. Second, physiological constants are needed for tissue and organ volumes and for blood flow through these. Third, biochemical constants are used to define the rate coefficients for important biotransformation pathways.

Although requiring detailed information on physiological and biochemical parameters, such PBPK models have also been used to predict the risk associated with exposure to some compounds. As an illustration, the physiological model used by Andersen et al. (1987) to describe the metabolism of methylene chloride (dichloromethane, DCM) is shown in Figure 3. The paths on the right hand side of the figure represent flows of arterial blood, whereas those on the left represent flows of venous blood. The lung has been divided into a first compartment in which gas exchange takes place and into a second compartment in which metabolism occurs. DCM administered in drinking water is assumed to pass through the GI tract directly into the liver.

The metabolism of DCM is complicated by the fact that there are two paths involved in the metabolism of DCM: the saturable mixed function oxidase path and the essentially linear glutathione-s-transferase (GST) path. Andersen et al. (1987) argued on the basis of bioassay data and other biochemical considerations that the GST surrogate is the most appropriate predictor of tumor incidence. To an extent depending on the particular assumptions made, the use of this PBPK model can appreciably lower estimates of human risk (Andersen et al. 1987; Krewski et al. 1987).

Chen and Blancato (1987) used a similar physiological pharmacokinetic model to assess the risks of exposure to perchloroethylene. Their model had no lung metabolism compartment, as one path in the liver was assumed to account for all metabolism and to produce the active metabolite. Species

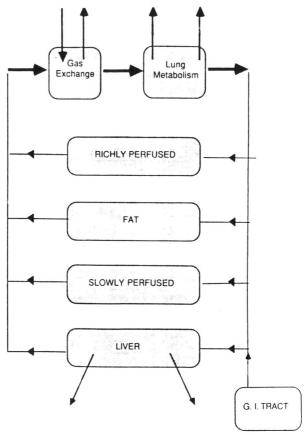

Figure 3
A PBPK model for methylene chloride.

equivalence on surface area, body weight, liver volume, and air concentration scales were all considered. In each case, the use of the metabolized dose produced estimates of human risks 5–10 times lower than calculations based on the administered dose.

Time-dependent Exposure

The prediction of carcinogenic risks from toxicological data requires the use of a mathematical model to relate the frequency of occurrence of neoplastic change to the level of exposure to the carcinogenic stimulus. Much of the previous work in this area has focused on situations where the level of exposure remains constant over time. In many cases, however, exposure will vary with time. For example, occupational exposure to agricultural chemicals is subject to seasonal variation, the ingestion of food contaminants varies in accordance with consumption patterns, and inhalation of manmade pollutants present in ambient air depends on emission rates and meteorological conditions.

To estimate the risks associated with such time-dependent exposure patterns, extensions to existing mathematical models of carcinogenesis are required. Crump and Howe (1984) extended the classical Armitage-Doll multistage model to allow for variable dosing regimens. This model is based on the premise that neoplastic transformation of normal tissue requires the occurrence in sequence of $k \geq 1$ fundamental biological events within a single cell, generally held to involve damage to genetic material such as mutations at specific gene loci (Armitage 1985).

Kodell et al. (1987) subsequently considered the consequences of using a simple time-weighted average dose to predict the risk associated with such variable dosing regimens. When only a single stage is dose-dependent, they demonstrated that this could underestimate the actual risk by a factor of at most k, the number of stages in the model. This bound also holds within the low-dose region when more than one stage is dose-dependent.

When only one stage of the model is dose-dependent, there exists a constant dose corresponding to a weighted average of the variable dose that will lead to the same risk as the variable dose, where the weight function depends on the number k of stages in the model and the particular stage affected ($1 \leq r \leq k$) (Murdoch and Krewski 1988). These results confirm that when an early stage is dose-dependent, early exposures will be more effective than later exposures, with the reverse being true when a late stage is dose-dependent (Day and Brown 1980).

To illustrate, consider the case of $k=6$ with $r=1$, and suppose that exposure occurs at a constant level d during the first quarter of an individual's lifetime and is eliminated thereafter (Fig. 4). In this case, the equivalent constant dose is $0.83d$ and exceeds the time-weighted average dose of $0.25d$ by more than threefold, since earlier exposures are more effective than later exposures.

A Biologically Motivated Model of Carcinogenesis

A more biologically motivated model of carcinogenesis than the multistage model is based on the notion that a tumor may be initiated following the occurrence of genetic damage in one or more cells in the target tissue as a result of exposure to an initiator. Such initiated cells may then undergo malignant transformation to give rise to a cancerous lesion. The rate of occurrence of such lesions may be increased by subsequent exposure to a promoter, which serves to increase the pool of initiated cells through mechanisms resulting in clonal expansion.

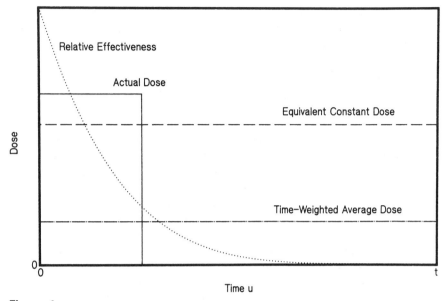

Figure 4

Equivalent and time-weighted average constant doses for a hypothetical time dependent dosing pattern in a 6-stage model with the 1st stage dose-dependent (weight function not to scale).

Mathematical formulations of this process have been given by Moolgavkar and Venzon (1979), Moolgavkar and Knudson (1981), and Greenfield et al. (1984). This stochastic birth-death-mutation model assumes that two mutations, each occurring at the time of cell division, are necessary for a normal cell to become malignant (Fig. 5). In the notation of Moolgavkar and Knudson (1981), initiating activity may be quantified in terms of the rate of occurrence λ_1 of the first mutation, with the rate of occurrence λ_2 of the second mutation describing the progression to a fully differentiated cancerous lesion. Promotional activity is measured by the difference $\delta = \alpha - \beta$ of the birth and death rates of initiated cells. In the absence of promotional effects and variability in the pool of normal cells, the two-stage birth-death mutation model reduces to the classical two-stage model. This model has recently been applied by Thorslund et al. (1987) to National Toxicology Program carcinogenesis bioassay data in conjunction with supplementary information on tissue growth. However, further concomitant information on the rate of cellular proliferation is necessary to identify all of the parameters of the model.

The birth-death-mutation provides a convenient context within which to quantitatively describe initiation/promotion (IP) mechanisms of carcino-

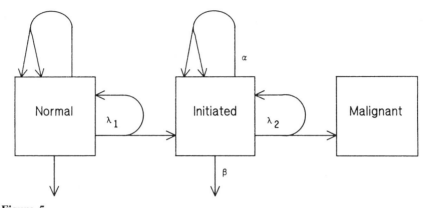

Figure 5
The M-V-K two-stage birth-death-mutation model. (λ_1 and λ_2 denote the transition rates from normal to intermediate cells and from intermediate to malignant cells respectively; α and β denote the birth and death rates of initiated cells.)

genesis (Moolgavkar 1986). An initiator is a substance that increases the rate of occurrence of the first mutation, whereas a promoter increases the pool of initiated cells. The term progressor has been used to describe an agent that increases the rate of occurrence of the second mutation resulting in malignant transformation to a cancerous cell (EPA 1987). Note that it is possible that the same agent may increase the rate of occurrence of both mutations, thereby enhancing both initiation and progression.

The experimental investigation of IP phenomena involves short term exposure to the initiator followed by longer term exposure to the promoter, along with other relevant treatment combinations to separate initiation and promotion effects (Gart et al. 1986). The subsequent administration of a second initiator that increases the rate of occurrence of the second mutation can markedly increase the production of neoplastic lesions (Scherer et al. 1984; Yuspa 1984). This so-called initiation/promotion/initiation (IPI) protocol, in conjunction with the more conventional IP protocol, offers a means of studying effects on the two mutation rates separately in the two-stage birth-death-mutation model.

Thorslund et al. (1987) also considered the two-stage birth-death-mutation model when the level of exposure varies over time. In the special case where the number of normal cells available for conversion to initiated cells is held fixed and promotional effects are constant over time, early dosing is most effective when only the first stage is dose-dependent (Murdoch and Krewski 1988). Conversely, when only the second stage is dose-dependent, dosing later in life is more effective. More importantly, the use of a simple time-weighted average dose can underestimate the risk associated with the variable dose by an arbitrarily large factor in both cases, depending on the net birth rate of initiated cells. This behavior cannot occur in the classical multistage model unless the number of stages k is allowed to be arbitrarily large.

Complex Mixtures

All of the approaches to carcinogenic risk assessment discussed to this point pertain to exposures to a single agent. Since people are often exposed to a number of environmental toxicants simultaneously, risk assessment techniques for multiple exposures are of interest. This question was recently addressed by the National Academy of Sciences Committee on Methods for the In Vivo Testing of Complex Environmental Mixtures (National Academy of Sciences 1988).

The issue of joint exposures is of particular interest because of the potential for synergistic effects among the components. Although the precise definition of interaction between toxicants is in itself a subtle issue, clear empirical evidence of interactive effects is available in a limited number of cases. For example, synergy occurs with lung cancer (excluding mesothioloma) following joint exposure to asbestos fibers and cigarette smoke (Hammond et al. 1979). Cigarette smoking and alcohol consumption may also lead to synergistic effects with respect to oral cancer (Rothman and Keller 1972).

Most of the cases in which interaction has been demonstrated have involved joint exposure to relatively high doses. At lower doses, conditions under which excess cancer risks may be generally expected to be additive have been identified (National Academy of Sciences 1987). For example, the additive background model of Crump et al. (1976), extended to the case of mixtures, predicts additivity of risks at low doses. Similarly, when the relative risks for two or more components combine multiplicatively (Siemiatycki and Thomas 1981), the excess risk will be nearly additive at low doses. For these reasons, the U.S. Environmental Protection Agency has recently stated that ". . . if sufficient data are not available on the effects of the chemical mixture . . .the proposed approach is to assume additivity (EPA 1986b)."

DISCUSSION

To estimate potential carcinogenic risks associated with low levels of exposure, some form of reasonably robust estimation procedure incorporating the assumption of low-dose linearity is desirable. Low-dose linearity may be a reasonable assumption in many cases and will provide an upper bound in cases where sublinearity occurs. This has led to the use of both the linearized multistage and model-free approaches to linear extrapolation.

Pharmacokinetic models may be used to obtain more accurate estimates of risk at low doses through the use of dose delivered to the target tissue as a surrogate for the administered dose in toxicological studies, particularly when the response of interest is roughly proportional to the delivered dose. Predictions of the internal tissue dose for other routes of exposure may be obtained using PBPK models, provided that measurements of the physiological and biochemical constants associated with the different routes are available. Extrapolation between species may also be facilitated using physiological models to predict the delivered dose in the species of interest. In those cases where all of the relevant model parameters cannot be measured directly in humans, however, these must be obtained by scaling the corresponding animal values.

It is clear from models of carcinogenesis that incorporate time-dependent dosing that the time at which exposure to carcinogenic substances occurs is an important determinant of the corresponding level of risk. In both the classical multistage model and the two-stage birth-death-mutation model of carcinogenesis, early (or late) exposures are more effective when an early (or late) stage is dose-dependent.

It is also clear that the risk predicted on the basis of a simple time-weighted average level of exposure will generally differ from the actual risk corresponding to the particular time-dependent exposure pattern experienced. Although limited to a factor of k (the number of stages) with low doses under the multistage model, this difference can be substantial in the presence of large promotional effects under the two-stage birth-death-mutation model.

The two-stage birth-death-mutation model of Moolgavkar-Venzon-Knudson (M-V-K) appears to accommodate many of the important components of carcinogenesis and provides a more biologically motivated approach to cancer modeling than the classical multistage model. Initiation corresponds to the occurrence of the first mutation, with progression to malignancy following a second mutation. Promotion involves increasing the initiated cell population by means of clonal expansion, thereby increasing the chance of a second mutation occurring. Application of the M-V-K model in practice will require information on tissue growth and cellular proliferation rates. Estimation of the two mutation rates separately will also require special IPI protocols rather than the more conventional IP protocols.

The quantitative assessment of carcinogenic risks posed by complex mixtures of environmental toxicants is a difficult issue, because of the potential for synergistic effects among the components. Nonetheless, conditions under which risks at low doses are predicted to be additive have been identified, including the multiplicative relative risk and additive background models. In the absence of evidence to the contrary, additivity of risks at low doses may thus be a reasonable working hypothesis.

ACKNOWLEDGMENT

This work was supported in part by grant no. A8664 from the National Sciences and Engineering Research Council of Canada to D. Krewski.

REFERENCES

Andersen, M.E., H.J. Clewell III, M.L. Gargas, F.A. Smith, and R.H. Reitz. 1987. Physiologically based pharmacokinetics and the risk assessment process for methylene chloride. *Toxicol. Appl. Pharmacol.* **87**: 185.

Anderson, E.L. and the Carcinogen Assessment Group 1983. Quantitative approaches in use to assess cancer risk. *Risk Anal.* **3**: 339.

Armitage, P. 1985. Multistage models of carcinogenesis. *Environ. Health Perspect.* **63**: 195.

Bickis, M. and D. Krewski. 1985. Statistical design and analysis of the long-term carcinogenicity bioassay. In *Toxicological risk assessment* (ed. D.B. Clayson et al.), vol. 1, p. 125. CRC Press, Boca Raton, Florida.

Bischoff, K.B. 1987. Physiologically based pharmacokinetic modeling. In *Drinking water and health*, vol. 8: *Pharmacokinetics and risk assessment,* p. 36. National Academy Press, Washington, D.C.

Chen, C.W. and J.N. Blancato. 1987. Role of pharmacokinetic modeling in risk assessment–perchloroethylene (PCE) as an example. In *Drinking water and health*, vol. 8: *Pharmacokinetics and risk assessment,* p. 369. National Academy Press, Washington, D.C.

Crump, K.S. 1984. An improved procedure for low-dose carcinogenic risk assessment from animal data. *J. Environ. Pathol. Toxicol. Oncol.* **6**: 339.

Crump, K.S. and R.B. Howe. 1984. The multistage model with a time-dependent dose pattern: Applications to carcinogenic risk assessment. *Risk Anal.* **4**: 163.

Crump, K.S., D.G. Hoel, C.H. Langley, and R. Peto. 1976. Fundamental carcinogenic processes and their implications for low dose risk assessment. *Cancer Res.* **36**: 2973.

Day, N.E. 1985. Epidemiological methods for the assessment of human cancer risk. In *Toxicological risk assessment* (ed. D.B. Clayson et al.), vol. 2, p. 3. CRC Press, Boca Raton, Florida.

Day, N.E. and C.C. Brown. 1980. Multistage models and the primary prevention of cancer. *J. Natl. Cancer Inst.* **64**: 977.

Environmental Protection Agency (EPA). 1986a. Guidelines for carcinogen risk assessment. *Fed. Reg.* **51**: 33992.

———. 1986b. Guidelines for the health risk assessment of chemical mixtures. *Fed. Reg.* **51**: 34014.

———. 1987. *Report of the EPA Workshop on the development of risk assessment methodologies for tumor promoters* (Report EPA/600/9-87/013). U.S. Environmental Protection Agency, Washington, D.C.

Gart, J.J., D. Krewski, P.N. Lee, R.E. Tarone, and J. Wahrendorf. 1986. The design and analysis of long-term animal experiments. *IARC Sci. Publ. no.* **79**.

Gibaldi, M. and D. Perrier. 1975. *Pharmacokinetics*. Marcal Dekker, New York.

Godfrey, K. 1983. *Compartmental models and their application*. Academic Press, London.

Greenfield, R.E., L.B. Ellwein, and S.M. Cohen. 1984. A general probabilistic model of carcinogenesis: Analysis of experimental urinary bladder cancer. *Carcinogenesis* **5**: 437.

Hammond, E.C., I.J. Selikoff, and H. Seidman. 1979. Asbestos exposure, cigarette smoking and death rates. *Ann. N.Y. Acad. Sci.* **330**: 473.

Hoel, D.G., N.L. Kaplan, and M.W. Anderson. 1983. Implication of nonlinear kinetics on risk estimation in carcinogenesis. *Science* **219**: 1032.

Kodell, R.L., D.W. Gaylor, and J.J. Chen. 1987. Lifetime dose rate for intermittent exposures to carcinogens. *Risk Anal.* **7**: 339.

Krewski, D. and C. Brown. 1981. Carcinogenesis risk assessment: A guide to the literature. *Biometrics* **37**: 353.

Krewski, D. and J. Van Ryzin. 1981. Dose response models for quantal response toxicity data. In *Statistics and related topics* (ed. M. Csorgo et al.), p. 201. North-Holland, Amsterdam.

Krewski, D., C. Brown, and D. Murdoch. 1984. Determining "safe" levels of exposure: Safety factors or mathematical models? *Fundam. Appl. Toxicol.* **4**: S383.

Krewski, D., D. Murdoch, and A. Dewanji. 1986. Statistical modeling and extrapolation of carcinogenesis data. In *Modern statistical methods in chronic disease epidemiology* (ed. S.H. Moolgavkar and R.L. Prentice), p. 259. Wiley, New York.

Krewski, D., D.J. Murdoch, and J.R. Withey. 1987. The application of pharmacokinetic data in carcinogenic risk assessment. In *Drinking water and health*, vol. 8: *Pharmacokinetics and risk assessment*. National Academy Press, Washington, D.C.

Moolgavkar, S.H. 1986. Carcinogenesis modelling: From molecular biology to epidemiology. *Annu. Rev. Public Health* **7**: 151.

Moolgavkar, S.H. and A.G. Knudson, Jr. 1981. Mutation and cancer: A model for human carcinogenesis. *J. Natl. Cancer Inst.* **66**: 1037.

Moolgavkar, S.H. and D.J. Venzon. 1979. Two-event models for carcinogenesis: Incidence curves for childhood and adult tumors. *Math. Biosci.* **47**: 55.

Murdoch, D.J. and D. Krewski. 198. Carcinogenic risk assessment with time-dependent exposure patterns. *Risk Anal.* (in press).

Murdoch, D.J., D. Krewski, and K.S. Crump. 1987. Quantitative theories of carcinogenesis. In *Cancer Modeling* (ed. J.R. Thompson and B.W. Brown), p. 61. Marcel Dekker, New York.

National Academy of Sciences. 1988. National Academy of Sciences Committee on Methods for the In Vivo Toxicity Testing of Complex Mixtures. *Methods for the in vivo testing of complex mixtures*. National Academy Press, Washington, D.C. (In press.)

Office of Science and Technology Policy (OSTP). 1985. Chemical carcinogens: A review of the science and its associated principles. *Fed. Reg.* **50**: 10372.

O'Flaherty, E.J. 1981. *Toxicants and drugs: Kinetics and dynamics*. Wiley, New York.

Rothman, K. and A. Keller. 1972. The effect of joint exposure to alcohol and tobacco on risk of cancer of the mouth and pharynx. *J. Chronic Dis.* **25**: 711.

Scherer, E., A.W. Feringa, and P. Emmelot. 1984. Initiation-promotion-initiation. Induction of neoplastic foci within islands of precancerous liver cells in the rat. *IARC Sci. Publ.* **56**: 157.

Siemiatycki, J. and D.C. Thomas. 1981. Biological models and statistical interactions: An example from multistage carcinogenesis. *Int. J. Epidemiol.* **10**: 383.

Thorslund, T.W., C.C. Brown, and G. Charnly. 1987. Biologically motivated cancer risk models. *Risk Anal.* **7**: 109.

Whittemore, A.S., S.C. Grosser, and A. Silvers. 1986. Pharmacokinetics in low dose extrapolation using animal cancer data. *Fundam. Appl. Toxicol.* **7**: 183.

Yuspa, S.H. 1984. Mechanisms of initiation and promotion in mouse epidermis. *IARC Sci. Publ.* **56**: 192.

COMMENTS

Beland: I have two comments. The first deals with the saturation about which you are talking. I assume you are concerned with low doses and not high doses. I wonder if it really is going to be a problem, because when you give single doses of benzo[a]pyrene and aflatoxin B_1 over many orders of magnitude, you seem to get a very nice linear response between the administered dose and the adduct formation. There was no indication of saturation occurring. I showed the same thing earlier today; there was no saturation in adduct formation when 2-acetylaminofluorene was administered to mice chronically at doses up to 150 ppm. The only time we have seen saturation in adduct formation with 2-acetylaminofluorene administered chronically is at doses above 200 ppm in the rat.

Krewski: If that's the case, then at best you can work with the administered dose level.

Beland: Yes. I think that's probably correct.

Krewski: There are, however, many compounds where you do get saturation.

Beland: However, we're on the low doses now. The impression that I got, was that you were concerned about what happens at very low doses.

Krewski: At very low doses, saturation effects will probably not be apparent because nonlinear kinetics generally reduce to linear kinetics in the low-dose region. However, we have to make our inferences on the basis of higher dose data, and that's where the saturation effects become important. We're interested in low-dose risks, but we must infer those risks on the basis of bioassay data obtained at higher doses where saturable kinetics can actually occur.

Beland: The second point I would like to make deals with what you said about formaldehyde. Bea Singer this morning spent a lot of time showing us very precise DNA adducts that were formed from various compounds. Other people have talked about benzo[a]pyrene adducts and have spent time doing the chemistry that is very important. If you go back to formaldehyde, we are still dealing with gross binding, and no one knows what that structure is. It has been called a cross-link, but that is based upon an enzymatic digestion. Ten years ago, gross binding data were probably acceptable, but I do not believe that they are today.

Until the chemistry is done to show what the structure of this formaldehyde product is, whether it's a protein-protein cross-link, a protein-DNA cross-link, a DNA-DNA cross-link, it is premature to talk about linear or nonlinear responses.

Neal: It is apparently a DNA-protein cross-link. The problem is that once you hydrolyze the DNA, then the adduct goes apart and you just release free formaldehyde. I think it is apparent that you are probably never going to identify an adduct in the context or polycyclic aromatic hydrocarbon adducts or diethylnitrosamine adducts. At best, it is going to be circumstantial evidence of a DNA-protein cross-link.

Singer: The only comment I wanted to make, since I represent aldehydes, particularly formaldehyde, which we started studying in 1941, is that there is an enormous literature on formaldehyde. One of the reasons you have a completely different dose versus adduct is simply the reversibility of a reaction. That is, you are continually making and losing and making and losing. Every once in a while, you are going to be forming a cross-link that will be a methylene bridge cross-link.

I do believe that one can get at that particular adduct. Let's not leave out my friend alcohol from this, too, because this is endogenously formed as well. So, the formaldehyde/alcohol story may also enter into something like this, because that's a stabilization reaction. So are thiols, as you realize.

So, I believe that the chemistry can be unraveled as to what is happening in vivo. There is so much background to it. Since everybody is interested in this because it's a model of a nonlinear response, I think it is worth doing.

Now, when you ask what can one do, this is one place that something can be done. Many things aren't as amenable, but this one is, particularly with modern methods. Perhaps 40 years ago or so, you couldn't have done what you can do today, but I assure you, Dr. Neal, that the chemistry could be done. Why do you say no?

Neal: It is a methylene bridge, undoubtedly, between probably the amino group of lysine and one of the exocyclic amino groups of a DNA base. However, the minute you hydrolyze the DNA, there is a dissociation. You don't really trap an amino acid base adduct.

Singer: We could talk about it separately, but you don't have to do it that way.

Neal: I think there is no other way to identify it.

Singer: They have been identified, and I'll quote you the paper.

Neal: I'll show you where that paper was wrong, too.

Krewski: Could I break into the middle of this debate here? This discussion is very important and very relevant. We have to understand what the various possible measures of delivered dose mean. What I tried to do today was say that *if* covalent binding in the case of formaldehyde is an appropriate measure of delivered dose, there is an effect on the estimates of risk. I hope you can tell me if that assumption is right or not.

Singer: We do have the problem of reversible reactions. We haven't mentioned this before. Reversible reactions make the interpretation of dose response difficult.

Krewski: I think we should perhaps leave this type of discussion for later.

Michejda: I'm not sure just where my question is going to lead, Dan, but you sparked a memory of a paper on teratogenesis that I had read, teratogenesis about folic acid inhibitor, specifically, that had been administered by various regimens. One of them was by a single pulse, another one was by continuous infusion, that integrated over time, was equimolar to the pulse dose. Yet, the physiological effects were dramatically different. In the pulse type of a regimen, one got teratogenesis; in the continuous infusion, one got fetal death. So, integration over a period of time won't be appropriate. You have to look at much smaller cells.

Krewski: I think what you're describing is a situation where something like an acute toxic effect is highly dependent on the peak exposure level. What I was talking about here was a situation of low-exposure levels, where the dosing cycle is relatively short compared to the time intervals (such as a lifetime) in which you are interested. Under the conditions that I just described, the area under the curve is probably going to be a reasonable thing to look at so that systematic availability will be a good indicator of exposure. However, for the case you described, this would not be appropriate at all.

Guengerich: The same thing happens, as I recall, with ethylene dichloride, too. In one case, you will actually get tumors, if you have the gavage dosing, whereas, if you have the same amount in the drinking water, you don't see anything. I think that has been related to metabolism. There are fairly low levels of adducts formed from ethylene chloride and dichloroethane.

Pfitzer: I think there are a lot of examples where peak exposure is critical.

Ahmed: Could I ask you to explain, Dan, what you meant by "physiological models?" What variables are you going to put into your model?

Krewski: Just the kind of physiologically based pharmacokinetic model that I discussed earlier, where we think of the body as comprising a number of relevant physiological compartments. The relevant parameters are the partition coefficients, allometric relationships, and metabolic constants.

Ahmed: Have you done any calculations using some of those parameters?

Krewski: Yes, we have.

Ahmed: What do you find?

Krewski: Depending on the assumptions that you make, you can get differences in risk estimates that vary quite a bit using delivered versus administered doses. That is known to be the case with methylene chloride, as many of you are aware. There are also other things that enter into this analysis. For example, how you scale pharmacokinetic constants across species is important. The issue is a bit complicated, and I didn't want to get into that level of detail today.

Panel Discussion

EMIL A. PFITZER
Hoffman-La Roche, Inc., New Jersey

Pfitzer: Both panelists were not able to make it to the meeting. I have volunteered to be the panelist.

There is one point I would like to present to you by way of discussion which I think brings together some of the questions about scientific approaches and modeling and will also include enzyme induction. It relates to the problem of thyroid tumors, a problem for many of us studying chemicals in the bioassay.

First of all, let me say there clearly are molecules that are genotoxic and cause thyroid tumors by mutagenic mechanisms. There are also a large number of compounds that appear to be primarily promoters of thyroid tumors by interfering with thyroid metabolism. Let me just give you an example of the situation that I think can be explored scientifically and can be used in many of the pharmacokinetic models.

Let's take a molecule that is an enzyme inducer in the liver and induces thyroxine glucuronyl transferase. Phenobarbital is such a molecule. By inducing thyroxine glucuronyl transferase in the liver, phenobarbital causes an increased elimination of thyroxine via the bile. This results in a decreased level of circulating thyroid hormone and a feedback stimulation to the pituitary to produce thyroid stimulating hormone (TSH). TSH stimulates the follicular cells of the thyroid gland to produce more thyroxine (actually, both T_3 and T_4). This is the body's homeostatic mechanism to maintain circulating thyroid hormone necessary for normal metabolism. When there is long-term repeated administration of phenobarbital to a rodent at enzyme-inducing doses, then this homeostatic mechanism is stressed to compensate for the abnormal loss of thyroid hormone via the bile.

A classic study to show tumor promotion with phenobarbital involves a short-term production of thyroid tumors in rats with nitrosamine followed by a marked increase in tumor incidence when the nitrosamine is followed by phenobarbital administration. The results are clear and dramatic. Dr. Michael McClain in our laboratory has shown that this promoting effect of phenobarbital can be blocked by administering thyroxine to the rat. Thus, the loss of circulating thyroxine caused by the enzyme induced by phenobarbital is replaced, and there is no feedback stimulation of the thyroid gland. The feature relative to carcinogenesis is that a rodent with a "genetic" susceptibility to "spontaneous" thyroid tumors of the follicular cells will have an increased incidence of these tumors when the thyroid gland becomes enlarged due to the stimulation for continued increased production of thyroid hormones.

This example shows the role of interference with homeostatic mechanisms that are secondary to the pharmacokinetics of the chemical or drug itself. Our challenge is to understand such secondary mechanisms in sufficient depth so that the appropriate extrapolation from rodents to humans can be assessed. There are other secondary mechanisms for the interference of thyroid metabolism, such as the enzyme that converts T_4 to T_3. Perhaps the best known mechanism for thyroid tumors in rats is that caused by several sulfa drugs. Here the mechanism is not induction but inhibition of the peroxidase enzyme in the thyroid gland that is necessary for production of T_3 and T_4. The end result is the same, i.e., decreased circulating thyroid hormone, feedback stimulation to the thyroid, an enlarged thyroid gland, and an increased incidence of follicular cell neoplasia in susceptible rodent strains.

As one seeks to improve risk assessment models for carcinogenesis, it is important to investigate the potential for abnormal stress to homeostatic mechanisms that can lead to neoplasia from endogenous sources. This is independent from pharmacokinetics of the chemical itself, although the dose-response data from a given experiment may appear to fit a pharmacokinetic model. It is possible that correlations between genotoxic screening data and rodent neoplasia would be better if such secondary mechanisms for neoplasia were understood and considered. There are other factors, of course, such as the apparent unique susceptibility of male rats to kidney neoplasia that is associated with abnormal urinary proteins. In addition the relationship of promotion of carcinogenesis to inhibition of gap junctions has presented new hypotheses to be explored.

Kraemer: There are some agents used that promote gap junctions and inhibit tumor promotion. One of them we have used in a small study with patients with xeroderma pigmentosum who have had high rates of skin cancer. We counted their tumor incidence, removed them all, and then put them on the drug, which was a retinoid 13-*cis*-retinoic acid, for two years, and their tumor rate fell substantially within several months. Then, when we stopped the drug, their tumors increased again within two months. So, this seems to be working to block the later stages of carcinogenesis in this human model.

Trosko: It increases gap junctions in epithelial-related type cells.

Pfitzer: Also, in the rat, it causes adrenal gland phaeochromocytomas.

Trosko: It also by itself will at high doses promote tumors, I believe.

Kraemer: That may be the first of many compounds with which we may be working that affect promotion.

Pfitzer: If there are no further questions, we will call this discussion to an end.

Implications for Policy
and Research

Perspective on Risk Assessment of Carcinogens

ELIZABETH L. ANDERSON
Clement Associates, Inc.
Fairfax, Virginia 22030

OVERVIEW

The broad practice of using risk-assessment approaches for the evaluation of suspected human carcinogens is about 12 years old. The primary departure point was the announcement by the U.S. Environmental Protection Agency (EPA), which adopted guidelines for assessing the risk of carcinogens and a policy to regulate suspect carcinogens based essentially on a risk management approach. The scientific basis was derived from the earlier experience of assessing the risk of health impacts from radiation exposure. From a practical standpoint, the use of risk assessment for carcinogens has received broad and general endorsement. The early use of risk assessment of carcinogens relied heavily on replacing the uncertainties in the risk-assessment process with very conservative assumptions to make sure that, in no case, would the risk be underestimated. As the practice of risk assessment has become widespread, considerable attention has been focused on improving the scientific basis for evaluating each step of the risk assessment: the weight-of-evidence indicating likely carcinogenicity, the dose-response relationships, and the environmental exposures. More attention has been focused on the scientific relationships that underlie the characterization of suspect carcinogens and their dose-response relationships, including extrapolation from animals to humans and from high dose to low dose. Far less attention has been focused on the exposure assessment, which can have an effect on the outcome of the quantitative risk assessment by certainly as much as the assumptions in the dose-response extrapolation part of risk assessment. This volume's focus has been primarily regarding the improved understanding of the mechanisms of carcinogenesis, based on current research and, by implication, the incorporation of progress in research into the risk-assessment process. The effect of these developments is being felt in the public policy area, where current attention is focused on using biologically based dose-response models to describe "more likely risks" in addition to "upper-bound" estimates derived from the linear, nonthreshold model, the model of choice for past risk assessments. Other factors, such as pharmacokinetic information, are also being factored into the risk assessment process. For example, EPA has just downgraded the potency of arsenic by ingestion by one order of magnitude and has proposed to do the same for dioxin, based on these and related

Banbury Report 31: Carcinogen Risk Assessment: New Directions in the Qualitative and Quantitative Aspects © Cold Spring Harbor Laboratory. 0-87969-231-6/88. $1.00 + .00

considerations. Of equal importance are the recent developments in exposure assessment, which are also leading to sharpened scientific tools for evaluating human exposure. All of these advances in the risk assessment of carcinogens should be kept in perspective when viewing new directions in the qualitative and quantitative aspects of carcinogen risk assessment.

INTRODUCTION

As in many forums, the focus of this conference has been heavily weighted toward biomedical issues involved in the qualitative and quantitative aspects of carcinogen risk assessment. Whereas these developments represent some of the more exciting scientific risk-assessment trends, this paper takes a broader overview, focusing on the significance of this work to the overall risk-assessment process. Included is a discussion of the recent advances in exposure assessment, which have at least equal importance to the quantitative outcome of the risk assessment of carcinogens. An overview of the risk-assessment process is presented, as previously practiced, and focuses on advances in the scientific basis for carcinogen risk assessment and related implications that are leading, on the whole, to less conservative risk outcomes.

RESULTS

Risk Assessment of Carcinogens: An Overview of the Process

In 1976, EPA adopted the first policy for the use of risk assessment of toxic chemicals that were suspected of being human carcinogens, and it accompanied this policy statement with guidelines for the scientific risk-assessment process (EPA 1976; Albert et al. 1977). These guidelines were adopted in response to the need for a major regulatory agency to develop a means for regulating the presence of hundreds of suspected carcinogens in the environment under numerous environmental legislative statutes, which had been adopted by Congress. In short, it was obvious that EPA could not regulate all suspected carcinogens, which were being identified in rapid succession as environmental contaminants, to a zero risk level as had been the risk goal of the Food, Drug, and Cosmetic Act's Delaney Clause. Such a goal had clearly been the objective of the strong environmental movement that characterized the first half of the decade of the 1970s. The adoption of guidelines for risk assessment, with the implication that EPA planned to accept residual risk as a regulatory policy, was initiated under the watchful eyes of the scientific community, the regulated community, and the environmental communities.

In short, there was considerable skepticism about the approach as a basis for public policy because of the substantial scientific uncertainties, particularly in quantitative risk assessment. After the EPA action, several other endorsements followed. The Inter-agency Regulatory Liaison Group adopted similar scientific principles in 1979 (IRLG 1979). These guidelines were followed by the report of the National Academy of Science, which endorsed the use of risk assessment and provided descriptive terms for each step of the risk-assessment process that have now been adopted as a common vocabulary (NAS/NRC 1983). In addition, the Office of Science and Technology Policy published similar scientific principles in 1985 (OSTP 1985), and EPA has updated its earlier guidelines (EPA 1986). In short, the application of risk assessment to toxic chemicals for the evaluation of scientific evidence, which indicates that a chemical might be a human carcinogen and also provides information as to the magnitude of current and anticipated public health impacts, has been endorsed and described in many forums and also has been the subject of discussion in many scientific conferences.

The process is generally described in four steps: hazard identification, dose-response modeling, exposure assessment, and overall risk characterization (NAS/NRC 1983). In practice, over the last 12 years the hazard identification step in risk assessment has relied on all of the available human, animal, and/or in vivo or in vitro data to describe the weight-of-evidence that indicates that a chemical might be a human carcinogen. At various times, the weight-of-evidence has been stratified according to either the International Agency for Research on Cancer criteria (IARC 1982) or the more recent EPA stratification scheme (EPA 1986) for assigning a category to the weight-of-evidence. Although these two categorical schemes are very closely related, the EPA scheme expands on the inadequate evidence labeled Category E in the IARC criteria to include three additional categories: C to indicate evidence that constitutes the category of "probable" carcinogen for humans, D to indicate inadequate testing, and E to indicate negative evidence.

Dose-response modeling has largely followed a linear nonthreshold hypothesis for low-dose extrapolation as a basis for defining a "plausible upper limit" on the risk, meaning that the risks are unlikely to be higher but could be considerably lower (Crump et al. 1977; Crump and Watson 1979; Crump 1981; OSTP 1985; EPA 1986). This model relies on the possibility that any suspected carcinogen can induce cancer by a single-hit phenomenon and makes no distinction for different biologically based mechanisms of cancer induction. To date, other models, which have variously been suggested for low-dose extrapolation from high-dose data, have been empirically based models that seek statistically to define the best shape to the dose-response curve. They have not been based on data that seek to describe the biological events that lead to cancer.

Other assumptions, such as those used to extrapolate animal responses to humans, have been adopted that also have been chosen to be protective where scientific information was lacking (e.g., surface area is often chosen as the conversion factor rather than body weight). Dose is assumed to be synonymous with exposure, unless there are data to the contrary. Other conservative assumptions have also been chosen including, for example, the interpretation of the significance of benign tumors that can lead to malignancy.

Exposure assessment, likewise, has followed a conservative trend. Generally, "maximum plausible levels" of chemical exposure have been used in risk assessments, sometimes in conjunction with "average exposure" estimates. An example of a frequently used conservative assumption is that an individual is exposed for a lifetime of 70 years unless there is evidence to the contrary. In practice, the overall risk characterization has relied on a ranking of the weight-of-evidence, which placed considerable weight on any tumor response in animals and sought to quantitatively describe the risk to current or anticipated exposed populations as an upper-bound risk based on maximum plausible exposure estimates. The first decade of experience with carcinogen risk assessment has been studied from both the scientific standpoint and the use of risk outcomes in public policy decisions (Anderson and CAG 1983). In short, if scientists have been successful in the past describing risk assessment as upper-bound estimates reflecting maximum plausible exposures, then as better science is developed to fill the gaps of uncertainty, risk assessments should be expected to become less conservative.

Risk Assessment of Carcinogens: Current Trends

Historically, protective assumptions replaced uncertainties; in some cases, uncertainty is now being replaced by improved scientific information. In the area of weight-of-evidence, fresh consideration is being given to the weighting of evidence at high dose and its appropriateness for low-dose weighting. For example, in the Carcinogen Assessment Group's risk assessment of ethylenethiourea (EPA/CAG 1977), the uniqueness of the observation of rate thyroid tumors was discussed in the context of having a threshold, namely that these tumors resulted from suppression of thyroid activity only after the administration of a sufficiently high dose. Currently, the rat response is being examined to determine whether environmental exposure levels are likely to approach those that could be expected to elicit the rat thyroid tumor response. If not, it may be appropriate only to factor the mouse liver tumor response results into the weight-of-evidence determination for environmental exposure levels. Other chemicals are similarly being reviewed for their relevance to human exposure because of mechanism of action, tumor type observed, dosing levels used, or metabolic and pharmacokinetic differences between humans and laboratory test animals.

The improvements in dose-response modeling probably represent the most dramatic departure from practices of the last 12 years. There is a clear effort by regulatory agencies to seek a biological basis for the development of more accurate estimates of risks expected to occur at environmental exposure levels. This effort represents a substantially different approach from applying empirical formulas to estimate low-dose responses from high-dose data. Rather, the attention is focused on the importance of research data that may guide low-dose modeling efforts. Such an approach provides, at a minimum, an indication of the extent to which the plausible upper bounds may be overestimating risk for particular chemicals. Early efforts to define more accurate estimates of risk began at EPA in early 1985 and have culminated in the development of a generic approach using a two-stage model. This model adapts the clinical observations of Moolgavkar and Knudson (1981) to parameters involving exposure to toxic chemicals. The effort was first undertaken by EPA's Risk Assessment Forum and was ultimately published in the Journal of Risk Analysis in early 1987 (Thorslund et al. 1987). Thus far, EPA has proposed two important decisions in line with the trend toward less conservatism in dose-response modeling. Both of these decisions were discussed in a recent *New York Times* article (Shabecoff 1988). For example, the Risk Assessment Forum has recommended lowering the arsenic ingestion potency by approximately an order of magnitude (Levine et al. 1987; Moore 1987), based on modifications in dose-response calculation methodology and better estimates of the exposure involved in the epidemiology studies that were the basis for the evaluation. There is a further consideration of reducing the potency of arsenic by ingestion by still another order of magnitude to reflect the fact that skin cancer caused by arsenic ingestion is less likely to lead to death than is lung cancer induced by inhalation. Considerations of the latter raise the issue as to whether or not treatability, survival, and severity should be routinely considered as a part of the risk-assessment process and, in particular, the potency evaluation. In addition, EPA has proposed to downgrade the potency of dioxin, based on several factors, but most importantly the use of the two-stage model of carcinogenesis for modeling the promoting activity of dioxin, which indicates that the potency of dioxin may be two or more orders of magnitude less than the potency defined by the linear nonthreshold model for low doses (T.W. Thorslund and G. Charnley, in prep.). This work was prompted by recommendations of the EPA Science Advisory Board and is still under consideration (EPA/OPTS 1986).

The two-stage model of carcinogenesis has also been applied to several other chemicals with similar outcomes. For example, the model has also been applied to chlordane and heptachlor and methylene chloride (T.W. Thorslund et al., pers. comm.). Although the mechanisms in each case differ, the outcomes of the model are to indicate most often several orders of magnitude lower potency at low dose than predicted by the linear nonthreshold model at the plausible upper bounds.

Additional applications of the biological model have involved the polycyclic organic compounds. Past practices have used the potency of benzo[a]pyrene as a unit equivalency to all other potentially carcinogenic polycyclic organic compounds, greatly overestimating risk. This practice has continued in spite of the fact that comparative potency methods have been developed for other chemical classes, such as the dioxins. When assembled in the aggregate, several laboratory studies provide a more substantial basis for developing a comparative potency approach for polycyclic aromatic hydrocarbons (Thorslund et al. 1986; M.M.L. Chu and C.W. Chen 1984, unpubl.). In addition, the shape of the dose-response curve for benzo[a]pyrene itself has been reevaluated. Benzo[a]pyrene is a genotoxic agent as indicated by a linear rate of DNA adduct formation that parallels exposure. The tumor dose-response data do not parallel DNA adduct formation, however, but appear to fit a quadratic equation, indicating that two events are probably necessary to induce the response. EPA's initial cancer potency estimate for benzo[a]pyrene does not reflect this relationship. The comparative potency approach for other polycyclic compounds, together with a revised dose-response curve for benzo[a]pyrene, has been used to accurately predict tumor outcomes in bioassays of chemical mixtures, which is not possible using upper-bound estimates (Thorslund et al. 1986). Another example of a chemical that may require two events to produce a cancer outcome is benzene. Current investigations are examining the mechanistic data, which indicate benzene causes chromosome damage, which is thought to be responsible for the chromosomal deletions and rearrangements observed in leukemia patients. This relationship implies that, although linearity may establish a plausible upper bound on human leukemia risk from benzene exposure, a quadratic relationship may be more appropriate to estimate the actual risk. Should this turn out to be the case, the risk from low-dose exposure to benzene would be considerably lower than previously estimated (T.W. Thorslund and G. Charnley, pers. comm.).

A great deal of attention is also being focused on the metabolic and pharmacokinetic data to estimate actual levels of chemical exposure to the target tissue. In extrapolating animal data to humans, the effective dose in the animal studies has always been assumed to be the dose that the animal was exposed to by route-administered dose. As our ability to describe the actual dose to the target tissue in the animal improves, so will our ability to extrapolate animal responses to humans. In addition, the importance of pharmacokinetic data to define the significance of human exposure in the environment is exceedingly important.

Of equal importance, trends in exposure assessment research are also leading to improved estimates of population exposures, which provide a better foundation for current and projected exposures. Traditional practices have relied heavily on generic models to describe exposure to human populations. EPA has developed generalized dispersion models for describing air transport and similar generalized dispersion models for surface and groundwater. The overall impact of these dispersion models has been to provide conservative estimates of exposure.

The use of generalized models provides a practical approach for widespread exposure estimation by regulatory agencies because it would be highly impractical for a national agency to evaluate site-specific parameters for every source. For important cases, however, it is possible to estimate actual parameters that may refine the estimates obtained by generic modeling. An example is the risk assessment of the ASARCO smelter in Takoma, Washington, which was conducted by EPA (Patrick and Peters 1985). The use of generalized dispersion modeling using the human exposure model (which assumes a flat terrain, an immobile population, and uses meteorological data from the closest weather station), when coupled with the dose-response curve, estimated a maximum individual risk of about 1×10^{-1} for populations living near the smelter. Subsequently, a local study was conducted that permitted the use of several site-specific assumptions, including a more accurate description of the actual terrain, local meteorological data, and better emissions information. The outcome was to lower the exposure assessment and the overall risk about an order of magnitude. This brought the risk into closer alignment with the limited monitoring data that were available for the ambient air.

The same phenomenon has been observed when comparing estimates using generalized dispersion models for groundwater with estimates that rely on site-specific parameters. For example, in the Equation 1 below, the generalized groundwater dispersion model, the vertical horizontal spread (VHS) model using EPA default values overestimates the risk by a factor of 5.7, when compared to the results from the more complex Equation 2, which incorporates measured site values (Domenico and Palciauskas 1982; EPA 1985):

(1) VHS model using simple equation, EPA fixed default values

$$\frac{C}{C_0} = \mathrm{erf}\left(\frac{Z}{2(DY)^{0.5}}\right) \mathrm{erf}\left(\frac{X}{4(DY)^{0.5}}\right)$$

$$= 0.34$$

(2) VHS model using complex equation, measured site values

$$\frac{C}{C_0} = \frac{1}{4} \left(\operatorname{erf}\left[\frac{z+Z}{2(D_zY)^{0.5}} \right] - \operatorname{erf}\left[\frac{z-Z}{2(D_zY)^{0.5}} \right] \right)$$

$$\times \left(\operatorname{erf}\left[\frac{x+X/2}{2(D_xY)^{0.5}} \right] - \operatorname{erf}\left[\frac{x-X/2}{2(D_xY)^{0.5}} \right] \right)$$

$$= 0.06$$

Another important area that has sharpened exposure estimates and practically has lowered the outcome from exposure assessment by several orders of magnitude, and thus the quantitative risk assessment, has been considerations of bioavailability. For example, dioxin was originally assumed to be 100% biologically available in soil. Recent studies, however, have demonstrated that dioxin is only partially available, $>0.5–85\%$ depending on soil type (Umbreit et al. 1986). In practice. it has been our experience that dioxin is mostly available in the range of 15–50% (P. Chrostowski, pers. comm.). Dioxin in fly ash also was originally assumed to be up to 100% available. Recent studies have found that this is not correct but rather that dioxin in fly ash is biologically available between 0.1% and 0.001% (van den Berg et al. 1986). The bioavailability issue is now being commonly investigated in many different situations where the availability in soil and fly ash is important to the outcome of the risk assessment. Other considerations that tend to lower exposure assessments may come from knowledge of the hydrogeology of an area. For example, work completed by our scientists at a site in California indicated an upper-bound lifetime risk associated with ingestion of water containing trichloroethylene (TCE) in an aquifer to be as high as 10^{-3} risk (Figure 1). This level is associated with a 70-year lifetime exposure via exposure to drinking water from the contaminated aquifer. Scenario 2 in Figure 1 describes the decline in risk associated when hydrogeology models are applied to the site; the model assumes that the source of contamination has been removed. In Table 1 and 2, the monitoring well data are displayed and, likewise, the risk comparison over time given the ability to model the area. In this particular circumstance, remedial action was being considered that would cost in the million dollar range and require a number of months to install. If the hydrogeology models are correct, the theoretical risk could be lowered considerably over the first 18-month period given the natural ability of the hydrogeology of the area to remove the contamination. Caution, however, should be exercised in assuming that the source has been removed because recent publications indicate that in some circumstances some chemicals may remain entrapped in soil micropores and, thereby, provide a slow, diffuse release (Sawhney et al. 1988).

Although improving the scientific information available for site-specific exposure assessment tends to lower the overall outcome of the exposure

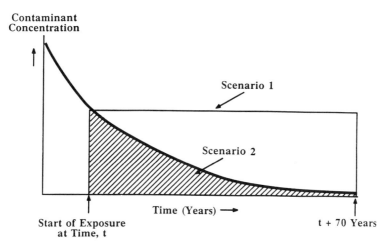

Figure 1

Scenario 1 assumes decay in contaminant levels until start of consumption and then a lifetime exposure to a constant concentration of the contaminant. Scenario 2 assumes decay in contaminant levels both before and during the period of exposure.

assessment and, thus, the risk assessment, there are important exceptions. For example, a recent paper, which addressed the issue of risk associated with inhaling volatile organic chemicals from contaminated drinking water during shower activity (S. Foster and P. Chrostowski, pers. comm.), indicated that as much as half or more of the total body risk could be associated with the shower exposure rather than with the drinking water exposure. In addition, recent improved methods for modeling the actual deposition of particulate matter from stationary sources tend to raise the risk compared with the earlier EPA air transport models that assumed that both large and small particles bounced from the surface of the earth in very similar ways and were carried from the site by air transport. The more recent models take into account that the small particles deposit on the surface and are not so readily transported (Sehmel and Hodgson 1979). Also, closer attention to chemical conversions may tend to raise or lower the risk; for example, TCE is converted under anaerobic conditions to vinylchloride, which has a higher potency value by ingestion than does TCE (Cline and Viste 1984; Parsons et al. 1984). Recognition of this conversion raises the overall risk assessment for circumstances that appropriately are evaluated by these methods.

Numerous other refinements in exposure assessment are also being incorporated in the risk assessment process, for example, use of human biological data to assist in exposure estimation, better descriptions of life style for subpopulation groups, the use of statistical methods to describe likely expo-

Table 1
Groundwater Monitoring Data

Well no.	Sampling date	TCE mg/l		Well average TCE mg/l
1	1/1/85 1/20/85 2/2/85	.100 .144 .127	} .124	
2	1/1/85 1/20/85 2/2/85 2/8/85	<.005 1.10 1.98 2.00	} 1.27	
3	1/1/85 2/2/85	<.005 <.001	} .003	
4	1/1/85 2/2/85	.005 .080	} .068	0.36
5	1/20/85 2/2/85	.210 .177	} .194	
6	1/1/85 2/8/85	.510 1.40	} .96	
7	1/20/85 2/2/85	.160 .305	} .23	
8	1/1/85 2/8/85	.070 <.005	} .04	

Table 2
Risk Comparison

Time of exposure initiation (years)	TCE at start of exposure (mg/l)	Lifetime upper bound cancer risk	
		scenario 1	scenario 2
t_0	.36	1.1×10^{-4}	3.5×10^{-6}
1	.23	7.1×10^{-5}	2.2×10^{-6}
2	.14	4.5×10^{-5}	1.4×10^{-6}
3	.09	2.8×10^{-5}	8.8×10^{-7}
4	.06	1.8×10^{-5}	
5	.04	1.1×10^{-5}	
6	.02	7.2×10^{-6}	
7	.01	4.6×10^{-6}	
8	.009	2.9×10^{-6}	
9	.006	1.8×10^{-6}	
10	.004	1.1×10^{-6}	

sure below detectable limits, and the use of pharmacokinetic data to describe the actual dose to target tissue. These developments rely on advancing research in multiple disciplines for use in the practical consideration of human exposure.

DISCUSSION

Implications of the Qualitative and Quantitative Aspects of Carcinogen Risk Assessment

The risk assessment process as applied to toxic chemicals for use in carcinogen risk assessment has been most criticized because of the enormous uncertainties involved in the process, and yet it is this very process that has encouraged the dialogue between researchers, risk assessors, and public policy officials who are increasingly involved in difficult decisions where the most accurate description of theoretical risk is of the utmost importance. As dialogues with an increasingly better informed public take place, the need to develop the most accurate risk assessments possible is also increasing. Other interested parties, including the regulated community and the environmental communities, will equally benefit as their programs can focus more accurately on the most important health problems in our society. The deficiencies in the risk assessment process are actually turning out to be benefits in the sense that the flaws in the process are stimulating better communications between scientists involved in risk assessment and those involved primarily in bench research on some of the most important issues in the public health arena. For the most part we are looking at increasingly improving the scientific basis for carcinogen risk assessment. The direct, practical applications for some of the most exciting research is immediately possible in the risk assessment process. In general, practices of the past, which tended to err on the side of public health, are becoming less conservative, although there are exceptions that have been discussed in this paper. The implication is that increasingly the risk-assessment process will be able to accommodate the exciting developments in research, which elucidate the mechanisms of carcinogenesis. Likewise, increasingly the part of the risk assessment that focuses on exposure is incorporating improved environmental data and is looking for improved techniques to use body-burden data and biological markers to better define the exposure basis for risk assessment. As our carcinogen risk assessments become better descriptors of reality, our public policy decisions can be focused to generate the greatest gains in public health resulting from social and regulatory sacrifices.

ACKNOWLEDGMENTS

I want to thank Luci Henry, my administrative assistant, for assistance in preparing the manuscript and Judy L. Fauls for technical editing of the manuscript. In addition, I would like to thank my colleagues, Gail Charnley, Paul Chrostowski, Sarah Foster, Todd W. Thorslund, and Judy Vreeland for their constructive comments and assistance.

REFERENCES

Albert, R.E., R.E. Train, and E.L. Anderson. 1977. Rationale developed by the Environmental Protection Agency for the assessment of carcinogenic risk. *J. Natl. Cancer Inst.* **58**: 1537.

Anderson, E.L. and The Carcinogen Assessment Group (CAG) of the U.S. Environmental Protection Agency. 1983. Quantitative approaches in use to assess cancer risk. *J. Risk Anal.* **3(4)**: 277.

Cline, P.V. and D.R. Viste. 1984. Migration and degradation patterns of volatile organic compounds. In *National Conference of Uncontrolled Hazardous Waste Site Proceedings*, p. 217. Hazardous Materials Control Research Institute, Silver Spring, Maryland.

Crump, K.S. 1981. An improved procedure for low-dose carcinogenic risk assessment from animal data. *J. Environ. Pathol. Toxicol.* **52**: 675.

Crump, K.S. and W.W. Watson. 1979. A Fortran program to extrapolate dichotomous animal carcinogenicity data to low doses. *Natl. Inst. Environ. Health Sci.*, Contract No. 1-ES-2123.

Crump, K.S., H.A. Guess, and L.L. Deal. 1977. Confidence intervals and test of hypotheses concerning dose-response relations inferred from animal carcinogenicity data. *Biometrics* **33**: 437.

Domenico, P.A. and V.V. Palciauskas. 1982. Alternative boundaries in solid waste management. *Groundwater* **20**: 303.

Environmental Protection Agency (EPA). 1976. Interim procedures and guidelines for health risks and economic impact assessments of suspected carcinogens. *Fed. Reg.* **41**: 21402.

———. 1985. Final exclusions and final vertical and horizontal spread model (VHS). *Fed. Reg.* **50**: 229.

———. 1986. Guidelines for carcinogen risk assessment. *Fed. Reg.* **51(185)**: 33991.

Environmental Protection Agency/Carcinogen Assessment Groups (EPA/CAG). 1977. *Preliminary report on ethylene bisdithiocarbamate (EBDC)*.

Environmental Protection Agency/Office of Pesticides and Toxic Substances (EPA/OPTS). 1986. *Report of the dioxin update committee*.

Inter-agency Regulatory Liaison Group (IRLG). 1979. Scientific basis for the identification of potential carcinogens and estimation of risks. *J. Natl. Cancer Inst.* **63**: 243.

International Agency for Research on Cancer (IARC). 1982. Chemicals and industrial processes associated with cancer in humans. *IARC Monogr. Eval. Carcinog. Risk Chem. Hum.* **4:** 7.

Levine, T., A. Rispin, C.S. Scott, W. Marcus, C. Chen, and H. Libb. 1987. Special report on ingested inorganic arsenic: Skin cancer; nutritional essentiality. Risk Assessment Forum. U.S. Environmental Protection Agency Science Advisory Board Review, Washington, D.C.

Moolgavkar, S.H. and A.G. Knudson. 1981. Mutation and cancer: A model for human carcinogenesis. *J. Natl. Cancer Inst.* **66:** 1037.

Moore, J.A. 1987. *Recommended agency policy on the carcinogenicity risk associated with the ingestion of inorganic arsenic—action memorandum.* U.S. Environmental Protection Agency, Office of Pesticides and Toxic Substances, Washington, D.C.

National Academy of Sciences/National Research Council (NAS/NRC). 1983. *Risk assessment in the federal government: Managing the process.* Prepared by the Committee on the Institutional Means for Assessment of Risk to Public Health, Commission on Life Sciences, National Academy Press, Washington, D.C.

Office of Science and Technology Policy (OSTP). 1985. Chemical carcinogens: Review of the science and its associated principles. *Fed. Reg.* **50:** 10372.

Parsons, F., P.R. Wood, and J. DeMarco. 1984. Transformation of tetrachloroethene and trichloroethane in microcosms and groundwater. *Res. Technol.*, p. 56.

Patrick, D. and W.D. Peters. 1985. Exposure assessment in setting air pollution regulations: ASARCO, Tacoma, a case study. Proceedings of the Society for Risk Analysis 1985 annual meeting. Society for Risk Analysis, McLean, Virginia.

Sawhney, B.L., J.J. Pignatello, and S.M. Steinberg. 1988. Determination of 1,2-dibromoethane (EDB) in field soils: Implications for volatile organic compounds. *J. Environ. Qual.* **17(1):** 149.

Sehmel, G.A. and W.H. Hodgson. 1979. *A model for predicting dry deposition of particles and gases to environmental surfaces.* Prepared for the U.S. Department of Energy by Pacific Northwest Laboratory (PNL-SA-6271-REV 1), Richland, Washington.

Shabecoff, P. 1988. EPA reassesses the cancer risk of many chemicals. *New York Times* (Monday, January 4) p. A1.

Thorslund, T.W., C.C. Brown, and G. Charnley. 1987. Biologically motivated cancer risk models. *Risk. Anal.* **7:** 109.

Thorslund, T.W., G. Charnley, and E.L. Anderson. 1986. Innovative use of toxicological data to improve cost-effectiveness of waste cleanup. In *Management of uncontrolled hazardous waste sites.* Hazardous Materials Control Research Institute, Silver Spring, Maryland.

Umbreit, T.H., E.G. Hesse, and M.A. Gallo. 1986. Bioavailability of dioxin in soil from a 2,4,5-T manufacturing site. *Science* **232:** 497.

van den Berg, M., M. van Greevenbroek, K. Olie, and O. Hutzinger. 1986. Bioavailability of PCDDs and PCDFs on fly ash after semi-chronic ingestion by rat. *Chemosphere* **15:** 509.

COMMENTS

Stevenson: Did you consider the possibility of using biological sample monitoring for establishing the exposure of, for instance, hair or blood. I would have thought you would have gotten a pretty a good estimate of exposure?

Anderson: Yes, we certainly have. We have done that for lead. We wanted to use it for the urine. I know this is something in which ATSDR has a keen interest. However, it has really been used very little, except in specific cases. Also, we get into the biological markers and the ability to use that kind of information. That, too, is potentially very important.

Priorities in Risk Assessment Research

CATHERINE ST. HILAIRE
ILSI Risk Science Institute
Washington, D.C. 20036

OVERVIEW

A survey of ten research organizations to identify and to characterize research aimed at improving carcinogen risk assessment was conducted. A substantial number of research projects were identified, especially in relation to the first two steps in risk assessment, hazard identification, and dose-response assessment. In contrast, research related to exposure assessment and risk characterization was significantly less. Analysis of research according to key assumptions (components) of risk assessment revealed that research is more actively related to several components, such as markers of exposure and effects of test variables on outcome, than others. In addition, analysis of research on those components identified by federal risk assessors as most significant revealed that some are essentially unstudied. Ideally, research planning in this area should include consideration of ongoing research as well as those areas identified as most significant by risk assessors.

INTRODUCTION

Regulatory actions are based on two distinct processes: risk assessment and risk management. According to the definitions developed by the National Research Council (NRC 1983), risk assessment is the characterization of the probability of potentially adverse health effects from human exposures to environmental hazards. Risk management is the process of evaluating alternative regulatory actions and selecting among them, guided by risk assessment information and other considerations.

Because of the current state of the science, the risks projected by the regulatory agencies generally include risk estimates derived with methods for which there is limited validation or for which no validation methods have been devised. Also, current methods used to collect information about harmful effects rely upon postulated exposure conditions that do not match and, indeed, are generally far in excess of actual environmental exposures.

Portions of this paper are derived from *Review of Research Activities to Improve Risk Assessment for Carcinogens* to be published by the International Life Sciences Institute (currently in press).

Banbury Report 31: Carcinogen Risk Assessment: New Directions in the Qualitative and Quantitative Aspects © Cold Spring Harbor Laboratory. 0-87969-231-6/88. $1.00 + .00
295

As a result the risks now projected by risk assessment cannot be confirmed as accurate. This discrepancy may be eliminated but only by research into the bases of the many forms of extrapolation needed to conduct risk assessments. Widespread recognition of the need to improve the scientific bases of the various extrapolation tools used by risk assessors has led to efforts to conduct research to improve the scientific basis of risk assessment. In order to assess the extent and types of such research, a survey of several organizations most likely to be involved in research on risk assessment was conducted. These organizations were the Department of Energy, the Department of Health and Human Services (primarily the Centers for Disease Control, the Food and Drug Administration, and the National Institutes of Health), the Environmental Protection Agency, and the National Science Foundation. Information also was collected from four privately funded organizations: the Chemical Industry Institute of Toxicology, the Electric Power Research Institute, the Health Effects Institute (which also receives government funding), and the ILSI Risk Science Institute.

RESULTS

A working definition of research on risk assessment was developed for use in discussions with key research personnel at each of these organizations: Risk assessment research consists of those activities aimed at developing and expanding risk assessment methodology in order to reduce the uncertainties in the risk assessment process. A broad definition was purposely used that would encompass laboratory and field studies as well as analytical work aimed at developing new approaches in risk assessment.
Three broad criteria to identify research on risk assessment were used:

1. The research had to be concerned principally with the development of new risk assessment methodologies.
2. The research had to be pertinent to at least one of the four steps of risk assessment or to development of test methods used to generate data relied upon in risk assessment (Fig. 1).
3. Research aimed primarily at developing information on particular chemicals was included only if the project was also designed to (or in some cases expected to) have general value in improving risk assessment methodologies.

Because risk assessment has most often been applied to questions about cancer-causing agents, the survey was limited to risk assessment research that focuses on cancer. Basic research in cancer, which is a vast enterprise, was not included in the survey unless a direct link with the current concerns of risk assessors could be identified.

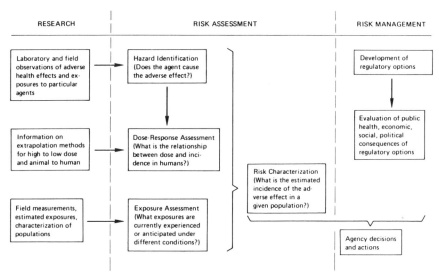

Figure 1

Diagrammatic representation of relation between research, risk assessment, and risk management.

Another effort, development of a comprehensive list of the uncertainties and assumptions inherent to carcinogen risk assessment, was conducted in parallel with the survey. An NRC committee (NRC 1983) identified points where insertion of assumptions is required as *components* of risk assessment, and this terminology was adopted for the survey. The list of components compiled here builds upon the list developed in the NRC report. More than 70 components of carcinogen risk assessment were identified. (This number is somewhat arbitrary. Some components on the list could be combined and some could be further subdivided, decreasing or increasing the number. The 75 were chosen because they provide reasonable detail for analysis.) Components identified in this survey are given in Table 1.

The results of the survey of ongoing research programs were then analyzed and categorized according to the components of risk assessment most likely to be influenced by each research project. The directors of the identified organizations or key directors of research were interviewed for this survey. In addition, all publicly available documents describing current (FY 1986–1987) research activities, including both intra- and extramural programs, were collected. Specific projects were characterized to determine the steps of risk assessment being studied (i.e., hazard identification, dose-response assessment, human exposure assessment, and risk characterization). In addition,

Table 1

Components Identified in Survey

(a) *Step 1. Hazard identification*

Epidemiology:

1. What criteria must an epidemiological study meet to identify a carcinogenic hazard?
2. What criteria must a epidemiological study meet to support a conclusion that no carcinogenic risk or no risk greater than a specific number exists at a particular exposure?

Short-term tests:

3. What criteria must a short-term test meet to identify genotoxic effects or to be used in prediction of carcinogenicity?

Structure-activity analyses:

4. What criteria must be met for analysis of structure-activity relationships to be used for predicting carcinogenicity?

Animal studies:

5. What are the effects of differences in life span and age at first exposure?
6. What are the effects of differences in body size?
7. What are the effects of differences in diet?
8. What are the effects of differences in genetic variability, species differences?
9. What are the effects of differences in population homogeneity?
10. What are the effects of differences in concurrent disease and stress?
11. What are the effects of differences in pharmacokinetics?
12. What are the effects of differences in metabolism?
13. What are the effects of differences in DNA damage and repair?
14. What are the effects of differences in routes of exposure?
15. What are the effects of differences in exposure regimen?
16. What are the effects of differences in sex and hormonal status?
17. What are the effects of exposure to other chemicals?
18. What are the experimental criteria for defining complete carcinogens, initiators, promoters, secondary mechanisms of carcinogenesis?
19. What is the degree of relevance of certain organ systems and tumor types to hazard identification?
20. How relevant to assessing hazard are increases in rare tumors?
21. How should an increased incidence of common tumors (tumors with a high and variable spontaneous incidence rate) be evaluated?
22. Should benign tumors be considered as evidence of carcinogenic effect?
23. How should negative trends in tumor incidence in animal bioassays be interpreted?
24. What is the significance of tumors in organs that have no human analog?
25. How should multiple comparison problems in statistical analysis of tumor incidence be addressed?

Analyses:

26. What factors should be considered in a weight-of-evidence approach to deciding the carcinogenic potential of a substance?
27. How should epidemiology, animal, and short-term results be combined in a weight-of-evidence determination?

(b) *Step 2. Dose-response assessment*

Epidemiology:

28. How should dose-response information from human studies be modeled and used?

Short-term tests:

29. How can quantitative information on genotoxicity be used to predict carcinogenic potency?
30. How can quantitative information from other short-term tests be used to predict carcinogenic potency?
31. How can quantitative information on DNA adduct formation be used to predict carcinogenic potency?

Structure-activity analyses:

32. How can quantitative structure-activity data be used to predict carcinogenic potency?

Animal studies:

33. Which low-dose extrapolation model should be used? What criteria should be applied to guide the selection of a model?
34. Should low-dose extrapolation be done differently for promoters? If so, how?
35. Which species and strains are most appropriate for dose-response assessment?
36. How should pharmacokinetic information be incorporated in extrapolation methods?
37. Can dose-response models be developed to adjust for differences in metabolism?
38. Can dose-response models be tailored to particular chemicals?
39. What effect does exposure to other chemicals have on dose response?
40. How does diet affect the relationship between dose and response? Can dietary differences and effects be accounted for so that risk estimates are relevant to the human situation?
41. What effect does dose rate and duration have on the dose-response relationship? What effect does experiment length have on dose response?
42. What data should be used to develop risk estimates? How should the data on pharmacokinetics be used to guide data set selection?
43. What variables should be used to determine potency—incidence, types of tumors, number of tumors per animal, time to tumor, combined incidences of benign and malignant tumors? How should these variables be weighted and combined?
44. How relevant are quantitative results from one route of exposure to other routes of exposure?
45. How can the relationship between administered and target-tissue (or effective) dose be identified and then used in establishing the dose-response curve?
46. How accurate are the standardized scaling factors used to extrapolate dose across species?
47. How should negative trends (anticarcinogenic effects) be considered?
48. Which risk estimates should be used: maximum likelihood or best estimate (average likelihood)?
49. Is there a threshold for carcinogenic effects?

(Continued on following page.)

(c) *Step 3. Exposure assessment*

General issues:

50. How can uncertainties in exposure modeling (that depend on the behavior of the chemical in the environment) be reduced?
51. Can structure-activity data be used to predict environmental mobility, fate, persistance, and bioaccumulation of chemicals?

Route-specific issues:

52. What is an appropriate value for dermal absorption of various compounds? Can a method be developed to predict this value based on chemical properties?
53. How much soil is ingested?
54. Information about specific routes of exposure: What factors influence bioavailability of chemicals absorbed to soil?
55. Information about specific routes of exposure: What are the patterns of tissue exposure following inhalation of pollutants?

Dose issues:

56. Can better estimates of food and beverage consumption be developed?
57. What is "effective dose" and how can it be evaluated? What is the effect of other chemicals on effective dose?
58. How should pharmacokinetic and metabolism data be used to refine human exposure estimates?
59. How do exposure variables affect the effective dose in humans?
60. What lifestyle factors influence dose? How should they be considered in risk assessment?
61. Should exposure be expressed as an average over a lifetime or should dose rate and age when exposure occurs be considered?
62. What dose measurements should be used?
63. Can markers be used to measure exposure? Can DNA adduct formation be used to estimate human exposure to a substance?
64. Can the target dose of inhaled substances be measured and predicted?
65. Can methods be developed that detect hazardous substances in human tissues and fluids?
66. Can information on exposure from one chemical be extrapolated to other chemicals?

Susceptible populations:

67. How should highly susceptible populations be identified and characterized?
68. Are there characteristics of routes of exposure that cause some populations to be highly susceptible?

(d) *Step 4. Risk characterization*

69. How should qualitative (i.e., weight of evidence) and quantitative determinations be combined and reported?
70. How should risk and exposure information be combined and reported?
71. Should risks from multiple exposures and multiple sources of a given carcinogen be considered to be additive?
72. Are risks from concurrent exposure to several carcinogens additive?
73. How should uncertainties be considered when developing risk estimates?
74. What are the demographics of susceptibility to the effect of carcinogens? How should this information be incorporated into the final risk estimates?
75. How should acceptable or tolerable risk be determined?

research aimed at test improvement in the following areas was also included in the survey.

1. Epidemiology studies.
2. Short-term tests: mutagenicity, short-term carcinogenicity assays, and analysis.
3. Structure-activity studies.
4. Chronic animal bioassays: statistics; route of exposure; dosing effects, dose selection, pharmacokinetics; diet effects; strain effects; new assays; effects of chemical mixtures; and analysis.

In most cases, project summaries received from the organizations were sufficient to identify the specific components of risk assessment under study, although in some cases descriptions were too general to allow for this. A best guess was made in such cases. Because of an intentional bias to be inclusive, the number of projects included in the survey probably exaggerates the number of ongoing projects directly linked to risk assessment.

Because of the brevity of this report, a compilation of findings is not presented here. In the full report of the survey (ILSI RSI 1988), research projects are tabulated according to the components of risk assessment affected or according to test improvement. If an individual project addresses aspects of more than one component, it is listed for each component. Details about the content of the projects and the general nature of the research conducted by each supporting organization are presented in the full report.

A sample entry from the complete summary table of the results of the survey follows (Table 2). Entries are in the following form: descriptor of the project and sponsoring organization in parentheses.

DISCUSSION

Based on the survey, the field of risk assessment research is not particularly well defined or organized (as evidenced by the difficulties encountered in trying to understand how specific projects or portions thereof might ultimately affect risk assessment). However, it is apparent that some investigators and research directors in most of the institutions surveyed are actively thinking about and encouraging research to improve risk assessment. This trend was apparent in almost every research document examined. Increasingly, investigators are attempting to conduct their experiments on specific substances using novel techniques in the hope that the data collected will provide better information for the risk assessor. Significantly more research projects were identified in this survey than in a similar one conducted approximately two years ago (ILSI RSI 1985).

Table 2
Sample of the Results of the ILSI Survey

Component	Research projects
What is the degree of relevance of certain organ systems and tumor types to hazard identification?	Mechanisms of carcinogenesis associated with thyroid neoplasia (EPA)
	Phenotypic differences and liver neoplasms in mice (FDA-NCTR)
	Relevance of rat leukemia to humans (NIH-NIEHS)
	Liver tumors—model development, assessment of significance (NIH-NIEHS)
	Relevance of hepatocellular preneoplastic lesions in rodents (CIIT)
	Relevance of mouse lymphoma as a model (CIIT)

Sponsoring organizations are in parenthesis: Environmental Protection Agency (EPA); Food and Drug Administration (FDA); National Center for Toxicological Research (NCTR); National Institute of Health (NIH); National Institute of Environmental Health Sciences (NIEHS); Chemical Industry Institute of Toxicology (CIIT).

General Observations

As seen in the results of this survey, certain areas of investigation appear to be particularly active. The first area includes studies of the effects of differences in animal test variables (hazard identification). Researchers are looking at the effects of variables such as differences in animal body size and exposure regimens on the outcome of animal tests. The second area includes studies of the relevancy to humans of dose-response data derived from animal studies (dose-response assessment). All of the organizations surveyed supported at least one project in this area.

In addition, two other areas are receiving a great deal of attention: studies of the relevance of certain organ systems and tumor types (test improvement, hazard identification) and identification of "biological markers" of human exposure (exposure assessment). In the first, the biology of certain tumor types (e.g., rodent liver tumors and mouse lymphomas) are under investigation to understand the reasons for the high and variable incidences of these tumors. The relevance of preneoplastic and benign lesions to assessing carcinogenic potential is also being investigated. In the second, there is strong interest in improving knowledge of human exposure by developing measures of exposure at critical biological sites in the body. Although most research in this area is in an early stage of development, there are a relatively large number of preliminary investigations under way. In addititon to the above areas, the number of studies dealing with chemical mixtures and the effects of other chemicals on dose response and on the use of pharmacokinetic data in extrapolation methods is increasing.

Relevance of Research to Risk Assessment

The survey provides a picture of the relative level of activity associated with major uncertainties in carcinogen risk assessment. The degree to which the areas being investigated are the most significant areas of uncertainty is less clear. One way to address this issue is to compare the results of this survey with a list of risk assessment components that were identified by federal regulatory agencies (at the request of the Office of Science and Technology) as the most critical for their risk activities. This comparison is presented in Table 3. Note that these components were set forth as the assumptions that are currently used by regulatory agencies when they conduct risk assessments. The agencies identified these as the most important assumptions needing experimental study. From the analysis presented in Table 3, all of the components identified in this summary are not equally important in their impact on carcinogen risk assessments, nor do these components that have been judged by agency risk assessors to be critical have equal research emphasis. For example, several areas identified by agency risk assessors are essentially unstudied (e.g., structure-activity studies, use of average doses, use of surrogate chemicals for exposure assessment, estimation of exposure from multiple sources, and quantifying uncertainty).

The greatest improvements in risk assessment methodology in the short run will result from studies having two important prerequisites: (1) potential for a great effect on risk assessments and (2) adequate technical approaches available. This approach for determining research agendas does not appear to be operative.

One additional observation is the relative absence of broad analyses of existing data relevant to risk assessment. Although most of the major research issues will require experimental work of one type or another, there is a large body of published scientific data, both basic and applied, that might provide important clues regarding some of the methodological issues. For example, careful analyses of the vast body of epidemiological literature on the causes of human cancers and of corresponding animal data on the suspect agents might reveal some new information of great value. In addition, analyses that use existing data to explore theories associated with carcinogenic mechanism, for example, the role of peroxisome proliferation, would also likely be beneficial. Such nonexperimental research requires understanding of the underlying scientific issues and creative syntheses of large bodies of information. Almost no work of this type was identified as being currently

Table 3
Comparison of Risk Assessment Components Identified by Federal
Regulatory Agencies with Research Activities Ongoing in Key Research
Organizations

Key assumptions	Number of studies
1. If a compound induces cancer in laboratory animals, it is assumed to have the capacity to induce cancer in humans.	37
2. Use of a battery of short-term tests to predict carcinogenicity requires careful consideration of the appropriateness of the chemical and the type of test.	6
3. In the absence of chemical-specific data, structure-activity correlations can be used to predict human carcinogenicity.	1
Dose-response assessment	
1. Observed experimental results can be extrapolated across species by use of standardized scaling factors.	7
2. In the absence of pharmacokinetic data, the effective or target dose can be assumed to be proportional to the administered dose.	18
3. Results from one route of exposure are relevant to other routes of exposure.	4
4. In predicting overall cancer risk to humans, risks should be derived from the most sensitive species, benign plus malignant tumors, and pooled tumor incidence.	6
5. A linear multistage model can be used for low-dose extrapolation.	6
6. Results of animal studies terminated early can be extrapolated to lifetime studies by use of an appropriate scaling factor.	6
Exposure assessment	
1. Average doses give a reasonable measure of exposure when doses are not constant in time or rate.	2
2. Structure-activity relationships can be used to predict the environmental mobility and bioaccumulation potential of chemicals.	0
3. Human exposure data from surrogate chemicals can be extrapolated to other similar chemical used in a similar manner.	0
4. Biological markers can be used as an indication of exposure.	6
Risk characterization	
1. The risks from multiple exposures and multiple sources of exposure are additive.	0
2. There are valid methods for quantifying uncertainty in the risk assessment process.	0
	0

underway, yet it is badly needed to form a bridge between the work of experimentalists and the ultimate needs of the risk assessor.

Finally, the step in risk assessment with the least amount of research underway was risk characterization. This final step in risk assessment, which combines all information and feeds directly into risk management decision making, requires additional research attention.

REFERENCES

International Life Sciences Institute (ILSI) Risk Science Institute (RSI). 1985. *Review of current research activities to improve risk assessment and identification of major gaps.* ILSI Risk Science Institute, Washington, D.C.

———. 1988. *Review of research activities to improve risk assessment for carcinogens.* ILSI Risk Science Institute, Washington, D.C. (In press.)

National Research Council (NRC). 1983. *Risk assessment in the federal government: Managing the process.* National Academy Press, Washington, D.C.

COMMENTS

Hoerger: Cathy, I think you have really teased the audience with some information here. I know you're quite willing to discuss this further.

Wilson: First of all, you have done a fantastic job, Cathy, and that report is both monstrous in size and depth and undertaking and in kind and quality. As you say, no one ever undertook before to do anything on that scale. It should hardly surprise anyone that there are lots of omissions. However, considering the size, it is still a remarkable achievement.

St. Hilaire: It can be improved, obviously.

Wilson: A couple of questions. The Science Advisory Board did a review of extrapolation research. The EPA Science Advisory Board recently published a review, *Extrapolation Research*. One question is: Are the conclusions you have come to very different from theirs? As to your 70 assumptions, are those also many of the same assumptions that people who worked on the Guidelines used?

St. Hilaire: To tell you the truth, I really started with the Guidelines. That was the way that we started to tease out where the assumptions are, because that's what the Guidelines are for. When you get to a point where the science doesn't give you the answers, there are your assumptions. So, I really started working from the Guidelines, in terms of listing out and fleshing out the list of components or assumptions. So, the Guidelines development and this kind of survey were very much related.

In terms of the Science Advisory Board study, they looked at EPA research and had presentations on EPA research. They did not catalog the research the way that I'm describing. They did reach some conclusions in terms of areas that they think should be emphasized. They are very similar to the kinds of things that would have come out of my report. Sitting where the Science Advisory Board does and sort of seeing what some of the real problems and major uncertainties are in risk assessment, they also have a sense of what the priorities should be. So, it is very similar.

Their report was not just on quantitative risk assessment, it was on extrapolation. I thought it must only deal with quantitation, but they were talking about all the kinds of things that I listed earlier: What are the effects of changes in diet, how do you go from one species to another, and that type of thing.

Hoerger: Thank you so much, Cathy. Earlier, we had reference to lumpers and splitters, and I think you have added a bit here by your categorization of the assumptions and the research.

Molecular Dosimetry Data in Humans: Implications for Risk Assessment and Research

FREDERICA PERERA
Columbia University School of Public Health
Division of Environmental Sciences
New York, N.Y. 10032

OVERVIEW

Human molecular dosimetry data have the potential to significantly improve qualitative and quantitative risk assessment for environmental carcinogens. Parallel studies in humans and experimental animals should improve interspecies extrapolation but have not yet been carried out. Few well-designed molecular epidemiological studies have been undertaken. However, data developed so far have implications for risk assessment and suggest important areas for research. These include the extent of interindividual variability in the biologically effective dose of carcinogens and the substantial "background" seen in control groups. Specific research recommendations are included.

INTRODUCTION

A number of biological markers are becoming available for quantitation of the biologically effective dose[1] of mutagens/carcinogens in humans with environmental exposures. These include carcinogen-DNA and carcinogen-protein adducts (as a more feasible surrogate), sister chromatid exchange (SCE), micronuclei in lymphocytes, and somatic cell mutation. Although these markers reflect a biological response that is qualitatively linked to tumor formation, in the absence of data illustrating their precise predictive relationship to cancer, they are most usefully construed as carcinogen dosimeters and as qualitative indicators of cancer risk (i.e., hazard). As such, markers of biologically effective dose have the potential to assist human cancer risk assessment in the following ways:

1. Markers assist by allowing timely identification of carcinogenic hazards. There is general agreement that elevated levels of DNA adducts or

---

[1]The biologically effective dose is defined as the amount of the carcinogen or its metabolites that has interacted with critical cellular macromolecules (DNA, RNA, or protein) in the target tissue or a surrogate.

Banbury Report 31: Carcinogen Risk Assessment: New Directions in the Qualitative and Quantitative Aspects © Cold Spring Harbor Laboratory. 0-87969-231-6/88. $1.00 + .00

chromosomal damage in well-controlled human studies indicate the need for surveillance and/or preventive measures (Vainio et al. 1983; Perera 1987).

2. Markers have the potential to increase the power of epidemiological studies to establish causal associations between particular exposures and cancer by more precisely classifying study subjects according to their biologically effective dose, rather than their estimated environmental exposure. Reduction of misclassification error is generally seen as an important advantage of available biological markers.

3. Markers assist human cancer risk assessment by improving quantitative risk extrapolation between rodents (whose chemical dose/tumor response relationship is established in the bioassay) and a human population exposed to lower levels of the same chemical and whose cancer risks have not been ascertained epidemiologically. This is a more controversial point with disagreement centering on whether parallel laboratory animal and human molecular dosimetry data are necessary to establish that the relationship between administered dose and biologically effective dose seen in the laboratory animals holds in the human population, or whether this assumption can be made a priori. In fact, a recent attempt to utilize data on putative formaldehyde-DNA-protein cross-links in the nasal epithelium of rats as a basis for revising downward the estimated risks of formaldehyde to workers (Starr and Buck 1984) has been criticized, appropriately in my view, for the posssible lack of relevance of the experimental results to the human situation (Expert Panel Report 1986). Occupational Safety and Health Organization also rejected the modified risk assessment as too speculative (OSHA 1985). Nevertheless, there is general agreement on the validity of the parallelogram approach in risk assessment, when it is supported by comparable human and animal data (Sobels 1981).

Despite this broad promise, no parallel human and laboratory studies of the same chemical exposure have been carried out and most human applications have involved small numbers of subjects with inadequately characterized exposures (for review see Perera 1987). Only a few molecular epidemiology studies have been conducted in which a hypothesis is tested regarding the causative role of an environmental exposure or agent. These investigations have incorporated biological markers into ecological or analytical epidemiological studies. For example, in an ecological study, excised aflatoxin-DNA adducts in urine were moderately correlated with liver cancer incidence rates for one ethnic group (Autrup et al. 1987). In another study, we are evaluating levels of polycyclic aromatic hydrocarbon-DNA (PAH-DNA) adducts in peripheral blood cells from lung cancer patients compared to controls (orthopedic patients without cancer), when age and cigarette smoking (a major source of PAHs) are adjusted for (Perera et al. 1988). The hypothesis tested is that the ability to activate and bind carcinogens such as PAHs may be a risk factor in lung cancer. In a related study, we are evaluating evidence of oncogene activation in lung tumor tissue from lung cancer cases studied and autopsy controls.

Although research is becoming more sophisticated in terms of laboratory methodology and study design, the biological markers are still somewhat crude indicators of molecular dose. For example, antibodies used in immunoassays to detect carcinogen-DNA adducts may cross-react with a number of structurally related compounds (as in the case of the antibody, produced in response to the benzo[a]pyrene-diol epoxide adduct, that recognizes a number of other PAHs). In addition, immunoassays provide a summation of all DNA adducts, rather than those at the critical site(s) on DNA. Moreover, markers are lacking to detect human exposures to nongenotoxic carcinogens such as promoters.

DISCUSSION

What implications can be drawn from human dosimetry data accumulated thus far? Taking the body of carcinogen-DNA and carcinogen-protein adduct data generated thus far in human studies as an example, three major implications emerge for risk assessment and research.

1. These measures should be interpreted as indicating potential risk of cancer on the group rather than the individual level. This is dictated by the lack of data on quantitative relationships to risk and by the observed overlap in levels of markers between "exposed" and "unexposed" groups (Shamsuddin et al. 1985; Perera et al. 1987).
2. There is substantial variability between individuals with comparable exposure. For example, in smokers of 1–2 packs per day, PAH-DNA adduct levels ranged from nondetectable to 0.5 fmole/μg of DNA, whereas 4-aminobiphenyl-hemoglobin (4-ABP-Hb) adducts in the same subjects ranged from 75–256 pg/g (Perera et al. 1987). Even in patients treated with the same cumulative dose of the chemotherapy agent cisplatinum (400 mg/m^2), cisplatinum-DNA levels varied from nondetectable to 0.18 fmole/μg (Reed et al. 1986).
3. There is a substantial background of adducts in so-called unexposed control groups. This has been reported by a number of investigators using various methods: immunoassays to PAH-DNA adducts in peripheral blood cells and lung tissue; gas chromatography/map spectroscopy (GC/ MS) to quantitate 4-ABP-Hb adducts; and the ^{32}P-postlabeling method to study DNA adducts related to environmental mixtures (IARC 1987; Perera 1988a; Poirier and Beland 1987).

4. Most experimental data on adduct formation suggest that these mac-romolecular effects at low administered doses generally follow first order kinetics: the degree of binding is usually proportional to administered dose (for review, see Perera 1988a,b). In humans, dose-response data are limited, but for ethylene oxide and propylene oxide a linear relationship was seen between carcinogen-hemoglobin adducts and estimated exposure (Calleman et al. 1978; Wright 1983). Human data on PAH and 4-ABP-Hb do not suggest a threshold.

Based upon the above brief review, important research initiatives include the following:

1. Parallel molecular dosimetry studies in laboratory animals and humans to investigate the persistence of adducts, the relationship of levels of markers in target versus surrogate tissue, and the adduct levels in various cell types (e.g., Clara cells of the lung or T-cell lymphocytes).
2. The use of combinations or batteries of markers, as well as confirmatory methods for the same end point (e.g., immunoassays and GC/MS to quantitate carcinogen-protein and carcinogen-DNA adducts).
3. Well-designed studies of model human populations: patients treated with chemotherapy agents which are themselves mutagenic/carcinogenic; workers with well-defined exposures to chemicals such as ethylene oxide, styrene, PAHs, vinyl chloride, butadiene, and to hazardous waste; and cancer patients compared with controls. Essential components in these investigations are adequate sample size, appropriate controls, control of potential confounding variables and detailed characterization of exposure using questionnaires, medical and employment records, and actual monitoring data. An optimal design that would explore the quantitative relationship between markers and cancer risk is the nested case control study in which biological samples are collected and stored at the start of a prospective study and are assayed at the end of the study to determine whether markers are elevated in cases compared with controls. This research should make an important contribution to the validation of biological markers in molecular epidemiology and risk assessment.

REFERENCES

Autrup, H., T. Seremet, J. Wakhisi, and A. Wasunna. 1987. Aflatoxin exposure measured by urinary excretion of aflatoxin B_1-guanine adduct and hepatitis B virus infection in areas with different liver cancer incidence in Kenya. *Cancer Res.* **47:** 3430.

Calleman, C.J., L. Ehrenberg, B. Jansson, S. Osterman-Golkar, D. Segerback, K. Svensson, and C.A. Wachtmeister. 1978. Monitoring and risk assessment by means of alkyl groups in hemoglobin in persons occupationally exposed to ethylene oxide. *J. Environ. Pathol. Toxicol.* **2:** 427.

Expert Panel Report. 1986. Expert review of pharmacokinetic data. In *Formaldehyde, final evaluation report* (prepared under program no. 1415 for work assignment no. 7, contract no. 68-02-4228, January 2, 1986). U.S. Environmental Protection Agency, Washington, D.C.

IARC. 1987. Detection methods for DNA-damaging agents in man: Application in cancer epidemiology and prevention. *IARC Publ.* (in press).

OSHA. 1985. Occupational exposure to formaldehyde. *Fed. Reg.* **50:** 50412.

Perera, F. 1987. Molecular cancer epidemiology: A new tool in cancer prevention. *J. Natl. Cancer Inst.* **78:** 887.

————.1988a. The significance of DNA and protein adducts in human biomonitoring studies. *Mutat. Res.* (in press).

————. 1988b. Biological markers in risk assessment. In *Carcinogen risk assessment* (ed. C.C. Travis), p. 123. Plenum Press, New York.

Perera, F.P., R.M. Santella, D. Brenner, T.-L. Young, and I.B.W. Weinstein. 1988. Application of biological markers to the study of lung cancer causation and prevention. *IARC Sci. Publ.* (in press).

Perera, F., R.M. Santella, D. Brenner, M.C. Poirier, H.K. Fischman, and J. Van Ryzin. 1987. DNA adducts, protein adducts and SCEs in cigarette smokers and nonsmokers. *J. Natl. Cancer Inst.* **79:** 449.

Poirier, M.C. and F.A. Beland. 1987. Determination of carcinogen-induced macromolecular adducts in animals and humans. *Prog. Exp. Tumor Res.* **31:** 1.

Reed, E., S.H. Yuspa, L.A. Zwelling, R.F. Ozols, and M.C. Poirier. 1986. Quantitation of *cis*-diamminedichloroplatinum II (cis-platin)-DNA-intrastrand adducts in testicular and ovarian cancer patients receiving cisplatin chemotherapy. *J. Clin. Invest.* **77:** 545.

Shamsuddin, A.K.M., N.T. Sinopoli, K. Hemminki, R.R. Boesch, and C.C. Harris. 1985. Detection of benzo(a)pyrene-DNA adducts in human white blood cells. *Cancer Res.* **45:** 66.

Sobels, F.H. 1981. The parallelogram: An indirect approach for the risk assessment of genetic risks from chemical mutagens. *Prog. Mutat. Res.* **3:** 323.

Starr, T.B. and R.D. Buck. 1984. The importance of delivered dose in estimating low-dose cancer risk from inhalation exposure to formaldehyde. *Fundam. Appl. Toxicol.* **4:** 740.

Vainio, H., M. Sorsa, and K. Hemminki. 1983. Biological monitoring in surveillance of exposure to genotoxicants. *Am. J. Ind. Med.* **4:** 87.

Wright, A.S. 1983. Molecular dosimetry techniques in human risk assessment: An industrial perspective. In *Developments in the science and practice of toxicology* (ed. A.W. Hayes et al.), p. 311. Elsevier, Amsterdam.

COMMENTS

Weber: I don't know if you know of the study done in Germany by Walther et al., where they actually phenotyped people for their acetylating capacity.

Perera: Yes.

Weber: Then you know the story. I won't go on, except to say that hemoglobin adducts were measured. Unfortunately, they didn't do any DNA determinations. It turns out that the slow acetylators were the ones that developed the adducts and, even under conditions of accidental exposure, the rapid acetylators didn't have a problem. So, there is apparently a very wide difference in sensitivity, at least on that measure. I agree, that your emphasis on the "promising tool" is a reasonable one to make.

Michejda: There is an interesting parallelism in the thought that the protein adducts and the DNA and RNA adducts were parallel. I wonder, do you think that is a general phenomenon?

Perera: Generally speaking, yes. The rationale for using hemoglobin as a surrogate is that it is so much more readily available.

Michejda: For one thing, you've got at least an order of magnitude more adducts with which to deal.

Perera: Exactly.

Michejda: Secondly, what is the meaning of measuring O^6 alkyl adducts in cancer patients? The fact of the matter is, these adducts are repaired extremely rapidly, and, even if they're not, you don't know what the rate of repair is but only that repair is occurring. It may be entirely fortuitous that you see anything. Those are difficult measurements to make.

Guengerich: Umbenhauer did actually measure rates of repair.

Perera: They concluded that the differences were not attributable to interindividual variation in activity of repair enzymes.

Michejda: For O^6 methyl?

Perera: They attributed it to some other factors that influenced the formation of adducts in these people.

Guengerich: Or the amount of nitrosamine ingested.

Michejda: Unless there is no repair, O^6 methyl residues are repaired with a half-life of about 48 hours?

Guengerich: Less than that.

Singer: It depends on the dose, but it has been measured down to a few seconds.

Michejda: Yes, but the cancer patients aren't going to be ingesting nitrosamine sources anymore, presumably.

Beland: The point of the paper was that they were assuming that the exposure in the cancer patient in China was the same as it had been throughout an entire lifespan. What I think they were saying is that the Chinese had a higher exposure to nitrosamines, and that was the reason they were getting tumors.

Perera: I think that's correct.

Panel Discussion

RONALD W. HART
National Center for Toxicological Research, Arkansas

ROBERT A. NEAL
Chemical Industry Institute of Toxicology, North Carolina

WILLIAM FARLAND
U.S. Environmental Protection Agency, Washington, D.C.

PAUL F. DEISLER, JR.
University of Houston, Texas

A. KARIM AHMED
Natural Resources Defense Council, New York

MARY F. LOWE
U.S. Food and Drug Administration, Maryland

Hoerger: Let's have Ron Hart continue the discussion.

Hart: I resisted the tremendous temptation to talk about the research interests I have pursued for a number of years in DNA damage and repair and its role as a biomarker, because Frederica (Perera) covered it so elegantly in the previous presentation. Hence, I would support that area as an important research field.

It is extremely important because, not only does it give you the possibility of a high-dose to low-dose extrapolation, it gives the possibility of a common denominator for comparing interspecies variations and differences, and, thirdly, it gives you the possibility of looking at the role of modulatory factors, such as sex, age, diet, and so forth. One would hope that if it was truly a biomarker for a given toxicological end point, as those conditions change or alter and alter the end point, that factor would also be reflective of those changes, for example, diet modulating that biomarker and, hence, the end point.

A second area that is going to be terribly important, one that I really did not appreciate fully prior to this conference, is the concept of gap junctions. To me, they were just funny little marks on an EM plate. I, of course, was raised in the environment pre-Setlow, that nothing important was outside the nucleus. Almost by definition, a gap junction is outside the nucleus, although I do believe they connect by some indirect pathway back to the nucleus and the DNA.

However, that entire area of alternate carcinogens, secondary carcinogens, promoters, cocarcinogens, enhancers, and all the other names

names that we have developed for these agents that do not appear directly to damage DNA, is becoming quite a problem for us. It is becoming a problem in regulatory agencies, it is becoming a problem in testing and screening, and it is becoming a public health problem.

It is becoming a public health problem because we don't know how to evaluate it. When you don't know how to evaluate something, you can't give any data; all you can give is speculation. That causes concern in a society such as ours.

I don't know whether or not what Jim (Trosko) has proposed will work, but I certainly do believe it is one alternative that is worth pursuing, and it is one that allows us to quantitate and test certain results and compounds to see if it is or is not predictive.

With the machine (the device that has been made up at Michigan State) and the baseline data that Trosko and others have put together, it would seem that that type of an approach would be amenable for a more definitive analysis of analogs of those substances that are not active in inducing the end effect.

A third area, which was touched upon by Kenneth Crump and by other individuals at the conference but was not discussed in detail by people within that particular area of expertise, is the role of cellular proliferation. I think it really goes beyond cellular proliferation. It goes to the idea of DNA replication and polyploid development, those functions that alter the state of the genetic material or cell in such a way that may actually lead to a higher probability of expression of a given end point.

Cells which do not divide are resistant to radiation. We have known that since 1916 or 1917. Cells that do not have a division potential tend to be less susceptible to spontaneous tumor occurrence. We all know that from our classical pathology. Yet, it has only been relatively recently that proliferation has started to be factored into many of our mathematical models.

That is a terribly important end point that requires us to do a better job. Curtis Travis mentioned this in his presentation. Proliferation is something we have tended to ignore. In fact, even though we have a great deal of biological data on it and it is now starting to be factored into some of our predictive models, I think proliferation is something on which we have now got to do quantitative research. That is a relatively easy thing to do because we have some very elegant cell-sorting machines available now that allow us to quickly analyze proliferation changes and differences in vivo as well as in vitro.

The fourth and final area is the role of modulatory factors. An example is Bea Singer's very short discussion of alcohol. That is certainly a major modulatory factor. As Betsy (Weisburger) pointed out, 7–8% of human cancers have been associated with alcohol. It is a major factor. It is a carcinogen at the very least and, perhaps, a modulatory factor as well.

Regarding diet, if you go through the literature of the last few years and you look at the role of diet on the ability of chemical compounds to induce cancer (Pariza, Newberne, and several others) you find a tremendous impact of minor modifications, such as 16% reduction in calories, on the ability of compounds to induce cancer. Even if you look at spontaneous tumor occurrence in various populations worldwide, you will find that diet also plays a major role on what types of cancer are induced and the occurrence of risk. This has been brought more to our attention in the last four to five years by people like Bruce Ames, even though, again, the classical animal physiological data and human experimentational data from the 1920s, 1930s, or 1940s were out there. However, it has been ignored as not the in-vogue field of science. Nutrition has not been in vogue for some time, but it is extremely important as an end point.

Other factors that appear to be terribly important are all the other modulatory factors because they do add a certain degree of uncertainty, and humans do tend to have a high degree of heterogeneity in their actions. I would say that, certainly, those are four broad categories of research, all four of which have been directly or indirectly touched upon at this conference.

I was somewhat delighted to see that we did not get into a debate, at least not too much of a debate, about male versus female mouse tumors. We have had several conferences on that over the years, as well as certain other topics that have normally been the mainstays as issues of burning importance. They are issues of importance. It's just that they have already been discussed extensively.

My concluding point is that this was a high-risk conference, as Jan (Witkowski) pointed out. It was a high-risk conference because, normally, conferences where you get a great diversity of talent, opinions, and backgrounds together, either are terribly successful or fall on their face. The probabilities are higher that they are going to fall on their face because everyone may be bored with everyone else. I think the interactions and discussions that have occurred indicate a great success, and I think most of the people here would concur.

However, I do believe that we have another thing that we must accomplish. Now that the ice has been broken between some of our most elegant basic research scientists and our regulators, policymakers, and our biostatisticians interacting with one another, these interfunctional discussions must be continued on more focused areas. What about the assumption of the interdependency of diet? What about the assumption of all routes of administration are equal in the absence of data to the contrary as long as the same total dose is maintained? What about single versus intermittent versus continuous dosing as long as the same total dose is maintained? These are things which are ripe for research. They are also ripe for further discussion and evaluation by interdisciplinary panels, groups, or workshops, that can then focus in on how one might address these issues in a more reasonable fashion. I hope that this will also be a result coming out of this conference.

Willy (Lijinsky) made a very cogent point earlier. Maybe we really do owe it to the taxpayers, who are paying our salaries and have paid for our research over the years, to address some of these issues. They are really not bad science. As a molecular biologist who turned risk assessor who turned policy person, I thought that was the true key of success of the conference, and I thank Willy for it.

Clayson: I was delighted to hear you mention the importance of cellular proliferation. I would like to add two facts that are new. The first one is that Martin Lipkin at Sloan Kettering in New York has stated in a paper that, as far as human colonic cancer is concerned, the rate of cellular proliferation in crypt cells may well be a biomarker. The second one concerns a piece of work which we have done in Canada, where we have looked at total dietary restriction. We do find that that has a marked effect on cellular proliferation in several tissues. I think these are pointers to the importance of what you said.

Hart: That's interesting. Where are you going to come out with the latter study?

Clayson: The latter study is in press. I would say we should be out in *Cancer Letters* in four months.

Trosko: Let me just follow up on what Dave (Clayson) said to points two, three, and four; namely, those zits that you referred to, the gap junctions; the cellular proliferation area, which you rightly pointed out is of concern; and, the modulating factors such as diet. I am saying that those are the contributing biomarkers, if you will, of the promotion phase of carcinogenesis. There may be those here who disagree. I didn't see them as differences, but you obviously do.

Hart: James, I've always split them up.

Stevenson: You just remarked on the importance of diet. One of the things that has impressed me is the dietary factors that alter tumor incidence in mice also affect gut bacteria in the same way. For instance, the dietary restrictions and the intermittent feeding have very remarkable effects on the bacteria of the gut. I just wondered if there is some work there. Basically, my point is that I don't think we understand our laboratory animals very well.

Hart: Exactly. You're right, Don. I was tempted to include that as one of the points. I did not do so because we are very fortunate at NCTR to have Carl Cerniglia who is a terribly gifted person in that area. He has found significant differences in the gut and gut flora. When I talk about dietary modulation, it includes the concept of changes in the gastrointestinal flora.

Hoerger: We have to move on. Bob Neal is next.

$$*\qquad *\qquad *$$

Neal: I would like to remind you again of the topic of the conference, "New Directions in Qualitative and Quantitative Aspects of Cancer Risk Assessment," and I am adding in parentheses "in humans" because that is the species in which we are interested. This particular panel is to address the implications for research directors, and so I have jotted down some remarks from the point of view of a research director with limited resources and, of the variety of things that one can examine, which are the ones with the highest priority.

I think in the qualitative region there are some areas where application of resources may be beneficial in a reasonably short period of time, in allowing us to arrive at some judgments about the qualitative relationship between cancer end points in some animal models and the relevance of those end points to humans. Regarding the male rat kidney tumors which are produced by the accumulation of α_{2u}-globulin in the kidney, there is reasonable evidence that these tumors may not be relevant to humans, but it is an area that is going to require additional study with additional compounds to establish this hypothesis with greater certainty.

I think some sets of rodent liver tumors, particularly those that are caused by the peroxisomal proliferators, which is a very important group of compounds, may lend itself to an understanding of the mechanism by which those compounds are producing rodent liver tumors, and with comparative studies, tumors in humans. Studies in humans are essential. The only way we are going to bridge between animal and human data is to do studies in exposed human populations or in human tissues if exposed human populations aren't available.

Another area is the mouse lymphoma. The concept exists that lymphoma in mice may result from a combination of the effect of a chemical and certain ectropic virus sequences that are inherent in murine species, rather than the chemical alone. I think that is something important. It may also be important relative to humans because of our increased understanding of the existence of a human thymic leukemia virus. This is a straightforward representation of the role of virus in human cancer. Does exposure to chemicals at certain levels predispose one to virus-induced cancer? I think that is an area that deserves additional attention.

Rat mammary tumors is perhaps another area that could lend itself to some information that would be useful in assessing the relevance of those end points to humans.

In the quantitative area, I am going to repeat largely what Frederica (Perera) and Ron (Hart) have said. I think the key to understanding low-dose cancer relationships is going to be based largely on a better understanding of the mechanism by which the chemical causes the carcinogenic effect and then using that information to devise measurements that are more sensitive than tumors as end points. To verify estimates of low-dose response, I think we have to identify preneoplastic biochemical changes that are more sensitive than tumors, that occur perhaps more frequently, and that we can measure easily. All of these lesions will not progress to tumors, but they have the potential to do so, and I think those are the kinds of measurements we are going to have to come up with if we are going to put low-dose risk extrapolation on a more scientific basis.

The human biomarkers that Frederica (Perera) mentioned are critical. I think we need to identify the biomarkers in experimental animals, understand what they mean relative to the production of cancer, and then go to human populations and look for them as well.

Cell proliferation rates are critical. I think, when this chapter is finally written, it may indicate that cell proliferation is as important a factor as initiation in cancer, and that the initiated cells may not express themselves unless there is a strong proliferative stimulus as well.

The target site dose is, of course, an important measurement as well. As an aside, there was some suggestion earlier that the target-site dose cannot be used unless there is a specific structure knowledge of the adduct. I think that is not true. I think you have to look carefully at what we are trying to do with target-site dose information. We are, in most cases, trying to look at the concentration of a particular carcinogen or its carcinogenic metabolite in the target site that is bound to DNA. In some cases, it is not going to be possible to actually determine what this adduct is because of instability and other factors. It is important to remember that, even if you can measure a specific promutagenic lesion in a genome, there are going to be thousands or tens of thousands of them, but it only is a rare event when that particular promutagenic lesion leads to the production of a cancer. So, you are measuring all of these adducts, but most of them have no relevance to the neoplastic process, and all you are measuring is an event that gives you a sort of a functional measure of the potential of hitting that one rare target and starting the neoplastic event. In measurements of initiating carcinogens bound to DNA, if you cannot measure the promutagenic adducts, remembering that it's difficult to define which are the promutagenic adducts, I think that one can use target site dose in a more general sense than knowledge of specific adducts in improving our ability to estimate low-dose risk.

We have to be careful not to oversell what we are doing to try to improve qualitative and quantitative risk assessment. In our frustration with the current risk assessment process, which is at best marginally scientific, we should not fall into the same trap and propose that particular data show that it is not relevant to humans if you cannot mount a substantial and compelling body of data to suggest that is the case. If we too often make those kinds of statements and the data really do not support that point of view, we are going to bring ourselves into the same trap as the current risk assessment process finds itself. The data will be considered as not compelling, and the whole process of trying to improve the ability to estimate potential carcinogenic risk in humans in both the qualitative and quantitative sense may be harmed. I think we have to be careful when we say that a particular body of data indicates that a certain cancer end point is not relevant to humans. We have to have a very compelling body of data that suggests that really is the case.

One final point, and that is the physiologically based pharmacokinetic models. They have gotten quite popular, and I think rightly so. They are a valuable addition to our ability to estimate low-dose responses. However, let me caution that we should not get enamored with them to the exclusion of other approaches. Why model the target site dose when, in fact, you can measure it? If I were a regulator trying to do a risk assessment on a particular compound and was faced with data that were determined by modeling or data that were determined by actual measurements, I certainly would have more faith in the actual measurements. In some cases, it is not possible to do the measurements, and we have to resort to modeling as a second choice. However, measured data means a lot more than data from models. PPK models have a role in our improvement of low-dose risk estimation, but we need to put them in proper perspective and not get so enamored with them that we adopt that methodology to the exclusion of other more relevant and more accurate measurements.

Singer: This doesn't necessarily refer to you at all, but I have listened as much as I can, trying to understand what people are saying. Nobody seems to have mentioned in any of these calculations genetic suscep-tibility. We know it exists. Is it anywhere a factor, or did I miss it?

Neal: I think the place at which it must be factored in is in this examination of biomarkers that Frederica (Perera) touched on. When we finally have a set of markers that we know mean something relative to clinical disease, I think we will be in a position to look at genetic variation and genetic susceptibility in certain populations. I think it is a critical factor, but the only way to approach it is through biomarkers in humans where you can measure preneoplastic events.

Singer: I am getting at something a little bit different than that. It isn't groups of people about which we are talking. The first question you often get asked is, "Does anybody in your family have heart disease, cancer, and so on?" They usually will have exactly the same type of tumor. However, they are just a family. They are not a large cohort of any nature. Those people know they are at risk. They don't know from what they're at risk, except that inherited susceptibility is playing a role. You inbreed mice for the same purpose. We don't do that with people. Now, should those people be in a different class from the general population? Someone asked are we trying to protect the most sensitive person, which essentially does impinge upon that subject.

Neal: Bea, I think it's a matter of identifying those classes, and the biomar-kers are a way of doing that.

Hoerger: That will apply to both classes and individuals.

Weber: Just a follow-up. I'm glad that Bea (Singer) brought up the subject. It is an important point. However, apart from the biomarker side, there is the effect of capacity to metabolize things at different rates, which shows up in pharmacokinetics. As I have sat here and listened, I wondered about why no one has mentioned genetic susceptibility ex-plicitly. I said to myself that it's in the pharmacokinetics, and you're talking about effect on pharmacokinetics. I'm just sorry that nobody has acknowledged it.

Neal: I think the comparative studies in humans and experimental animals are going to have to take those kinds of differences into account.

Weber: It's clear that there are certain traits that have an effect.

Ahmed: Ron (Hart) mentioned earlier that no one talked about mouse liver tumors, so I'm not sure whether I should open this up for discussion. You mentioned peroxisomal formation in liver. Could you tell us, Bob, some of your own feelings about peroxisomal proliferation?

Neal: I'll do it in a couple of sentences. The peroxisomal proliferation seems to be at least phenomenologically related to the tumor production, but the degree of peroxisomal proliferation does not seem to be related to the tumor incidence. What seems to be more related is the degree of oxidation that takes place in the tissue. That seems to be more related to the carcinogenic potency.

Ahmed: Is there a sex difference between male and female mice in terms of peroxisomal proliferation?

Neal: I'm not aware that there is.

Ahmed: Yet, their tumor rates are much different.

Michejda: There is no generality in this. There are some that are. Willy (Lijinsky) has some very interesting data in that regard, on peroxisomal proliferators and cancer.

Lijinsky: Not really peroxisomal.

Michejda: And also, mitochondrial proliferation.

Lijinsky: They don't show a sex difference.

Hoerger: I think we better move on. Earlier, we heard a lot about EPA and their approaches. I think it is time that we give Bill Farland a chance to give his views here. He has been very patient.

*   *   *

Farland: I am going to keep my remarks short, given that the previous speakers have covered a lot of ground that certainly applies to the types of things that I would want to say on behalf of a research director from EPA. We are talking in this conference about new directions in risk assessment and the implications on research. I guess I look at that in two ways.

First, there are very practical implications for me, as a director of research, the practical implications being that I am asked to get ahead of the curve. I am being asked by scientists, by risk managers, by people who use the work that we do, whether we will continue to use the assumptions that people frequently give us a hard time about, and what we are doing to try and get better at what we do.

That practical consideration has sort of pushed us in the direction of trying to institute a research program that is very much the second step about which Cathy St. Hilaire was talking: Having identified the areas that will help to reduce uncertainties in risk assessment, where do you focus the first barrage, where do you first get into the research, and on what types of things do you try and focus?

Two years ago, we started a program internally in my group to try and address some specific questions. We addressed some of these questions as essentially research scientists initiating proposals within our own group that was funded through contracts, cooperative agreements, and interagency agreements. That was a fairly small start, but we felt like we were going in the right kind of direction.

Some of you may be aware that this has taken on a much larger implication for the Agency. In budget discussions this past year, we had a situation where the House giveth and the House taketh away. The House decided that they were going to reduce the overall research and development budget in the EPA by $10 million. With a stroke of the pen, they established a program of $10 million in reducing uncertainties in risk assessment. At the point where that becomes part of the budget, our program becomes directed that way.

Needless to say, we began a scramble to determine how we were going to approach this and what type of a plan we were going to provide, so that we could deal with this directed funding, and deal with it in a way that would be saleable to our scientific supporters and also saleable to our funding supporters.

In terms of the scientific issues, there is a purpose behind our pushing in terms of what subjects on which we are going to actually work over the next couple of years. As I said, this is something on which we wanted a little bit of a start. We also have some information that we can build into our decisions as to the areas on which we are going to focus.

First, there are things that we have talked about for a long time within the Agency, a long time within our interagency groups, with our industrial colleagues, with our basic science colleagues. These are the areas that we feel are going to be most important for us to take a look at. I am not going to run through them. Suffice it to say that, among all of the things that we have wanted to take a look at, there are probably four areas that we think are particularly important right now.

One area is exposure. That is something that has not been talked about a lot here. When you start getting into exposure and reducing uncertainty in exposure, one thing that we have found is that you have to deal with exposure scenarios and try to use those scenarios to predict exposures to humans. What we don't know much about is the effect of human activity patterns on exposure. How do you build the way a human lives into a reasonable scenario of exposure to environmental chemicals? That is one of the important areas for us to take a look at.

The reason that I think it is particularly important is that, if we apply models to estimate exposure, that essentially gives us a maximally exposed individual at a fenceline. That person is expected to have lived at that fenceline for the last 40 years and to have spent all his time sitting on his front porch. We are not really providing the type of exposure scenario that is going to be useful to us, especially when we have to deal with essentially an upper bound estimate of the risk. So, that is one area on which we are concentrating. We have found that the development of these exposure scenarios with much better estimates of human activity patterns built into them may very well help to reduce some of the uncertainty in our exposure assessment.

The second one is physiologically based pharmacokinetic models, and I couldn't agree more with Bob Neal. If I can measure something to determine whether a total metabolite is going to be at a particular level in order to be built into my risk assessment, I couldn't agree more that that is the way that I should do it. However, my ability to do that is limited.

So, what I am faced with is modeling things that I can't measure, developing parameters that help me do the comparative physiology between the experimental animals, for which we have end point data, and the human, and collecting as much data as I can on important parameters to make that model as realistic as possible. We are looking at the parameters that are used, and how we do a sensitivity analysis on the model that we use. Then we can actually select data to build into the model.

The third area is in biologically based dose-response models. I am not going to go into that. We have heard a lot about that here. The promising areas there appear to be proliferation, a surrogate measure for what we have long termed initiation of cells, and, hopefully, some sort of an understanding of implications of what we now call promotion and progression of this process. We have heard some very interesting things at this conference as to where we might go with that.

The fourth area is probably one of the most important ones from the perspective of the development of a longer term research program for reducing uncertainties in risk assessment. The real application of sensitivity analysis, the application of techniques that have been used in a number of other fields, is to determine the areas that contribute the most to the uncertainty in the risk assessment. Therefore, that's a direction where additional resources should be focused.

We have a number of people in this field that are very interested in applications to health risk assessment, particularly cancer risk assessment. We have seen some very promising approaches. We think this is going to be an area that is going to be immediately applicable to our program of understanding where the major uncertainties lie and communicating that to our risk managers and to the public.

I don't have anything else to say with regard to the directions for research. I would just like to express my thanks to the organizers. I think that this was a tremendous opportunity for me, immersed in this sort of thing, to be in a position to interact with the basic science community and to look at some very specific areas. These are exactly the areas in which I am particularly interested. I think we have all had an opportunity to learn and grow in this conference. Thank you.

Hoerger: Thanks, Bill. We appreciate your comments.

Tennant: One thing that concerns me a bit is, in terms of the issue of the dose-response model, if we are dealing with an increasing number of substances that don't adduct, that generate specific biomarkers, and whose effects are the product of prolonged exposures, then I think we have to think fundamentally in terms of concentration-over-time responses. That involves a fundamentally different approach to modeling. We have been driven by the mutagen/adduct/direct interaction phenomenon that grew out of virtually everything that had been done previously in radiation biology, but there is a class of substances that is probably fundamentally different and is going to require fundamentally different concepts to evaluate.

Farland: I think that you're right, and building the biology into the models is going to be very difficult. Statistically, some of those issues have been addressed. Dan Krewski briefly talked about that earlier, in terms of the sorts of differences you might expect if you had a chemical that impinged on a certain stage in a multistage process and on windows of susceptibility. How would that affect the total outcome over the course of a lifetime of an animal, and so on? There have been a number of papers published on that topic that try and estimate those differences.

In terms of actually trying to take the biology and explain tumor results, or development of foci, or those sorts of things, I would agree, we are going to have to find ways to build those results into the model to take account of them. Remember, what we do right now is to count tumors and to model those tumors statistically. We are able to modify that slightly in terms of time to tumor analysis and some of those other things, but at this point that is the only piece of biology that we build into that particular model, other than assumptions that go into the mathematics that make up the model.

Kraemer: This is along the lines of what Dr. Singer and Dr. Hart had mentioned with DNA repair. In looking for new directions for research, particularly with regard to humans, there are presently identified certain populations at high risk of cancer that we have a feeling may be also at greater risk for environmental carcinogens, such as patients with a disease like xeroderma or ataxia telangiectasia. They are rather rare. However, carriers of these autosomal recessive diseases, heterozygotes, are much more frequent in the population. They may represent several percent of the population.

There is a paper by Michael Swit in the May *New England Journal* showing increased risk of breast and other cancers, particularly breast cancer, in family members of patients with ataxia telangiectasia. The heterozygote carriers presumably are at increased risk. There is no indication of what the mechanism of this increased breast cancer development is in these patients. For instance, in measuring certain adducts, if you had a theory as to why their development occurs, these would be the people to look for first. They are at greater risk. They could be considered a sentinel population of human data that is just sitting there waiting to be explored.

Wilson: Newson has said the same thing.

*   *   *

Hoerger: I would like to thank all of the speakers on the panel. They did an excellent job and have underscored a number of directions for research emphasis. We will now hear from three other distinguished speakers. May I introduce Paul Deisler.

Deisler: I will be fairly brief. First, I would like to comment on the meeting itself. I am not a life scientist. I am a chemical engineer, a physical chemist with a wrench. This meeting, frankly, has been a truly broadening experience. The diversity of viewpoints and the gaps between the backgrounds of the people attending have made for a very interesting meeting.

I also appreciated the fact that some of our speakers, Jim Trosko, John Graham, and others indulged in what I would call "constructive iconoclasm." Taking a look at things from a different perspective and challenging some of our conventional thinking is extremely useful. I think we have all felt that there is a tremendous ferment going on in an attempt to bring a little more science into quantitative risk analysis in some logical, reasonable, and hopefully scientifically based way.

My first recommendation is this. The first EPA Guidelines on carcinogens came out in 1976. A decade later, we had the current Guidelines. That's an awfully long time between Guidelines. A lot happened in that period, although not that the first Guidelines were all that bad. They are not as specific as the current ones, but they still make good sense. However, in terms of the accelerating accumulation of knowledge, of understanding the mechanisms, and of the methods of expressing some of those mechanisms in useful quantitative forms, I think that ten more years is way too long.

So, my first recommendation is that the Guidelines should be a living document, not a monument set in stone. There should be a deliberate effort, almost a policy, if you wish, to reexamine them in the light of new science and of experience in using the Guidelines. Change, modification, and additions should be considered. That's a rather simple, but I feel a fundamental, recommendation. It wouldn't surprise me if modifications appeared in the *Federal Register* yearly from now on.

A second very important point is to stress the need for examining and understanding the qualitative observations and factors involved in assessing risk before attempting to quantify risk, and not only for relevance to humans. I think the nonleaded gasoline case is a good example. There was a case, if I may digress for just a moment, where we had excellent dose-response data from a well-conceived, well-carried-out experiment. At the lowest dose level, which was 6–7 ppm, there was roughly a 5% excess response of kidney carcinoma. When you compared just that crude information with the fact that a full-time service station attendant was exposed to somewhere in the 7–8 ppm level, it was too close for comfort. The automatic, traditional calculation of risk verified that, not surprisingly.

It was only because some literature indicated that the male rat might be unique that further work was done. The Science Advisory Board's view was to wait before really applying the male rat data. It was possible to decide what identifying experiments to do next and then to get the CIIT to do some very fundamental work. We finally came to the conclusion that the male rat was unique and that it was not a model for people. There are other reasons for regulating gasoline, such as coming into conformity with the National Ambient Air Quality Standards, but the bioassay result was not one of them. This may be a rare case, but it illustrates the worthwhileness of first looking at qualitative information.

Qualitative analysis of factors could and should also be used in considering alternative models. Are there factors that say this kind of mechanism or that type of model, perhaps modifying the existing multi-stage model, would give a directionally better result? Another area in which I think it can be important is when you have decided that you have a model and you now estimate the risk for the 70 kg rat or 70 kg mouse. Perhaps one could make arguments saying, "Well, I would expect the human, because of the factors we have talked about, to be either more sensitive or less sensitive," and get some idea of where the risk might truly lie.

Finally, I think that a careful examination of the qualitative information, starting at the very beginning of the process in hazard identification, can be very useful in recommending what experiments might be done to assist in the risk analysis. Too often, one thinks that one has to just take the data that are available and do a "risk analysis." Historically, it frequently takes a long time to go from the initial impetus to eventual regulation. Had you thought about what experiments you could do, as in the case of nonleaded gasoline, you might have actually gotten them done in time to influence your decision one way or another.

So, my third recommendation then is this: Frequently there is time to do additional work, and one should not ignore the possibility of some such work of a critical nature in the course of doing a risk analysis. Why not put that into the Guidelines?

The fourth recommendation is that the Guidelines should indicate that any model is simply a simulation, to use an engineering term. It ain't how it really happens. The better the simulation, perhaps, the better your risk estimate is.

If you go back to the original paper by Doll and Armitage some 30-plus years ago in which they first discussed the multistage nature of the carcinogenic process, among the things they discussed very clearly is that the coefficients attendant upon each stage differ from person to person, from animal to animal, and from time to time. Yet, of course, even in applying that model to say they are constants and then fit for them is all we can do, but it's a simulation to that extent. Conceivably, if we knew how to deal with those individual constants, we could build some of the anticarcinogenic effects into that model, or we could do it otherwise.

We have heard at this meeting Dan Krewski and Todd Thorslund speak about alternative ways of modeling carcinogenesis. The one that Todd Thorslund talked about yesterday was a very nice exposition of what you might call the kinetics of cell transformation. One would want to add to that some of the kinds of things that Hoel, Kaplan, and Anderson dealt with in thinking about the kinetics of metabolism to activate or inactive molecules (or detoxification) for more complicated cases.

There are many other models being developed nowadays, some of which I am sure you are all aware. The model we heard about yesterday is basically a kinetic model.

There is another one that is being developed that we didn't talk about, what I would call a "descriptive simulation," and that is the one that Bob Sielken is working on that has a lot of interesting properties. It compiles a number of things and describes general classes of activity without always getting into the mechanism. That has real practical utility. I might mention, by the way, that this model has one interesting feature, which has been brought up here. That is, that you can formally calculate from the model the most susceptible 5% or the most susceptible 10% of the population, etc. Whether it is a true calculation remains to be seen, but it can formally be done.

The next recommendation I would make is to give positive encouragement in the Guidelines to examining the possibility of more applicable simulations and models than is now done. In other words, by default, one might use the multistage, but first look at the other possibilities. What is done now, of course, is what I call negative encouragement. In effect, you use the multistage model unless you prove that something different is better. You might say, "Well, is this the difference between a glass that is half full of water and one that is half empty?" The answer is no, because that is the difference between an optimist and a pessimist. Attitudes make a lot of difference in what you do and how you do it.

John Graham mentioned judgment. One would hope that in future editions of the Guidelines, making stronger allowance for scientific judgment in the model will be encouraged. When you look at a risk assessment, you are not looking at a nice, neat theorem with a QED at the bottom. You are looking at something like a mosaic that has been dug up from some ancient ruin. You have a piece here and four pieces there and some others, and you think you have the outline of an animal, but you're not sure. You fill in the blanks as best you can. Some of those blanks must be filled in with scientific judgment.

If you don't allow for that sort of judgment, then the temptation on the regulator's part must be to do the arithmetic and to deal with toxic substances as though you were dealing with income tax: Here's the form, the 1040, fill it out, there's the final number. I don't think the regulators really want to do that. I don't think that risk analysis should be an automatic calculation like the Internal Revenue Service uses in its activities.

I also hope that in the future no court will really have cause to say, as they apparently did in the recent vinyl chloride case, that they would characterize the current risk assessment process as reaching decisions by the rules of arithmetic rather than of knowledge. I really hope we can do a little better than that. I think keeping the Guidelines alive is one way to help move in that direction.

Hoerger: Thank you, Paul. Let's go ahead with Karim Ahmed, coming from a slightly different perspective perhaps.

*   *   *

Ahmed: One way of looking at cancer risk assessment is to see what has happened in this field, i.e., how we were doing it before in the mid-1970s, and how we are doing it today, and to ask why we are doing it differently today, and why we want to move to a different plateau.

Another way of looking at it is to see how the debate on risk assessment occurred in the late 1960s and 1970s, say on pesticides, when the newly formed EPA took steps to cancel registration of some pesticides. At that time, I think the only way we were doing cancer risk assessment was based upon our knowledge of radiation biology–we used a one-hit or a simple linear model. Most of our judgment was based on qualitative assessment of risk. The question, which is embedded in the Delaney Clause of the Food, Drug and Cosmetic Act, was whether we knew from the toxicologists that a substance, particularly if you had animal data and not human data, caused cancer and whether you believed that it could be a potential carcinogen.

Once you were able to establish that a substance was an animal carcinogen, then you were left in a quandary. If you had the Delaney Clause, then you obviously had a policy tool. You could say, "Okay, this is a bad product, this goes off the market." On the other hand, if you had to regulate a compound under a different statutory provision, where you had to do benefit-risk analysis, then you really didn't have any guidance as to how to proceed.

Thus, at that time, we were basically dealing with qualitative approaches. Then began the period when we started to do some semiquantitative work. The Mantel-Bryan model, I guess, was the first to bring about some kind of quantification and a different approach than the simple linear radiation biology approach.

The uncertainties we had at the time of the 1950s and 1960s led to the adoption of the Delaney Clause. The reason why we have the Delaney Clause today is because at that time no one believed we could really develop any kind of a model that considered either threshold or non-threshold effects. Because you did not have a basis for deriving any quantitative hold on risk, you basically said, "A carcinogen is a carcinogen and, therefore, it should be off the market."

What happened after the 1970s, I think, since the environmental movement and public health concerns became stronger, was a move away from what I call the simple approach of risk assessment to today's more complex approach. Two things happened.

One was that we developed better methodologies, both in terms of modeling, but, more importantly, our data base started to improve. Remember the time when there was a big scandal about development of a data base from a testing laboratory that led to a concern about a number of commercial pesticides on the market? That led to the development of the Good Laboratory Practices regulation.

Also at that time, a number of people in the toxicological field decided to develop better protocols, i.e., standardized protocols. The agencies developed better testing Guidelines. The FDA, the EPA, and other regulatory agencies provided better guidance as to the kind of data that should be submitted by a manufacturer before a product could be registered or approved. So, we were improving our methods of analysis and we were developing a better data base. We could not have dreamed about doing any kind of pharmacokinetic modeling back in the early 1970s. There was not the data base to do that. Very few compounds even had simple metabolic data base.

Now we come to the present situation. In listening to all the discussion we've had the past few days, I am hopeful that we have come to the point where we can possibly improve our methodology in some areas, but I remain very pessimistic about some other areas which we haven't really touched on very much in our discussions. I think Betty Anderson mentioned some of them today, and I will try to focus a little bit more on them.

First of all, on quantitative risk assessment, we certainly have now developed some kind of reasonable consensus on our approach. Of course, Paul (Deisler) would like to see changes more quickly on the present EPA's Cancer Guidelines, so that other factors could also be considered. However, if you remember, Paul, it took a very long time to even develop the present Guidelines. There was a long process of building up consensus in the regulatory community to have come to this juncture. So, to suggest that we have yearly changes, unless you do it by fiat, it is not going to happen very quickly.

The linearized multistage model was accepted almost by default, if you will. Often, the multistage model and the one-hit model were essentially identical, but they sort of sugar-coated the linear approach by calling it a multistage model. In many ways, it has become the state-of-the-art approach today, so that anyone who has access to a computer can easily use it to generate risk numbers.

An area that concerns me is the approach that has been promoted by people like Richard Wilson and Bruce Ames, and that is the idea of ordering carcinogens by developing some kind of a ranking scheme. This approach raises a number of questions in terms of regulatory priorities, standard setting, etc.

The controversy here obviously lies in how to use toxicological data. Let us look at the Ames approach. What he has done is take cancer bioassay data of a number of carcinogens, derive what he calls a TD_{50} number, which is the calculated dose that produces 50% tumors. Then he takes certain exposure levels of the substance that he considers to be reliable, with which I don't necessarily agree, and then he says, "This is the relative risk to an individual if they were exposed at this level."

What is missing here, obviously, is a population risk number. If you have a compound that may pose a high intrinsic risk, but when exposure occurs to a small population of people who say drink comfrey tea or eat raw mushrooms every day, obviously you've got to be concerned. However, on the other hand, if you have a compound that has a relatively low risk but is consumed by a large population, such as trichloroethylene in drinking water, the risk becomes larger in a given community. Ames has completedly missed that aspect of risk in his ranking scheme.

Richard Wilson's system, on the other hand, does take population into account in his most recent papers. However, Wilson is very much interested in comparative risk assessment, for example, comparing the risk from dying in an automobile accident to carcinogenic risk, i.e. comparing apples and oranges.

The feeling I get from both Bruce Ames and Richard Wilson is that, if you put risk in a proper perspective, somehow cancer risks become trivialized, and therefore we shouldn't worry about them, and we can all go home and stop doing all the research work that we are supposed to be doing in the risk analysis field.

Now, the thing that has happened that is very promising in risk assessment, however, is what I call qualitative risk assessment. It is finally coming back into fashion once again, and it had been lost to the biostatistician and the quantitative risk analysis people.

When I talk about qualitative risk assessment, I mean in terms of how the IARC monograph defines it, i.e., in terms of the weight-of-evidence approach. It is also embedded in the present EPA Cancer Guidelines. That is, it takes into account what some people consider to be a bit of scientific judgment. Now, there are two ways of looking at scientific judgment. One is to think about it being something where an experienced person with a disinterested approach to the cancer data base can make judgments and come to a conclusion. The other is to sort of leave a big fudge factor somewhere, which allows you to make any kind of conclusion you wish. I try to believe that our process of making risk assessments avoids that fudge factor approach and uses the right kind of scientific judgment.

For example, because of the improved data base, we have much more data on metabolism of compounds. I'm not just talking about for purposes of pharmacokinetic modeling. We now know the difference between rodents, primates, and humans. To the extent the information is available, we can draw better conclusions as to the biological relevance, not just the statistical relevance, of the data base that one examines. This requires a judgment call in deciding whether a carcinogen is really one of higher priority concern or of lesser priority concern.

This information, unfortunately, is not easily available in the published literature. The few places I have gotten good quality metabolism data, particularly for proprietary chemicals, have come under discovery in a lawsuit or through FOIA requests, which public interest groups can obtain through the EPA. There are tons of data out there in industry. They have developed an incredible data base, but it is not readily available to the scientific community to look at. Metabolic pathways, characterization of metabolites, it is all out there in the so-called proprietary literature. I hope there is a way of getting access to the data so that more scientists can look at the data, analyze, and understand them. The regulatory agencies do have access to them, and they do draw their conclusions based on some of that information.

The thing that concerns me most is the poor state of exposure assessment. If you think that there are problems about dose-response modeling, you're basically talking about an order of magnitude difference in these models, although I have seen some dose-response models that can be different by many more times than one order of magnitude. From what I have been able to gather from talking to people at this meeting is that there may be about one or two orders of magnitude difference between pharmacokinetic modeling and conventional modeling. However, when you start looking at exposure assessment, you can sometimes calculate differences of six or more orders of magnitude, depending upon the assumptions used in one's models and the way one collects data and evaluates the data base. I think, as a matter of priority, EPA should develop exposure assessment as a high-priority research area.

There are two things wrong with the present system of exposure assessment. First of all, I don't think we have the proper methodology in place and not enough people in the scientific community helping develop that methodology. Maybe some hydrogeologists are working a little bit on modeling for ground water, but that's about it. Air modeling we do have: the EPA's Air Office has been air modeling for many years. But when you start going into the food chain, for example, with municipal incinerator risk assessment, you can go all over the map on exposure analysis.

The second thing that is wrong is there is no peer review going on in exposure analysis. When, for example, the Agency publishes a criteria document, there is a lot of peer review on the quantitative risk assessment, the cancer data, and so on. Very seldom do I see a really good peer review on how well the exposure assessment was done and how strong the data base was. It's almost like a whole different discipline of people within the staff that collect and analyze the data, and do the modeling. It seems to me that the agency has to do a little bit better in the way it presents the information on exposure assessment to the public and to the scientific community.

The one thing that I also am concerned about in the scientific process, and this is something that John Graham addressed, is how to insulate the scientific peer review process from political pressure. The perchloroethylene issue right now is a classic example of how science and politics have gotten so enmeshed that it's hard to separate one from the other. This is not the way an agency should have to make decisions, when people from an affected industry go directly to Congress and try to change a classification from B-2 to C carcinogen. That's not the position in which Congress should be placed, trying to decide on a scientific question while under pressure from an affected industry.

What John Graham said yesterday, with which I take great issue, is that one of the weaknesses he finds in our present approach is that since we cannot verify our risk calculations, our approach is unscientific. I don't think we want to wait to verify how good our risk assessment models are. We don't want to have legions of people exposed to carcinogens, particularly before the fact. So, I take issue with him about the way he defines the process of peer review. Peer review on carcinogens should only be done before the fact. To the extent that we have occupational and environmental risk data, we can certainly go back and look at a problem, but that should not be the norm.

Lastly, I want to quickly mention the necessity for harmonizing nomenclature and terminology in the cancer risk assessment field. I served for several years with Howard Rafia on a Committee of the National Academy of Sciences on Risk and Decision Making. John Graham was on the staff at that time. At times, it was funny, because you had Bill Ruckelhaus on that committee, and Richard Wilson, and Rosalyn Yarrow. That is, people from the natural sciences were sitting down with people from the social sciences, like Howard Rafia, and we couldn't even speak the same language. We were talking about totally different things. When some of us were talking about risk analysis generally, others were talking about quantitative risk assessment specifically. The distinction between risk assessment and risk management was not clearly delineated at that time. Later, another Academy panel finally defined and separated the process conceptually, although our committee had suggested it in the first place.

Thus, it is important to have some kind of a common nomenclature. For example, at times in this conference I have heard people asking each other, "What do you mean by a promoter?" and answering different things. We need to have a better definition of the terms we use, and we need to have better communication between research workers and policymakers. Unless you have a common terminology, you will never be able to really communicate what you are trying to tell each other. That is the first step in trying to harmonize those two communities of professionals.

Hoerger: Thank you, Karim. You and Paul (Deisler) have certainly covered a lot of ground. Are there any questions for Karim?

Weber: Maybe I show my ignorance here, but this whole conference is aimed at risk assessment, and to me risk is something that is floating around in the air and is in the water. What we are talking about to an equally great extent is the susceptibility of individuals to these things. For a given risk, the susceptibility of people will differ. I tend to think in terms of susceptibilities. I wonder if we're talking about the same or different things.

Ahmed: It depends. I don't know if you are familiar with the Clean Air Act. The Clean Air Act mandates that we develop criteria air standards based upon the most susceptible individuals. If you want to use that statutory standard, then your standards should be based upon the susceptible population, not upon the average population. If you really want to go after susceptible individuals, be warned that from a policy perspective the standard is not going to be based on average people. It might, in fact, be the marginal people upon whom the standard will be based.

Weber: I am not surprised at that. It's just that I am wondering about these two words, risk and susceptibility. Risk is something that confronts the individual, so many ppm of something in the air. The susceptibility is the way you respond to it.

Ahmed: I think many of the statistical models take the 95% upper confidence level. Whatever the shortcomings of that, it in effect takes in a larger population size. In a sense, it implies that the susceptible individuals will be factored in, but we also extrapolate from one species to the other in these models.

Wilson: In fact, the low end of the dose-response curve reflects exactly the most susceptible fraction of the population that you have studied. The people who respond first are those who are most susceptible.

Weber: You have more than one dose-response curve.

Wilson: There are very large numbers of dose-response curves. There is also the fundamental problem of knowing what animal species or strain most nearly resembles humans.

Weber: I mean within a species. I'm talking about within a species.

Michejda: Ken (Kraemer) was saying earlier, that the XP heterozygotes are predisposed to more than just skin cancer. Breast cancer is known to run in families. Pancreatic cancer is beginning to be recognized as being a family-oriented cancer. A large number of these things are being recognized as that, also. These are sensitive populations that need to be identified.

Weber: I'm really bringing this up as a matter of definition of two words.

Wilson: They are identified. They are the ones who died first, in fact. You can show the susceptibility to lung cancer in cigarette smoking. The susceptibility as a function of age decreases once you get past 70, because those who are most susceptible have already succumbed.

Singer: I thought you were going to comment on the 1986 California Water Act known as Proposition 65.

Ahmed: I was. Our organization is involved in a lawsuit on that issue, as you know.

Singer: Does everybody in the room know about it? Please explain.

Ahmed: I guess basically what it really amounts to is that Proposition 65 directed the Governor of California to come up with a list of known carcinogens that would be subject to special regulation in the state of California. The dispute is how extensive was the list that the Governor chose in the first go-around. His approach was to first come up with a small list that included only known human carcinogens, and then he set up a committee to suggest what other compounds should be added.

The people who pushed Proposition 65 argued in court that the mandate was to have a larger list, which was to start from the IARC list, and then from that list to throw out substances that they didn't believe posed carcinogenic risk. So, it's a matter of how one interprets Proposition 65. That question is still under appeal, I believe, in the courts.

Do you have a specific question to ask of me, Bea?

Singer: I didn't put in the second half of my question. It relates to labeling of the listed toxic substances. If you all don't know, mandatory labeling of every single consumer item at point of sale will be implemented shortly. In the grocery store, it will mean every apple and every orange, etc., will be labeled with what it could contain or has been exposed to. We'll never see the price, there will be so many of these signs. I just brought it up to say what happens when you overregulate.

Hoerger: Now to Mary Frances Lowe.

* * *

Lowe: I really have appreciated the opportunity to listen and learn at this conference. No doubt a lot of what I have heard will not be fully digested and used until much later.

I am very much in the "promising tool" camp. Based on the work that you have presented, I am very optimistic about the future of risk assessment. We can't be complacent, of course, and the complexities we have discussed really are dazzling, but we have come very far, both in terms of risk assessment science and risk management policy.

I can see real progress just looking back on my own relatively brief lifespan in the field. My experience began with a real bang when the first proposal to ban saccharin hit. I was working on Capitol Hill at the time. We heard from scientists, doctors, parents of diabetics, parents of cancer patients, and a broad spectrum of the American public, all wanting to know what the risk was. We didn't have very good answers then. I think we may have somewhat better answers now.

At FDA, in recent years, we have seen the development of a number of risk-assessment based policies. We are working to finalize what used to be called the "sensitivity of method" regulation, using risk assessment to help ensure animal drug safety, setting forth procedures to evaluate the potential risk posed by carcinogenic animal drug residues in edible tissues. We also have our "constituents policy," governing carcinogenic constituents in food additives, when the additive as a whole is not carcinogenic. Most recently, we have enunciated a *de minimis* policy interpretation with respect to food and color additives regulated under the Delaney Clause itself. None of these initiatives would have been possible without evolution in the scientific basis of risk assessment, as well as increasing sophistication and willingness to exercise what we, at this conference, have been calling scientific judgment.

Once a regulatory policy decision is made to go forward with risk assessment, with common sense and reason, we still face some very difficult issues in dealing with specific subjects of regulation. We need the best available scientific expertise to help sort out these issues. Some of the people in the room, such as Dr. Hart and Dr. Weisburger, can testify to the complexity of the issues addressed by the two color additive scientific review panels on which they recently served with distinction.

We have had to deal with the fact that nothing is a simple compound; everything is a complex mixture. We have to look at issues of contaminants, identified and unidentified. We have to make reasonable judgments about the likelihood that contaminants could be responsible for toxic effects observed in animal studies. We have to make sure that what is tested and found safe is the same thing that people will be exposed to when a substance is marketed. We try to control that with tight specifications, limiting the amounts of potentially troublesome impurities under our constituents policy to levels that we are confident are safe.

We are also working to address issues related to structural similarities and whether it may be possible to extrapolate relative potency from one substance to a related substance for risk assessment purposes. It's not clear how far we can go in this area, but it certainly raises some very interesting issues for us.

This brief review of just a few of the policy issues FDA has considered shows we are making progress in utilizing the science of risk assessment in policy development. It has been evolutionary. In deference to our gap junction presentation, there is such a thing as punctuated evolution.

I also want to respond to Paul's (Deisler) remarks about the need to be open to scientific refinement. We don't have all the answers. When we get better data, we need to be able to accept and incorporate them into our decision making. I think, by and large, the regulatory agencies have done so. Our methods are not set in stone.

So, all this is good news. As risk managers, and as scientists, though, we are still not satisfied. Ron (Hart) can tell you that I am even uncomfortable with some of the terminology, when risk assessors use words like "best guess" to describe their work. I just don't like the sound of it.

Hart: "Best hope."

Lowe: I like "best estimate" better than "best guess." It makes me more comfortable.

We need to test the assumptions underlying risk assessment. We need to understand mechanisms. Some of the last panel's suggestions for directions in research could help us to define better what is an appropriate test for assessing carcinogenicity and how test results can best be interpreted in terms of human safety.

Of course, as regulators, as some of my colleagues know, we can't wait for the results of these new directions in research. At FDA, we have a greater degree of luxury than our friends at EPA, in terms of new product introductions, because our premarket approval authorities allow us to ask for more data in many cases. However, there are practical as well as statutory distinctions in the standards that apply to new versus old substances, and we still need to act on less than perfect data.

In addition to testing the assumptions and developing better data, we also need to make very clear the assumptions that we are using. Much of the assumption-making process is not pure science. Although grounded in science, the choices we make among alternative assumptions are, to a degree, policy judgments. The risk manager's decisions about acceptable risks are societal judgments.

We should keep our progress in cancer risk assessment in perspective compared to related fields, however. Despite the gaps in our knowledge, we are ahead of many other areas of risk assessment. Murray (Cohn) said that in some sense initiators could be considered relatively easy–or easier. We have working hypotheses to deal with them. Dr. Graham cited the predictability of carcinogen risk assessment in general as a strength. I think, in a sense, we do have it easier than some other areas of risk assessment. We can argue about the models and assumptions we use, but at least we have models. We are not just counting tumors and feeding all the numbers into computers, of course. We are using judgment in both the interpretation of data and selection of model assumptions.

I am very encouraged by the areas that you are exploring, the data that were presented here, and the questions that are being asked: epidemiology questions; the possibility that we can get some relevant data from human populations with certain genetic susceptibilities; and recognition of the need to do sensitivity analyses varying the assumptions in our risk assessment models.

Let me conclude by coming back to a couple of questions. The first is the one Dr. Hart kept nagging us with earlier, which is: How do the data and the types of scientific issues we have been discussing affect regulatory policy? The simple answer is that we in the regulatory agencies try to use all the data we can get in making policy decisions.

One example with which I know Dr. Flamm is very familiar, is FDA's consideration of the safety of food irradiation. There was a misperception by some that we only had four or five studies to go on in our review and evaluation. In fact, there was a tremendous body of data going back to the 1960s. There may have only been four or five studies that met today's state-of-the-art criteria, but FDA's decision was based on examination of all the data, much of it imperfect. This reliance on the totality of information available is key to the "weight of evidence" approach, which is gaining increasing acceptance.

It is of course important that we work to improve the data upon which assessments are made, and that we understand the limitations of available data. I would also add that, for both regulators and scientists, it is also important to our own credibility that we learn how to comunicate very complex risk assessment and management concepts more effectively, both to policymakers and to the American people.

There is another question that I wanted to ask you all, and I hope we can discuss it a bit: How *should* the data affect regulatory policy? Are there kinds of data that you are developing that you think we ought to be cranking into the policy process but are not? We have heard many intriguing findings and possible directions for the future over the last few days. My impression is that it is still a little too soon to tell how and if we will be able to crank them all into risk assessment and risk management decision making, and I welcome your observations on that point.

In summary, we still have to make a lot of less than totally satisfying assumptions in risk assessment. We need to work, I think everyone here agrees, to elucidate those assumptions and test them when they're testable, to continue to make them clear, and to focus on communicating them a bit better.

Ahmed: Do you have a rule of thumb about what that cut off point would be, or is it on a case-by-case basis?

Lowe: *De minimis* is based on the legal doctrine that "the law does not concern itself with trifles." If, using conservative risk assessment assumptions, the level of theoretical risk that is calculated is so low as to effectively pose, in our view, no real risk at all, we would regard the risk as insignificant or trivial. We could conclude that the law, the Delaney Clause, does not require a ban in such circumstances, invoking a *de minimus* interpretation.

Ahmed: Do you have a rule of thumb about what that cut off point would be, or is it on a case-by-case basis?

Lowe: It's case-by-case. I think that the rule of thumb, first developed in the animal drug safety area, is a figure around one in a million lifetime risk. I think Curtis (Travis) has a paper indicating that regulatory agencies have tended to use that figure as a kind of benchmark. We haven't said, "This is the line, it's set in stone: 1.01×10^{-6} is unsafe, whereas 0.99×10^{-6} is safe." I don't think we can draw such a precise line. Again, we have to use judgment.

So far, under the *de minimis* policy, we have not set a single risk number. Some of the numbers have been much lower than others.

Michejda: How is that level dictated by political considerations, by pressure considerations? It really opens up a potential of tremendous variation depending on people's perception of what an "insignificant level" is.

Lowe: Again, we don't know where the line is, but we feel confident that the additives we have called *de minimis* are on the safe side of it. You may differ with us. As I understand the comments that came in on the animal drug safety/sensitivity of method rule, however, which had the one in a million benchmark figure in it, none of the commenters suggested that number was too large or represented significant risk.

Now, we do have people who disagree with us on whether or not the

Delaney Clause itself permits a *de minimis* interpretation. That legal issue is before the courts at this time.

Benson: All the comments that we got, as you said, more or less said, "Surely, one in a million is a very low risk over a lifetime." Some people said maybe a risk higher than that should also be considered insignificant, but nobody was willing to say what that number was.

Lowe: I heard a former FDA Commissioner speak to the issue of trivial risk in the context of toxic shock syndrome and tampon use. Someone raised their hand in the audience and said, "Oh, come on. This isn't really nearly as bad as cigarette smoke." I think we can all agree that smoking is not the appropriate benchmark for judging what's trivial, but there are people to whom it does seem appropriate and relevant. We feel our policy errs on the side of caution. To my knowledge, there is consensus at least that a lifetime risk of 1×10^{-6} is very low.

Weisburger: I really wanted to make a comment. I have seen over the past, say, 12 or 15 years a great evolution in the regulatory agencies' attitude toward risk assessment. I think they are using much more scientific data, not just fitting points into an equation somewhere.

Lowe: I was trying to get to that point, too. I don't think it is a fair characterization that any of the agencies just pump numbers into a computer model and have it spit out a number. Then, if it's 1 in a million it's okay, and if it's 1 in 1000 it's not. We are all more sophisticated than that, I think. As I said, we try to use all the data we can get and consider biological plausibility and the weight of the evidence.

Hoerger: Thank you.

Concluding Remarks

RONALD W. HART
National Center for Toxicological Research, Arkansas
FRED D. HOERGER
The Dow Chemical Company, Michigan

Hoerger: What does one say when so much has been said already? I would like to ask you to consider characterizing yourself in terms that I heard Dr. Bill Thilly of Massachusetts Institute of Technology use last week. He used the term "revolutionary centrists." I thought you might want to latch onto the concept. It seems to me that for the last three days we have all gained new perspectives, new questions that need answers, some issues that we now have a better answer to or a partial answer to, and, I hope, all of us are charged up to go out and give one or two strong nudges for the betterment of health protection and for risk assessment. Being revolutionary centrists, pick the idea or task that really makes sense to you and be an advocate for getting something done.

In concluding the conference, I would like to speak to one particular topic that has only been alluded to so far. I refer to what can be termed institutional approaches. All of us as scientists and regulators have our personal network of professional interchanges which catalyze our thinking. I hope that this conference has been a step in enhancing those networks for each of us.

When I refer to institutional approaches, I would like to go one step further than personal networks. Approaches to risk assessment are not only interdisciplinary, but also interfunctional in terms of different institutions with different functions. So I would like to encourage all of us in our own way to give more thought to new institutional approaches, such as new collaborative research initiatives between institutions. Collaboration among researchers is important and is one way to foster broader institutional cooperation. Bea (Singer) indicated that she and another person were debating ideas, but suddenly they decided to collaborate on a research project to test the ideas under debate.

More collaboration between institutions can be fostered. The federal government, through a recent law, is encouraging information transfer by the national laboratories through collaboration with the industrial sector. Another area of institutional approach exemplified by this conference is that the different sectors can get together to discuss these issues from the standpoint of making improvements. To me, it is really gratifying that we have had policy-oriented people and scientists here.

Banbury Report 31: Carcinogen Risk Assessment: New Directions in the Qualitative and Quantitative Aspects © Cold Spring Harbor Laboratory. 0-87969-231-6/88. $1.00 + .00   **345**

However, one can also characterize the conference as consisting of a number of institutions: the federal government, universities, the private sector, and some of the public interest groups. All really have been working constructively toward problem solving.

Many people are familiar with the Science Advisory Board at EPA and some of the Ad Hoc review boards at FDA; these are institutional approaches to foster scientific consensus. The Banbury Center provides an institutional approach in this meeting where we have merged science and policy on complex issues.

Very pragmatically, one could extend institutional approaches to early identification of data needs, where I think more could be done. There are some good examples from past experience. When regulators or industry recognize that there may be a regulatory decision to be made one or three years hence, it would be opportune to get several relevant disciplines together to identify those experiments that need to be done. Paul Deisler mentioned that often there is time to get research done before regulatory decisions are made. I would only amend his suggestion by saying that, perhaps, several scientists and several policy people from involved institutions could frame the questions to be addressed by research and fact gathering.

I do not have specific suggestions here, but I would encourage you to think of the new institutional approaches. We drift into some automatically and constructively in much of our professional networking, but across institutions I think there is an opportunity, too.

I would like to again thank all the speakers and all of you who participated throughout the conference. When we started, I said this was an outstanding group of people. To me, the conference has verified that in many, many different ways.

Ron Hart, I have really enjoyed working with you on this conference.

Hart: It has been mutually pleasurable. I'm glad I had someone to share the work.

Summary

FRED D. HOERGER[†] AND RONALD W. HART[*]
[†]The Dow Chemical Co.
Midland, Michigan 48674
[*]National Center for Toxicological Research
Jefferson, Arizona 72079

Both qualitative and quantitative risk assessments are being relied on increasingly by regulatory agencies in decision making on carcinogenic substances. Qualitative carcinogen classification schemes serve as priority triggers at both the federal and state levels. Quantitative estimates of risk are important aspects of the degree of exposure control prescribed in regulations. Over the past decade, risk assessment of carcinogens by regulatory agencies has become more formalized. Somewhat understandably, it has evolved with both the advances in science and the generation of more empirical data. Perceptions of the possibility of a widening gap between science and policy led David G. Hoel, in *Banbury Report 19*, to observe that risk assessment should incorporate as much relevant information as possible. Also, since each chemical or group of closely related chemicals will be essentially unique in its risk analysis, Hoel cautioned against overreliance on an algorithm or set of rigid guidelines that might be applied broadly to most chemical agents.

The purpose of these proceedings is to provide a contemporary analysis of this interface of science and regulatory policy, to examine recent research advances relating to carcinogenic risks, to describe recent approaches to integrating biological research findings into the risk assessment, and to summarize directions for future research and policy development. The conference participants generally concluded that risk assessment, as currently practiced, is a useful input tool for decision making and that current limitations can be improved, both by generic research in molecular biology and by generation of chemical-specific information.

The first section of the proceedings is on structure-activity relationships and includes a paper on nitrogen-containing alkylating carcinogens (Lijinsky). Extensive studies of nitrosamines and nitrosoalkylureas illustrate important distinctions in structure-activity relationships within a class. For example, the two classes give rise to differing types of tumors, and dose rate also affects tumor type. The results suggest that alkylation of DNA by these carcinogens may be an important event in carcinogenesis, but that other properties of the carcinogen determine whether or not tumors arise in a particular organ.

Auer's paper and the commentary by Farland illustrate the application of structure-activity relationships in evaluating hazard potentials of new chemicals by EPA. Enslein's commentary typifies recent advances in compiling a

Banbury Report 31: Carcinogen Risk Assessment: New Directions in the Qualitative and Quantitative Aspects © Cold Spring Harbor Laboratory. 0-87969-231-6/88. $1.00 + .00

data base correlating structural units to activity measured in two-year bioassays. Generally, conference participants concluded that data base correlations, knowledge from detailed studies of classes of compounds (such as nitrosamines, nitrosoalkylureas, and polycyclic aromatics), and expert judgment from experienced scientists, taken altogether, can provide a valuable tool for screening substances to develop priorities for extensive short-term or long-term bioassay investigations.

Papers and commentary in Section 2 relate to metabolism, mechanism of carcinogenesis, pharmacokinetics, and measurement of DNA adducts. Pharmacologically based pharmacokinetic models can be utilized in four aspects of dose-response assessment: extrapolation from one route of exposure to another, extrapolation of variable dosing time patterns to chronic dosing, high-dose to low-dose extrapolation, and extrapolation across species. Data on a limited number of compounds, such as methylene and perchloroethylene, are now available for reducing uncertainty in risk estimates. Available data vary from compound to compound, and use of information in cross-species extrapolation is still undergoing data development and debate.

Evidence from a variety of animal models supports a working hypothesis that differences in the metabolism of procarcinogens influence susceptibility to risk. A limited number of epidemiological and chemical studies have been conducted to explore the working hypothesis. For instance, an association has been shown between a slow acetylator phenotype and arylamine-induced urinary bladder cancer; whereas, in contrast, the rapid acetylator phenotype is associated with coliorectal cancer and breast cancer in women.

Guengerich suggests promising directions for future research: development of more information along the lines of specific molecular probes and catalyst specificity; searches for new variants, development of in vivo/in vitro relationships; and development of in vivo models that utilize in vitro data for interspecies extrapolation. Much chemical specific research is needed, as exemplified by the findings of Weber et al., of three different acetylation activities in the bioactivation of certain arylamines to carcinogens.

Commentary on mechanisms underscored views that (1) the significance of results from maximum tolerated dose bioassays must be addressed on a case-by-case basis; (2) more systematic and comprehensive empirical analysis of the bioassays showing only tumors in mice would be desirable; and (3) the magnitude of DNA adduct formation, although important in association with tumor formation, was certainly not the sole detriment of the associations.

Section 3 addresses molecular biological data from two widely differing, but supplementary perspectives. One is an overview of varying mechanisms involved in DNA adduct formation, and the other is the role of inhibited intercellular communication in tumor promotion and progression.

Singer reviews the literature and current studies on N-nitrosamines, N-nitrosourea, vinyl chloride, formaldehyde, acetaldehyde, asbestos, and ethanol. The lack of uniformity in the mode of action of these substances leads Singer to the conclusion that no single DNA adduct can be used as an indicator of risk.

Trosko and Chang examine experimental results from known tumor promoters as inhibitors of intercellular communication and suggest that current bioassays and short-term mutational test protocols have extensive limitations for nongenotoxic substances. Furthermore, no single in vitro cell system or single technique to measure gap junction function can be used as a universal screen for potential tumor promoters for all species. Results of gap junction studies suggest the need for an additional paradigm for incorporating biological factors in a number of risk assessments. The exact mechanisms by which chemicals can block gap junctions in various cell types from various species need further research. So far all tested inhibitors of intercellular communication seem to have no-effect levels, and tumor promotion may be a rate-limiting process in carcinogenesis. Trosko concludes that there is indirect evidence for threshold levels of tumor promotion if one assumes that inhibition of gap junctions plays a role in promotion.

Extensive commentary by discussants underscores the future importance of molecular data in elucidating the mechanism of action for specific chemicals, especially those believed to act largely by nongenotoxic mechanisms, for example, those nongenotoxic agents with steep dose-response relationships in the observed range, such as saccharin, formaldehyde, and butylated hydroxyanisole. A new era involving more up-to-date science is beginning to effect regulatory judgments in assessing risk. Study of adduct formation in relation to tumor formation is now in exploratory stages as well as a new shuttle vector plasmid system for studying ultraviolet photoproducts.

Several empirical correlations between short-term mutagenicity tests and tumor formation are presented. Concordance between a battery of short-term tests and a group of some 200 NTP-NCI bioassay results is about 60%. In contrast, the vast majority of human carcinogens are mutagenic in short-term tests.

Section 4 includes an introductory paper by Allen et al. based on a comparative analysis of carcinogenic potencies in animals and humans. Positive correlation is based on a model that mimics current Environmental Protection Agency extrapolation techniques but which relies on the median dosage for the combination of animal species/strains and the dosage expressed in terms of body weight rather than surface area. This analysis sets the stage for four papers presenting approaches to improving risk assessment.

Munro describes qualitative criteria for a weight-of-the-evidence analysis of animal data for relevancy to humans. Criteria include appropriateness of experimental designs relative to human exposure conditions, the characteristics of the species/strains of animal studies, the nature of the tumor response, dose-response relationships, and mechanistic considerations.

Graham et al. describe the prevailing approach to risk assessment practiced by U.S. regulatory agencies and outline strengths and weaknesses. Needed research can be divided into three strategies, mechanistic and pharmacokinetic studies, statistical modeling, and inclusion of expert scientific judgment. Eliciting the expert judgment of practicing scientists can help guide the use of data, help build models related to the specific biology, and help convey plausible ranges of uncertainty.

Papers by Thorslund and Charnley, Krewski and Murdoch, and Allen et al. describe recent approaches to extrapolation models with a biological basis. A model based on a two-stage paradigm of initiation/promotion has been applied to the putative promoters, TCDD and chlordane. Predicted tumor rates fit bioassay data quite well; predicted human cancer risk is two to three orders of magnitude lower than that predicted by the currently used multistage model. Broad application of the model will require development of information on tissue growth and cellular proliferation rates. Physiologically based pharmacokinetic models are currently receiving considerable attention when information is available on partition coefficients, physiological constants (tissue/organ volume of blood flow), and biochemical rate constants. Time dependent exposure models indicate that time of exposure to a carcinogen is an important parameter of resultant risk and that use of time-weighted average level of exposure generally oversimplifies the resultant estimate of risk.

The final section of the proceedings deals with future directions, in terms of research needs and recommendations for policy direction. The section is introduced with three prepared papers. Anderson emphasizes the importance of exposure data and modeling as a means of reducing uncertainty in risk estimates. St. Hilaire presents a novel analysis of current research by governmental and nongovernmental institutions correlated to a large number of specific assumptions frequently employed in risk assessment. Perera highlights biomarker research, exemplified by studies of DNA and protein adducts and facilitated by currently evolving experimental methodology. Biomarkers are regarded as promising tools for high-dose to low-dose extrapolation, to provide a common benchmark for interspecies comparisons, for study of modulating factors, and for examining past exposure of population groups.

Conclusions on research needs are drawn from a panel of research directors who participated in the conference. Studies of intercellular communication warrant continued research, as well as the role of cellular proliferation. Greater emphasis in exploring modulating factors also appears warranted.

Research that would provide more qualitative determinations of the relevancy of animal models to humans was also emphasized. This is exemplified by questions relating to the significance of male rat kidney tumors (e.g., unleaded gasoline), mechanisms of peroxisome proliferation, and lymphoma in mice. The key to low-dose extrapolation was felt to be a better understanding of mechanisms and the design of measurements of relevant preneoplastic biochemical changes. The many unresolved questions concerning individual susceptibility appear to be dependent on advances in identifying relevant human biomarkers and perhaps on comparative pharmacokinetics. From a regulatory perspective, important directions include: building realistic human activity patterns into exposure scenarios, obtaining pharmacokinetic data on more chemicals, continued development of biologically based dose-response models, and emphasis on sensitivity analysis to direct resources.

The proceedings are concluded with commentary from a panel of policy-oriented participants. Regulatory policies that encourage development, interpretation, and incorporation of elucidating information into risk assessment are emphasized. Periodic updating of risk assessment guidelines to reflect advances in scientific information and experiences in applying the guidelines seems important. There was some feeling that in some cases, the data bases can accommodate greater consideration of reasonably probable alternative models, qualitative consideration of relevancy of data sets and models to humans, and more consideration of which species most closely resembles humans. For a sense of priorities, qualitative and comparative assessments of activity and metabolism data were felt to be useful.

It was pointed out that there is relatively limited peer review of exposure protocols, models, and assessments. Greater peer review might stimulate advances in these areas. Harmonization of nomenclature and terminology would facilitate interaction between scientists and policymakers and facilitate communication with various public sectors.

From a policymaker's standpoint, risk assessment is viewed as an essential and evolving tool, which is dependent on continuing scientific refinement. Most policymakers now accept the concept of weight-of-the-evidence as a key part of assessment; best characterizations of risk are desired but a clear articulation of assumptions is critical. Credibility of risk assessment hinges on the ability of scientists and risk analysts to communicate complex scientific concepts to policymakers and various public sectors.

Research aimed at improving risk assessment, if aimed at improving decision making by risk managers, will not only improve the public good but also will contribute to a more complete and comprehensive understanding of the basic processes involved in evaluating risk and in understanding the biology of humans. In the immediately forseeable future, risk assessment will increasingly draw on expert judgment for weight-of-the-evidence considerations of qualitative information and biologically based quantitative models, increasing distinction between scientific consensus and generic policy, and characterizations of uncertainty.

Author Index

Subject Index

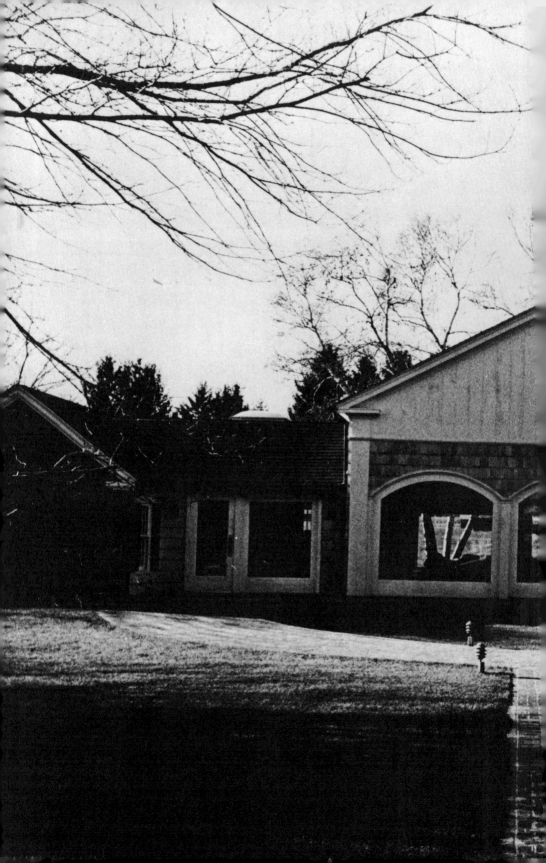